THE SUPERVISORY PROCESS IN SPEECH-LANGUAGE PATHOLOGY AND AUDIOLOGY

ELIZABETH S. McCREA

Indiana University

JUDITH A. BRASSEUR

California State University—Chico

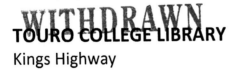

d on the Seminal Work of
Jean L. Anderson

Boston   New York   San Francisco
Mexico City   Montreal   Toronto   London   Madrid   Munich   Paris
Hong Kong   Singapore   Tokyo   Cape Town   Sydney

MW

Executive Editor and Publisher: *Stephen D. Dragin*
Editorial Assistant: *Barbara Strickland*
Marketing Manager: *Tara Whorf*
Editorial-Production Service: *Omegatype Typography, Inc.*
Manufacturing Buyer: *Andrew Turso*
Composition Buyer: *Linda Cox*
Cover Administrator: *Kristina Mose-Libon*
Electronic Composition: *Omegatype Typography, Inc.*

For related titles and support materials, visit our online catalog at www.ablongman.com.

Between the time Website information is gathered and then published, some sites may have closed. Also, the transcription of URLs can result in unintended typographical errors. The publisher would appreciate notification where these occur so that they may be corrected in subsequent editions.

Library of Congress Cataloging-in-Publication Data

McCrea, Elizabeth.
  The supervisory process in speech-language pathology and audiology / Elizabeth McCrea, Judith Brasseur.
     p.   cm.
  Includes bibliographical references and index.
  ISBN 0-205-33662-0
     1. Speech therapy—Study and teaching—Supervision.   2. Audiology—Study and teaching—Supervision.   I. Brasseur, Judith.   II. Title.

RC428 .M38   2003
616.85'506—dc21

2002028212

Printed in the United States of America

10   9   8   7   6   5   4   3   2   1   07   06   05   04   03   02

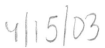

To the men in our lives—
David, Rob, Michael, and Ben, who gave us their patience
and support and the space to complete this work.

And most of all,
To Jean L. Anderson.

CONTENTS

CHAPTER THREE

Components of the Supervisory Process   37

CHAPTER FOUR

Understanding the Supervisory Process   50

CHAPTER TEN
Accountability   276

CHAPTER ELEVEN
Supervision across Settings   286

FOREWORD

In the 15 years since the publication of the first edition of this book, many highly motivated and dedicated professionals in speech-language pathology and audiology have directed their attention to the significance of high quality supervision in educational programs and in the work setting. In conjunction with the efforts of individuals, the American Speech-Language-Hearing Association has continued the work begun in the late 1960s. The organization and operation of several conferences on various components of supervision led to the establishment in 1974 of a Committee on Supervision in Speech-Language Pathology and Audiology. Since that time, the output of conferences, sets of guidelines, and research reports on this complex process have increased in quantity and quality.

We have made much progress since 1988 in recognizing the importance of studying the supervisory process, of upgrading its quality, and in accountability. There is much more to be done.

In the preface to the first edition I detailed my long and challenging journey to the book. I am grateful to Elizabeth McCrea and Judith Brasseur for continuing that journey. They were two of the many thoughtful, inquisitive, questioning doctoral students who were willing to experiment along with me, who could tolerate uncertainty and recognize the need that I saw. I am proud of all my former students who participated in my search. I am especially grateful to these two for making this tremendous effort to perpetuate my thoughts and words and bring their own into the equation.

I also stated that we were "in a wonderful period of evolution in the study of the supervisory process." I trust that this book will be another step in that evolution.

Jean L. Anderson, 2003

PREFACE

The supervisory process in speech-language pathology and audiology continues to challenge those who practice it. In the intervening fifteen years since the first edition of this book was published, research findings and reports of conceptual application of Anderson's Continuum of Supervision Model have found their way into the literature of the profession. The purpose of this book is to summarize, as completely as possible, the substance of the model for a new generation of supervisors and supervisees and to integrate the information of the last decade and a half into their consideration of it. Chapters One through Eight address each aspect of the model in detail, from both a theoretical as well as a practical application point of view. In the final chapter of this edition, several case problems are included in an effort to suggest how the dynamics of the model can be brought to bear to meet the demands of a variety of different supervisory encounters. Chapters Nine through Twelve address issues attendant on the full consideration of the process and its implementation, including preparation for the supervisory process, accountability, supervision across settings, and the supervision of speech-language pathology assistants.

The profession has recognized supervision as a distinct area of professional practice with a set of tasks and competencies, or in the language of the new millennium, knowledge and skills, that are fundamental to it (ASHA, 1985b). It is our hope that *The Supervisory Process in Speech-Language Pathology and Audiology* will inform and support the supervisory practice of both supervisors and supervisees as they work together to enhance their skill in this fundamental professional activity.

ACKNOWLEDGMENTS

As Jean L. Anderson indicated in the 1988 edition of this book, it is a pleasant but difficult endeavor to attempt to acknowledge the many people who have been important to us and whose influence can be found in this book. The importance of Jean Anderson's work and its impact on the professions of speech-language pathology and audiology is substantiated by the fact that she was one of three individuals who received the Honors of the American Speech-Language Hearing Association (ASHA) in 1997. We are indeed fortunate to have studied under her twenty-five years ago—and to continue to benefit from her wisdom, mentoring, and love.

We are grateful to Ruth Becky Irwin of The Ohio State University, Betty Ann Wilson of Purdue University, Adah Miner of the University of Washington, and Bill Diedrich of the University of Kansas, who along with Jean pioneered the study of the process of supervision and paved the way for it to become recognized as a distinct area of expertise and practice. Their vision, insights, and early collaboration provided a foundation for the growth of this essential component of our professions.

We want to express our appreciation to the faculty and our former fellow doctoral students in the Department of Speech and Hearing Sciences at Indiana University, which still holds the distinction of offering the only doctoral-level program in communication sciences and disorders with primary emphasis in the study of the supervisory process. Special thanks to Jean for her creativity, initiative, and leadership in developing the model program and finding a way to support it—and to all of her students. We also thank Rita C. Naremore, who shared her expertise and assisted so many of us with the research design and the statistical analyses of our dissertation studies.

Judy extends her appreciation for the special talents of two early supervisors, Helen Sapp and Diane Buethe, who not only encouraged her to go to I.U. to study with Jean but who also believed in her ability to successfully complete a Ph.D., and her sister, Susan, who has always championed every life endeavor and sensed when a dose of love and encouragement was exactly what was needed. Liz would also like to recognize several people: Marguerite Edmonson, who taught her in the spring of 1966 that data analysis is the crucible of behavior change; Ruby Davis, who taught her that leadership is not only creativity and productivity but also humor and warmth as well; and Fred and Sara Statts, who gave her a sense of herself and the gift of the notion that nothing is impossible. Both of us want to thank all of the supervisees with whom we have worked over the years for helping us grow and sustain our passion for the incredible professional growth process we know as supervision.

We thank the following reviewers for their helpful comments: Elizabeth Gavett, Boston University; Sara Elizabeth Runyan, James Madison University; Kristine V. Sbaschnig, Wayne State University; David A. Shapiro, Western Carolina University; and Shelley J. Victor, Nova Southeastern University.

Finally, to all of our wonderful, inspirational, supportive CSSPA colleagues, we owe you so much! Susan Bartlett captured the emotion when she said, "CSSPA is the central nervous system of supervision. It stimulates ideas, it connects people, and it innervates its members to promote the principles of excellence in supervision." It did exactly that and more—it gave us early opportunities for leadership and the gift of lifelong personal friendships.

Elizabeth McCrea
Judith Brasseur

PREFACE TO THE ORIGINAL EDITION

Although supervision has long been a component of the profession of speech-language pathology and audiology, the study of the supervisory process has been largely ignored until recently. In the past few years, however, there has been a surge of interest that has resulted in published articles, convention presentations, continuing education offerings, books, and activities of the American Speech-Language-Hearing Association (ASHA). This book makes a statement about where the profession stands in its implementation of the supervisory process as a major influence in the preparation of future speech-language pathologists and audiologists and the delivery of service to clients. It proposes a continuum of supervision, offered as a framework on which supervisors and their supervisees may place themselves as they work together, and through which they can examine, "dissect," and discuss the process. It is hoped that the presentation of the continuum and the accompanying material will encourage members of the profession to view the supervisory process as an important and appropriate area for self-study. Additionally, it is hoped it will help make clearer the many questions that exist about the effectiveness of supervisory methodologies and will stimulate active research to seek answers to those questions.

This book has been written mainly for the many people in speech-language pathology and audiology who have been or may be plunged into the role of supervisor without opportunity to think about it or study it. Speech-language pathologists and audiologists often become what I call "overnight supervisors"—one day a clinician, the next a supervisor. Many are thrust into the role without preparation, sometimes without much choice, and nearly always without much role definition from the organizations for which they work or within themselves. Often they have little opportunity to talk with anyone about supervision and are forced to draw on their own past experiences as supervisees, positive or negative, as a source for the development of their own techniques and methodologies. I hope that this book will help them and all the other supervisors make supervision manageable. I hope that it will encourage them to think about the process and to increase their knowledge of themselves and their supervisory procedures. I hope supervisors will perceive supervision as a process that can and must be studied, just as we expect our clinicians to study the clinical process. I hope, too, that student supervisees in educational programs will study the book and that it will serve two purposes for them—to help them understand their role as supervisees, and to prepare them for the time in the not-too-distant future when they will probably be supervisors themselves.

This book has been "happening" to me since long before I began seriously to put the words on paper. A series of events led to my interest in the supervisory process, but a few of them stand out as probably the most significant. The first was my own introduction into supervision, when I, too, became an overnight supervisor of a student in a school practicum assignment that was not defined and for which there were no guidelines.

The second experience, and possibly the most significant, was the opportunity to serve as a state supervisor of speech-hearing-language programs in a department of education. In this position I was able to spend several days a week for several years observing and talking with speech-language pathologists in the schools, program supervisors, and administrators as well as university personnel. Often I talked with clinicians who were serving as supervisors of "student teachers" with little or no guidance from universities about their responsibilities, and I heard about their questions. My experiences in this position led me to be concerned about the number of "leaderless" programs, that is, those in which there was no leadership from a person within our discipline. My attention first focused on this administrative aspect—what the ASHA Committee on Supervision was later to call *program management*. However, that attention soon turned to the *process,* later termed *clinical teaching* by the ASHA Committee. My interest in the process came as a result of the dawning realization that, when visiting and observing first- or second-year or even more experienced clinicians, I could often guess correctly where they had done their "student teaching," as the school practicum experience was then called, because of the obvious modeling that took place. Through this realization, I became aware of the impact that the teaching aspect of supervision has on the development of professionals and the significance of that impact on their future clients. In other words, I began to ask myself these questions: If each generation of clinicians does exactly what its supervisors do, where are we going in terms of the kind of service we will deliver to our clients in the future? Is there something in this teaching aspect of supervision that makes the difference between clinicians who become clones of their supervisors and clinicians who are able to go beyond their supervisors and become independent, autonomous clinicians that we profess to produce in our educational programs? Is there something in the supervisory experience that makes the difference and, if so, what is it?

The third important influence on my developing concern about how we, as a profession, were dealing with the supervisory process came when I had the privilege of becoming the chair of the first ASHA Committee on Supervision of Speech Pathology and Audiology. It was through the data-gathering done by the Committee that I fully realized the magnitude of the profession's lack of recognition of the importance of this process that affects all of us at some time. Further, the enormity of our neglect of the dedicated and frustrated members of the profession who were serving in the important role of supervisor became clear and was well documented by the first position statement of the Committee (ASHA, 1978a).

The fourth event was the opportunity to develop a doctoral-level program at Indiana University in which students could study the supervisory process, learn to prepare other supervisors, and conduct research on supervision. The interaction with the students in that program and the research we completed have been an important dimension of my own development.

Thus, a long journey that began with the sudden assignment of a student in the school practicum those many years ago has culminated in the struggle to produce this book. In the words of Alice in Wonderland, I have become "curiouser and curiouser" about the dynamics of the process, and about what I call the professional/political issues that have prevented, or at least not encouraged, the study of this important facet of our profession.

I make no claim for having found the answers to all the questions. Certainly I do not wish to proclaim that this book provides the answers for everyone. I only hope that it provides some encouragement for others to ask more questions about supervision—individually as supervisors or collectively as a profession. The book has become a statement of what I believe to be important in the supervisory process. Some of it is supportable by data, some by consensus, some by common sense. Not everyone will agree with what I say. None of it should go unchallenged, for we have only begun to scratch at the complexities of the process.

It was my somewhat nebulous objective at one time to produce a book that would bring together a spectacular review of what has been written in all the helping professions about supervision. This effort would have resulted in a lengthy tome that would not necessarily have been definitive because, alas, I have learned that many of those disciplines to which I had thought to turn—assuming that they had discovered the answer to the mystery of supervision—are not much better off than we are. Therefore, I have included only that material from other professions that is pertinent to specific points. I have drawn particularly, as will be seen, on the work in education by Blumberg, Cogan, and Goldhammer. But…a funny thing happened on the way to getting this book on paper! We have begun to develop a body of literature of our own over the past few years. It is literature that ranges over a broad continuum of importance and quality, but nevertheless it is ours, and it is developing rapidly to answer our own questions.

A few clarifications are necessary for the reader. One is related to the title, which includes "audiology." Why, you may ask, is a speech-language pathologist writing about supervision in audiology? The answer is that I believe the supervisory *process* is the same for the two areas of practice within the discipline. Differences, if they exist, will be more related to the position of supervisor and supervisee on the continuum, or to such factors as the differences between the needs of supervisees in the diagnostic process and in the therapeutic process. Not all audiologists will agree with me, but nevertheless I hope there will be much in this book that they will find useful.

Another clarification is necessary in relation to some of the examples provided in the book. My own professional background is in the schools, the school practicum, and the university program, so many of the examples come from those settings. I wish to emphasize here, however, as I do throughout the book, my unwavering belief that the *process* of supervision has more commonalities than differences across sites and situations. Therefore, readers are invited to apply the examples to their own experience.

The reader who is looking for statistical validation for the effects of any method of supervision will be disappointed with this book. So will the reader who is looking for unequivocal support for "*the* way to supervise." Neither will be found here, nor in any other source. Despite my confidence in the value of the approach to the supervisory process presented in this book, I am the first to acknowledge that it has not been validated. It is an approach that makes sense to me and that is actually used by many supervisors now, whether or not they conceptualize it in the same way I do. The methodology proposed herein should be weighed and measured carefully, however, to determine its validity.

We are, I think, in a wonderful period of evolution in the study of the supervisory process. It is my wish that this book contributes to that evolution.

Jean L. Anderson, 1988

CHAPTER ONE

INTRODUCTION

Speech-language pathologists and audiologists have been involved in supervision since the beginning of the profession. Indeed, supervision seems to have been the one component that has affected everyone in the profession at some time.
—ASHA Committee on Supervision in Speech-Language Pathology and Audiology, 1978a

In spite of the fundamental impact of supervision on the lives of the members of the professions of speech-language pathology and audiology, the ASHA Committee on Supervision stated, "We have no data to indicate that supervision makes a difference in the effectiveness of clinicians at any level of training or in the employment setting. We also have no knowledge of critical factors in supervision methodology" (ASHA, 1978a, p. 480). However, during the time period between the early 1980s and 1990s, the knowledge base in supervision in speech-language pathology and audiology enjoyed a flurry of development. A primary and motivating influence on this development was the Council of Supervisors in Speech-Language Pathology and Audiology (CSSPA), which, following the leadership of Jean Anderson, sponsored five national conferences on supervision and the supervisory process; a highlight of each of these conferences was the presentation and discussion of research by members of the council. Paralleling these conferences, doctoral students who studied the supervisory process with Jean Anderson at Indiana University were completing dissertations that also contributed to the body of basic research.

This body of research began to define the knowledge base in supervision in the professions. It was these research projects that began the refinement of the understanding of the critical factors in supervision methodology in speech-language pathology and audiology and their relationship to supervisory effectiveness. The underlying purpose of this book is first, to integrate these research results with the conceptual model of the supervisory process presented by Anderson in the first edition of *The Supervisory Process in Speech-Language Pathology and Audiology.* A second purpose is to suggest tools and strategies for ways this information may be brought to bear in the solution of practical supervisory problems that will be presented through exemplar case studies.

DESCRIBING SUPERVISION AND SUPERVISORS

Even though the two are tightly woven together, it is important to differentiate the clinical process from the supervisory process. The **clinical process** is defined in the report of the Committee on

Supervision of the American Speech and Hearing Association (ASHA, 1978a) as "that interaction that takes place between the clinician and the client" (p. 479). The **supervisory process** is defined as the "interaction that takes place between the supervisor and the clinician and may be related to the behavior of the clinician or the client or to the program in which the supervisor and clinician are employed" (ASHA, 1978a, p. 479). Thus, this interaction between clinician and supervisor is superimposed on the clinical process. At some point in the total process the clinician changes roles and becomes a supervisee and engages in a process that requires different objectives, insights, and behaviors. The clinician must play two roles interchangeably—clinician to the client, supervisee to the supervisor.

Tasks of Supervisors

The ASHA Committee Report (ASHA, 1978a) divides the tasks of supervisors into two categories: **clinical teaching** and **program management.** The report defines each category as separate aspects of the role while stating that each supervisor's professional activity may include behaviors from each category.

> Clinical teaching is defined as the interaction between supervisor/supervisee in any setting which furthers the development of clinical skills of students or practicing clinicians as related to changes in client behavior. Traditionally this interaction has consisted of observation and conferences. The conferences may include such components as objective setting, positive or negative feedback, information giving, questioning, joint problem solving, and planning for clinician and client change. Program management is defined as those activities that relate to the administration or coordination of programs, for example, scheduling, budgeting, program planning, employing, or dismissing personnel. (p. 479)

Emphasis on Clinical Teaching. The discussion in this book will center mainly on clinical teaching, although many of the principles to be presented are applicable to program management as well. Clinical teaching as it has been defined should be at the center of the supervisory process in any setting. It may receive a greater emphasis in the educational program, but is also the procedure through which continuing growth and development of clinicians is implemented after they enter the work force. Clinical teaching is certainly a crucial component of any program, even though program management may become the predominant responsibility of the supervisor of a service delivery program.

A further reason for concentrating on clinical teaching is the renewed interest in this category of supervision and the fact that despite the body of research in supervision a decade ago, supervision continues to receive little substantive attention from the professions. This is true even though clinical teaching appears to be the major responsibility of a large percentage of the professionals who are supervisors of speech-language pathology and audiology—those who supervise in educational programs, in off-campus or externship practica, Clinical Fellowship (CF) situations, or who supervise speech-language pathology assistants. In addition, the revised standards for the accreditation of academic programs in speech-language pathology and audiology imply a significantly greater emphasis on clinical teaching within training programs through their requirement for ongoing formative (and summative) assessment which evaluate critical thinking, decision making, and problem solving "for the purpose of improving and measuring student learning" (ASHA, 2000a). The new standards also require that supervision be appropriate to the level of knowledge, experience, and competence of each student clinician/supervisee. These new standards are promulgated at a time when there is not training in the supervisory process routinely available to those who will need to competently implement them.

For these reasons, this book concentrates heavily on the goals, objectives, and methodologies inherent in the clinical education/supervision process.

Titles of Supervisors

The Committee on Supervision also clarified terminology about the people who supervise. The Committee's report stated that, although the individual who carries out the tasks of supervision "may be called supervisor, coordinator, consultant, head clinician or clinical teacher, among other titles," the term **supervisor** was used in their report as a generic label for individuals who may operate under any of those titles in any of the places where speech-language pathology and audiology takes place (ASHA, 1978a, p. 479).

Currently, as the complexities of professional education and training in clinical disciplines continue to grow due to more diverse students in training, rapidly changing workplace demands, and increased public and employer expectations of graduates, a gap between current educational outcomes and workplace demands has grown. McAllister (2000) suggests that the persistent use of the term *supervision* may contribute to this dynamic. Indeed Chomsky, in his work *Language and Mind* (1968), suggests that what one thinks and perhaps how one behaves can be influenced by the semantics with which one communicates. The use of supervision by the profession connotes direction and evaluation of performance of supervisees by their supervisors. It suggests supervision to ensure compliance with standards or to assign a grade in a practicum experience. This point of view was underscored by Halfond (1964) who wrote, "More specifically, supervision is a process in which the direct application of information about communication disorders is reviewed by the supervisor and student clinician. Supervision also implies the giving of directions and maintenance of controls" (p. 442). Although this is certainly a part of a supervisor's responsibility, the exclusive use of this term may, in fact, constrain the perception of supervisors toward the range of their activity that is necessary to achieve "…professionally competent individuals…capable of self-analyzing, self-evaluating, and independent problem solving" (Casey, Smith, & Ulrich, 1988, p. 5). McAllister (2000) suggests that the terms **clinical education**

and **clinical educator** are more appropriate to characterize the skills and applications necessary to close the gap between current clinical training outcomes and those necessary for contemporary professional practice as they are captured by the revised training program accreditation standards. The use of these terms implies the transmission and application of knowledge from the clinical educator to and with the student clinician. In addition, Fish and Twinn (1997) suggest that the clinical educator has the responsibility to function across a wide range of educational interactions with students, each of which requires the use of different combinations of knowledge and skill by the clinical educator.

Historically, the term **supervisor** has been a generic label for individuals who may operate under this title in any place where speech-language pathology takes place (ASHA, 1978a, p. 479). This title has also been used in most of the literature up to this time as well as in official position statements of the profession. For exactly these reasons, the term will continue to be used in this work as well. However, the reader is cautioned to understand that the writers use **supervision/supervisory process/supervisors** in deference to history only and that the focus of this book is more fully captured in concept of **clinical education** and the work of **clinical educators.**

SETTINGS FOR SUPERVISION

The primary mission of speech-language pathologists and audiologists is the provision of clinical services to communicatively disordered individuals. These professionals are prepared by colleges and universities where their experiences include clinical work with communicatively disordered individuals. This clinical phase of their preparation is supervised by certified professionals in programs operated on-campus or in cooperative off-campus settings. The professionals prepared in this way ultimately provide services to communicatively disordered persons in a variety of settings—schools, clinics, acute care hospitals, sub-acute/

rehabilitation centers, long-term care/skilled nursing facilities, private practice, homes, and other agencies and institutions. At any point in their career in any of these settings, a speech-language pathologist or audiologist may also become a supervisor.

Educational Programs

In college and university programs, supervisors facilitate, support, and monitor students' application of academic knowledge to the solution of problems of disordered communication and service delivery in the interest of optimal service to current and future clients. Most of this applied teaching takes place in clinical programs operated by colleges or universities in conjunction with their academic programs. Supervisors in such programs operate within a number of different frameworks, depending on the particular organization and structure of the program in which they work. Some are full-time supervisors employed for this purpose alone, while for others, supervision is only a part of their responsibilities, which may also include clinical work, academic teaching, administration, or research.

Off-Campus Practicum

The off-campus practicum, where students are assigned to a service delivery setting to obtain clinical experience, is part of the total educational program. Some colleges and universities use off-campus sites more extensively than others in order to meet the ASHA (CAA) standards requiring experience across the spectrum of communications disorders and the lifespan. Two types of supervisors are typically involved in these off-campus experiences. One is the on-site supervisor whose primary responsibility is the provision of clinical services to the clients being served by the employer. This person assumes the additional role of supervisor for a particular student(s) from a college or university for a specified period of time. The other type of supervisor involved in the off-campus practicum is employed by the college or university to serve as a liaison between the campus program and off-campus personnel. The university supervisor performs a variety of tasks, ranging from site selection and assignment of students to on-site observations, and has a different degree of responsibility for the supervision and education of the student, depending on the structure of the total education program and the nature of and proximity to the off-campus site.

Service Delivery Settings

In settings where the main objective of the organization is the delivery of services to clients, supervision is the process through which these services are planned, monitored, improved, and evaluated. The functions of supervisors in these settings vary greatly and may include, among other duties, maintaining the quality of services to clients through program organization and management, monitoring and evaluating services, and being responsible for the on-going professional development of the speech-language pathologists employed by the facility. Such supervisors may also be directly or indirectly involved with students who are assigned to their programs by the college or university for off-campus practicum experience, with persons completing the Clinical Fellowship Year, or with speech-language pathology assistants.

The Clinical Fellowship

Many speech-language pathologists and audiologists supervise their colleagues during the Clinical Fellowship (CF). The CF is nine months of full-time professional or equivalent part-time practice after the Master's degree is obtained and in which a speech-language pathologist or audiologist is supervised by an individual who holds the Certificate of Clinical Competence (CCC) from ASHA. The CF is assumed to be a capstone experience during which the clinical fellow is supervised and mentored by the supervisor and is one of the requirements for granting a CCC. Program supervisors or other speech-language pathologists who hold the CCC may be asked to supervise persons who are completing a CF in their own facility or in another program. In these cases, contact between supervisor and supervisee is usually more intermittent than in situations in which the clinical fellow is on site.

Other Types of Supervisory Settings

Some supervisors function at the state or regional level, mainly in education and health departments. Their roles may be administrative, regulatory, or consultative, and may affect the individual speech-language pathologist and audiologist more indirectly than directly.

Another supervisory setting exists where speech-language pathologist assistants are employed to support and/or extend the delivery of services by the speech-language pathologist. When assigned an assistant, a speech-language pathologist assumes the role of supervisor in relation to the work done by the assistant. ASHA has adopted guidelines for the training, credentialing, use, and supervision of speech-language pathology assistants (1996) to guide the supervisor in these situations.

Some speech-language pathologists, and perhaps audiologists, may find themselves in a supervisory position with professionals from other disciplines. For example, speech-language pathologists may become supervisors in rehabilitation centers where they are responsible for physical and occupational therapists and their work, or they may find themselves in interdisciplinary settings where their function is to work with supervisors from other disciplines to meet organizational objectives.

COMPLEXITIES OF THE SUPERVISORY PROCESS

Everyone in speech-language pathology and audiology participates in the supervisory process at some time, certainly as a supervisee and frequently as a supervisor as well. The "web of supervision" is a complex one in which professionals may be involved in many different types of supervisory interactions throughout their careers or at any one time. The nature of these interactions varies greatly across situations and time.

For example, student clinicians may be engaged in the supervisory process at any one time with several different supervisors in their educational programs. The supervision may be done on a one-to-one basis or in a group. At the same time, they may be assigned to an off-campus site, adding the site supervisor and the university coordinator of the practicum to the mix of individuals with whom they interact. Or the off-campus site may be the single assignment for a particular period of time, often becoming the most intensive supervisory experience of the student's entire program.

In the service delivery setting, a variety of supervisory relationships are possible. In some programs a speech-language pathologist or audiologist may be appointed supervisor of other professional staff. Such supervisors may work with beginners or with professionals who have had many years of experience with practicum students, CF candidates, professionals in other disciplines, or assistants. In all settings, however, there is a high probability that speech-language pathologists and audiologists will work in settings where their immediate supervisor or administrator is from another profession. The range of possible interactions in such places is broad. For example, a speech-language pathologist or audiologist working in a school program may interact with one or more of the following: a program supervisor, a CF supervisor, a state/regional supervisor, several principals, and a director of special education. In medical settings, speech-language pathologists may be directly supervised by a member from another healthcare profession, such as physical therapy or neuropsychology. Realistically, it must also be stated that speech-language pathologists and audiologists often work in places where little or no supervision or support is provided, thereby creating another set of issues.

In summary, before becoming certified professionals, speech-language pathologists or audiologists will have been supervised by many different persons across several kinds of settings. Even after obtaining the CCC, they will interact with a variety of persons who will have supervisory or administrative responsibility for them. They may, in turn, supervise individuals during a CF, students in off-campus practicum, or assistants, and may at some point become a supervisor in an educational program, medical service delivery setting, state or regional agency, or interdisciplinary situation.

An additional aspect of this supervision web is that nearly every person who is a supervisor is also a supervisee to someone, thus necessitating another change of roles. The web of supervision is one that has different subtleties and dynamics associated with the variables inherent in each of its strands, and it is important for those involved in it to have a reasoned approach to the spinning of it.

CHARACTERISTICS OF SUPERVISORS— DEMOGRAPHIC DATA

It has always been difficult to obtain demographic data about supervisors in speech-language pathology and audiology. Although ASHA annually asks members to indicate their primary and secondary activity on their membership survey, the total number of professionals who are participating in some form of supervision has never been clearly documented. On June 30, 2001, ASHA figures documented a total certified membership of 100,087 (ASHA, 2001b). Of the 76,206 who responded to questions about their primary professional activity, 1.5%, or 1,143 members, indicated that their primary activity was as a "supervisor of clinical activity." However, this is only part of the picture. Currently, there are 242 (Council of Academic Programs in Communication Sciences and Disorders, 2000) accredited training programs in speech-language pathology and/or audiology in the United States. Assuming an average enrollment of 25 students each year, each of whom must accrue 350 supervised clinical contact hours, of which 25 to 50% must be observed, training programs need to generate a *minimum* of 539,375 supervised hours each year out of a total 2,157,500 clinical hours. Furthermore, in 2000, 5,207 (ASHA, 2001d) Certificates

of Clinical Competence were awarded at the end of the Clinical Fellowship. Each of these experiences required 18 supervisory contacts for a total of 93,726 supervisory activities. Clearly, these numbers speak to the intensity of the contribution supervisors make to the education and training of new members of the profession and imply involvement of more than 1.5% of the membership, probably in part-time supervisory situations (e.g., off-campus practicum, CF year).

Although the size of the membership has doubled since the original edition of this book (when it was 49,878), these data about the numbers of professionals engaged in supervision are unfortunately slightly less positive than those reported by Anderson (1988) 15 years ago. She indicated that in 1986, 3.1% of 39,769, or 1,233, professionals indicated that their primary professional activity was supervision. There are 90 fewer professionals functioning as supervisors today than in the late 1980s. This attrition occurred during the intervening decade of the 1990s when training standards that govern the amount and nature of student clinical practicum became more rigorous and increased the need for productive supervisory practices.

PURPOSES OF SUPERVISION

Supervision is not a process that is unique to speech-language pathology and audiology. Supervision exists whenever individuals work together in any type of hierarchical structure where one person has authority, power, or influence over another to accomplish the objectives of the organization in which they work, including quality of service to clients. Professionals in the helping professions—psychologists, counselors, medical educators, and social workers among others—also utilize supervision in their training programs as they facilitate the acquisition of the knowledge and skills associated with best practices by students. Historically, due to the lack of attention to supervision in the speech-language pathology and audiology literature, those interested in the process have often turned to other areas for guidance.

A perusal of the literature from education, business management, counseling, social work, and other disciplines where supervision is utilized reveals various perceptions about its purpose. Blumberg (1980) identified the goals of supervision in education as the improvement of instruction and the enhancement of the personal and professional growth of teachers and stated that these two goals are interdependent. Mosher and Purpel (1972), also writing about supervision in education, said that the goal is a very simple one that is common to all professions and occupations—to make sure that other persons do a good job.

Statements of the purpose of supervision are often embedded in discussion of roles, tasks, or components. Van Dersal (1974) believed that the goal of a supervisor is to work "with a group of people over whom authority is exercised in such a way as to achieve their greatest combined effectiveness in getting work done" (p. 10). Tannenbaum (1966) stated that the components of supervision in business organizations are (1) planning, (2) organizing, (3) controlling, (4) communicating, (5) delegating, and (6) accepting responsibility.

These statements refer mainly to the organizational-based supervisor in the work setting. Others have looked at the purposes of supervisors in preparing people to work in their professions. Mosher and Purpel (1972) called it "teaching teachers to teach" (p. 3). In discussing what they call *applied training* in such fields as education, counseling, social work, and psychiatry, Kurpius, Baker, and Thomas (1977) proposed that the supervisor conceptualizes, implements, controls, and manages this application of information. Brammer and Wassmer (1977) said that supervisors assist students in applying counseling theories, principles, and methods to their own clients. For Dussault (1970), the purpose is both teaching and evaluation, which are formally different although they may be accomplished by the same person. Vargus (1977), in reviewing many years of literature on supervision in social work, said that nearly all writers describe the roles of the supervisor as administrator and teacher and generally mention one of the following goals of supervision: (1) to ensure that agencies provide adequate service, (2) to help

workers function to fullest capacity, and (3) to help workers achieve greater professional autonomy.

PURPOSES IN SPEECH-LANGUAGE PATHOLOGY AND AUDIOLOGY

References to the purposes of supervision in speech-language pathology and audiology are also found in the statements of role and task. Villareal (1964), in reporting on a conference called by the American Speech and Hearing Association to discuss guidelines for supervision of clinical practicum, cited the report of one subcommittee at the conference when he wrote, "The role of an effective supervisor should transcend the mere monitoring of the student's clinical activities. It should include the informal teaching of clinical content, the demonstration of clinical techniques, and the mature counseling of the student in relation to his clinical training" (p. 14). Van Riper (1965) said that students are turned into clinicians through supervision. Anderson (1970), in a meeting of school program supervisors, stated, "The major roles of the supervisor are to manage, evaluate, and innovate programs for the communicatively handicapped children and youth within the community. At all times the welfare of children with speech, hearing, or language disorders is the reason for the supervisor's activities" (p. 152). Turton (1973) said, "Supervision can be viewed as a process wherein one person is responsible for changing the knowledge and skill level of another" (p. 94).

Ward and Webster (1965b), in discussing the training of clinicians, said that "Clinical supervision is conceived as an interactive process between student and supervisor in which both are working together to find the most productive ways of effecting the diagnostic or therapeutic relationship" (p. 104).

Writing about supervision in audiology, Rassi (1978) defined clinical supervision as clinical teaching and said, "Its aim is to teach a student in a one-on-one situation how to apply his academic knowledge in a practical clinical setting as he functions in that setting. The ultimate goal is to transform the student into an independent clinician" (p. 9).

A DEFINITION FOR SPEECH-LANGUAGE PATHOLOGY AND AUDIOLOGY

It is clear that there are a variety of personal concepts built into all of the statements about the purposes of supervision and the role of the supervisor, with some common threads running throughout. To add to this array, the following definition of the supervisory process is offered as the basis for the remainder of this book.

> Supervision is a process that consists of a variety of patterns of behavior, the appropriateness of which depends upon the needs, competencies, expectations, and philosophies of the supervisor and the supervisee and the specifics of the situation (task, client, setting, and other variables). The goals of the supervisory process are the professional growth and development of the supervisee and the supervisor, which it is assumed will result ultimately in optimal service to clients.

Despite the fact that this description of the supervisory process was first introduced in 1988, it is consistent with the notion of clinical education and of the goals of clinical educators that McAllister identified in 2000. Even more importantly perhaps, the goals of the process explicated in the first edition of this work are now embodied in the new standards for the accreditation of academic programs, which require that supervision of students be "appropriate to the student's level of knowledge, experience, and competence" (ASHA, 2000a) and must help students develop critical-thinking, decision-making, and problem-solving skills across the knowledge base of the professions. Furthermore, the dynamics of this definition of the supervisory process provide a platform for lifelong learning and refinement of one's own knowledge and skill as a supervisor.

SUMMARY

Supervision in speech-language pathology and audiology is a pervading and complex activity within the professions. Although it is accepted that many individuals are involved in supervision, complete demographic data are limited. The stated purposes of the supervisory process vary among individuals; however, this book is based on the premise that the objective of supervision is to develop independent professionals who, by means of their own professional knowledge and self-awareness as a service provider/supervisor and/or supervisee, can think critically, solve problems, and provide optimal services to communicatively disordered individuals.

CHAPTER TWO

ANDERSON'S CONTINUUM MODEL OF SUPERVISION

Each of us has his own strengths and weaknesses. Therefore, we would hesitate to insist that all of us should supervise in the same way.
—Van Riper, 1965

IS THERE A METHODOLOGY?

Perhaps the most reliable fact about supervision in speech-language pathology and audiology is that the vast majority of supervisors are operating without preparation for the supervisory process and that they have expressed the need for knowing more about how to supervise (Anderson, 1973b, 1974, 1980; ASHA, 1978a; Schubert & Aitchison, 1975; Stace & Drexler, 1969). Very few training programs offer coursework in the supervisory process as part of their curricular offerings for the Master's degree. Similarly, despite the continuing education activities—first of the Council of Supervisors in Speech-Language Pathology and Audiology (CSSPA) and now Special Interest Division 11—Administration and Supervision as well as individual convention contributions from members of the profession—there have been few formal and virtually no ongoing professional development opportunities sponsored by the American Speech-Language-Hearing Association itself. Therefore, it seems reasonable to assume that current supervisory practices continue to be derived in a variety of ways, not necessarily based on a conceptual or theoretical foundation, and possibly not thoughtfully planned or rationally decided.

The search for a methodology for supervision is a will-o-the-wisp, as elusive as a methodology for clinical interaction. Clients are different; clinicians have divergent needs; supervisors vary. Validation data on effectiveness of supervision methods in any field are sparse, and are almost nonexistent in speech language pathology and audiology.

Butler (1976), in a discussion of competencies in speech-language pathology and audiology as they relate to supervision, said:

Interaction between client and clinician in the therapeutic process reflects an almost kaleidoscopic matrix of events. Such interactions must take into account the nature and degree of the client's speech, language, or hearing disorder, the age and sex of the client, the age and sex of the clinician, the degree of sophistication and experience of both client and clinician in the therapeutic process, certain identifiable learning behaviors, and certainly, the professional persuasion of the supervising clinician. If you have ever been a supervisor in a college or university clinic, you know of the perils and the problems of quantifying such a complex matrix. (p. 2)

The supervisor of a service delivery program is no less vulnerable to these complexities. Fisher (1982) addressed the issues in supervising professional personnel in the schools and stated, "This responsibility requires a multitude of skills in human interaction, motivation, and leadership in developing professionals. The role of the supervisor is vastly different from the role of a speech-language pathologist in this respect. In essence, when a person becomes a supervisor, this person changes professions" (p. 54). Although most supervisors in the profession probably see themselves as speech-language pathologists foremost, Fisher's quote underscores the range of skills that are important to the process of supervision and that are important to supervisors' ability to mediate knowledge and skill as clinicians with their supervisees.

Gouran (1980) recognized the fact that supervision remains something of an art and said, "Recommendations related to the practice of supervision should be viewed in probabilistic terms" (p. 87). He further noted that there would be a number of exceptions for any set of recommendations and it would not be prudent to develop or implement standard operating procedures for all situations. Weller (1971) asserted that a single methodological approach is impossible; rather, supervisory functions related to problems should be identified and methodologies appropriate to each should be proposed.

DEVELOPMENT OF SUPERVISORY BEHAVIORS

In the presence of so many situational variables and relatively little "how-to-supervise" information, what forms the basis for the actions of professionals when they become supervisors? How do supervisory behaviors or styles develop? Ob-

viously, past experiences in human interactions influence behaviors toward people in all situations. A major focus in the way supervisors interact with those in less dominant positions in the supervisor/supervisee relationship may be the way in which they have been dealt with by others who have held dominant positions over them—parents, teachers, siblings, or others. Similarly, much of the perception of the role of the supervisor and the behaviors of persons who find themselves in that role probably have come from their interactions with their own supervisors, if not directly modeled from behaviors of those supervisors. They may reflect the style of a significant supervisor, their style may have become a potpourri of behaviors from many supervisors, or they may have learned "what not to do" from those supervisors with whom they did not have a positive and productive experience.

In addition to personal experiences, supervisory behavior may be influenced by a variety of other means. Popular media, both print and visual, have often depicted stylized characterizations of those with supervisory responsibility: the army sergeant, dad's department head, mom's boss, the newspaper editor shouting orders to reporters. Rarely are these portrayals examples of positive, cooperative interactions. More often than not, they are examples of highly directive, controlling behavior. Some supervisors may have read books and articles from other fields about leadership and management and tried to apply the content within the dynamics of their own situation. Policies or organizational structure of the workplace may also influence the way in which supervisors develop their style. Productivity pressures, organizational philosophy, delegation of responsibility, and other organizational variables may directly influence the way in which supervisors perceive and carry out their roles. Lastly, each supervisor's personal characteristics and interpersonal relationships will determine to a great extent the kind of supervisory interaction that each person adopts; they will reflect his or her approach to dealing with people in any setting. Generally speaking, then, individual styles of supervisors may have developed in response to a variety of experiences rather than as a result of a study of the supervisory process, reflection on one's own behavior as a supervisor, or the application of theoretical models and research findings. The development of supervisory behaviors and individual style likely occurs more by happenstance than by strategic design.

MANAGEMENT LITERATURE FROM OTHER DISCIPLINES

The study of supervision is made more complex because of its existence in so many arenas of endeavor. However, there is significant overlap among the helping professions, which makes it important to consider the contributions of each. A complete review of this literature would result in multiple volumes of text and so isn't possible here. Rather, substantive areas of thought will be identified below and will be highlighted by a literature citation, which can then be found in the References section of this work.

> **Scientific Management:** Taylor, 1911
> **Hawthorne Studies:** Mayo, 1933
> **Human Relations Management:** Tannenbaum, 1966; Kelly, 1980; Pascale & Athos, 1981; Reitz, 1981; Hampton, Summer, & Webber, 1982; Hersey & Blanchard, 1982; Peters & Waterman, 1982
> **Motivation and Personality:** Maslow, 1954
> **Participative Management:** McGregor, 1960; Argyris, 1962

Situational Leadership

Gouran (1980) implied that there is not one best way to supervise. This concept of adaptive leadership behavior or **situational leadership**—that is, not one best style but the most effective style for the situation (Gouran, 1980; Hersey & Blanchard, 1982; Reitz, 1981)—is probably the most significant theoretical model from other disciplines when the variables inherent in the definition of supervision in speech-language pathology and audiology are considered. The "leadership contin-

gency model" developed by Fiedler (1967) stated that, although there are more- or less-effective styles of leadership, they are not effective in every situation. The three major situational variables identified by Fiedler in determining the appropriateness of a style of leadership were (1) leader–member relations, (2) degree of structure in the task, and (3) the power and authority their position provides.

Gouran (1980) also suggested that too many people who have supervisory responsibilities function "within narrowly and stereotypically conceived notions of what constitutes 'good supervision'" (p. 93). He maintained that practices based on this erroneous conception are "injurious to the task of clinical supervision." He presented the work of Farris (1974), who identified four supervisory styles: **collaboration, domination, delegation,** and **abdication.** The appropriateness of each style is dictated by the relative capabilities of the supervisor and supervisee to deal independently with a specific kind of demand.

Gouran further stated several principles that are applications of Farris's ideas about the relationship between supervisory style and circumstantial influences:

1. No one style of supervision is best.
2. A supervisor must be prepared to deal differently with different supervisees.
3. Within any given supervisor/supervisee relationship, circumstances may require periodic changes in style.
4. Adoption of an inappropriate style in relation to a particular situational demand will reduce chances for achieving the supervisor and supervisee's mutually shared goals.
5. The measure of success in effective supervision is not the extent of the supervisor's influence on the supervisee, but the extent to which their interaction contributes to the achievement of specified objectives.

Hersey and Blanchard (1982) proposed a "situational leadership theory" utilizing the terms **task behavior** and **relationship behavior** to describe leadership style. Any leadership style is made up of some combination of task or relationship behaviors. *Task behavior* is defined as the extent to which the leader provides direction, organizes roles and activities, and specifies how they are to be achieved; *relationship behavior* is the extent to which the leader establishes and maintains personal relationships with the follower(s) that are supportive and facilitative. It is the interaction of style and environment that makes leadership effective or ineffective; therefore, no style is appropriate to all situations. Hersey and Blanchard further proposed that the level of maturity (Argyris, 1962) of the follower is a variable that must be considered in relation to task. Maturity is defined by Hersey and Blanchard as the ability to set high but attainable goals, the ability and willingness to take responsibility, and having the education and experience to complete a task or job effectively. Because maturity will vary among people or within a group, the leaders must know the level of maturity in determining the appropriate style.

Hersey and Blanchard's model includes four behavioral styles and presents an important parallel to the continuum of supervision proposed in this book.

- **Telling** (high task/low relationship)—leader defines roles and tasks
- **Selling** (high task/high relationship)—direction is still provided but it is accompanied by more two-way communication and socioemotional support to encourage communication
- **Participating** (high relationship/low task)—facilitative, shared decision making
- **Delegating** (low relationship/low task)—follower "runs own show"

Thus, they proposed that when the follower is immature in relation to a task, the appropriate style will be High Task/Low Relationship, that is, the leader will be more involved in organizing and directing in relation to the task. "As the individual or group begins to move into an above average level of maturity, it becomes appropriate for leaders to decrease not only task behavior

but also relationship behavior (p. 163). In other words, the follower works more independently, socioemotional support is not so necessary, and there is less direction and more delegation by the leader. **Style, then, changes as followers become more able to set goals and accomplish the task independently.**

LEADERSHIP AND SUPERVISION IN EDUCATION

At the time that this research on leadership and supervision was developing in the management area, a parallel stream of supervision theory and research was emerging in education. Often borrowing from the management literature, but frequently more related to the teaching aspect of supervision, this parallel development has probably had an even stronger impact on supervision in speech-language pathology and audiology than that of the business literature.

Until the 1970s, the bulk of the writing on supervision in education was related to curriculum development, instruction, in-service, parent and community relations, and similar issues pertinent to the total operation of the educational system rather than to the critical elements of supervisory behavior. Underscoring the lack of evidence about effectiveness of supervision in education, Alfonso, Firth and Neville (1975) stated, "Much attention has been directed toward the tasks that supervisors perform; little has been directed at the critical element of supervisory behavior. Few professional roles in education have had as little intelligent study done" (p. 32).

Research on behavior of teachers in the classroom during the 1970s influenced attitudes toward the study of supervision. Flanders (1967, 1969) was among the first to maintain that direct behavioral styles are less productive in problem-solving activities in the classroom than indirect styles. Generally, Flanders concluded from his various studies that children learned better from teachers who did not dominate but were flexible in their behaviors and those who could be direct or indirect as indicated by a particular situation.

Studies of Indirect and Direct Behavior

The direct/indirect concept was applied to the study of the supervisory process by Blumberg (1968), Blumberg and Amidon (1965), Blumberg, Amidon, and Weber (1967), Blumberg and Cusick (1970), and Blumberg and Weber (1968). Influenced by Flanders (1967) and Bales (1950, 1951), Blumberg and his associates maintained that the exclusive use of direct behaviors in supervision increased defensiveness on the part of supervisees. Blumberg (1974, 1980) also recognized that most texts on supervision did not address what happens between supervisor and supervisee in the supervisory interaction. He and his associates conducted extensive inquiries about the human relationship aspect of supervision, particularly the direct and indirect dimensions of the supervisor's behavior. Blumberg's investigations were based on Gibb's (1969) work on defensive communication, in which he identified six bipolar communication behaviors that were either **support-inducing** or **defense-inducing.** Behavior that was support-inducing, Gibb said, was oriented toward problem solving, spontaneity, equality, provisionalism, empathy, and description. Behavior that was defense-inducing was oriented toward control, strategy, superiority, certainty, neutrality, and evaluation.

Blumberg (1974, 1980) equated Gibb's defense-inducing behaviors with **direct** supervisory behaviors, including such behaviors as telling, giving opinions and suggestions, directing, criticizing, suggesting change, and evaluating. Support-inducing behaviors were equated with **indirect** supervisory behavior and included accepting and clarifying the teachers' questions, praising teacher behavior, asking teachers for their own opinions and suggestions, involving them in problem solving, accepting their ideas, and discussing teachers' feelings about the relationship between the supervisor and the supervisee. In other words, Blumberg contends that these direct/indirect styles communicate a totally different attitude about the teacher/supervisee. Direct behaviors communicate that the supervisor wishes to control the teacher, excludes the teacher from problem solving, sees evaluation by the supervisor as the main function of observation, and does not value the worth of the teacher in the teaching role. Indirect behaviors communicate a concern for the teacher as a person, a desire for collaborative problem solving, and a recognition of the teacher's personal and professional growth.

Using these categories of direct and indirect behaviors, Blumberg and Amidon (1965) investigated whether teachers could discriminate between specific types of behavior of their supervisors. Results of this study made it clear that a one-dimensional approach to supervisory behavior was too simplistic. From this study, the authors developed the following set of four supervisory styles that Blumberg and his colleagues used in subsequent studies:

- **Style A**—High Direct/High Indirect (supervisors are perceived by teachers as emphasizing both direct and indirect behavior, telling, and criticizing but also asking and listening)
- **Style B**—High Direct/Low Indirect (supervisors are perceived by teachers as doing a great deal of telling and criticizing but very little asking or listening)
- **Style C**—Low Direct/High Indirect (supervisors are perceived by teachers as rarely telling or criticizing but emphasizing the asking of questions, listening, and reflecting back the teacher's ideas and feelings)
- **Style D**—Low Direct/Low Indirect (supervisors are perceived as passive and not doing much within the interaction)

Blumberg and his associates also found that perceptions of these supervisory styles made a difference in the way teachers viewed their interaction with their supervisors. The results present support for a mix of the two styles of behavior but with a strong tendency to prefer high amounts of indirect behavior, and are an important base for the study of supervisory methodologies. Teachers in these studies perceived more positive interpersonal relationships with their supervisors under the two styles containing the most indirect behavior (Styles A and C). Teachers gave positive evaluations of their interpersonal relationships with their supervisors when they perceived the interaction to consist of telling, suggesting, and criticizing as well as reflecting and asking for information and opinions (Style A) or when there is little telling and much reflecting and asking (Style C). Negative attitudes resulted from perceptions of supervisory behavior as predominantly telling with little reflecting or asking (Style B), or when the supervisor was perceived as passive (Style D).

Teachers in these studies also indicated that they were able to obtain more insight about themselves, both as teachers and as persons, if supervisors used high amounts of indirect behavior with some direct (again a combination of Styles A and C). Thus, Blumberg (1980) stated, "This finding suggests that hearing about oneself is probably most productive, not only when the supervisor (or other helping agent) questions, listens, and reflects back what he hears, but also when he does a bit of telling and gives feedback" (p. 67). Behavioral Styles D (Low Direct/Low Indirect) and B (High Direct/Low Indirect) were not seen by teachers as contributing to learning about themselves. According to Blumberg, even Style B, which does include indirect behavior, was not seen as contributing to insight, perhaps because the presence of the direct was so potent that not only did it not enhance the teachers' feelings of worth and acceptance, but it also made it difficult for them to accept the indirect.

When supervisors were perceived to use Style B (High Direct/Low Indirect), the teachers understandably perceived their supervisors to be more oriented toward control than problem solving. Teachers under this treatment felt the need to be more strategy oriented and less spontaneous, and they felt that supervisors were more oriented toward superiority than equality and more oriented toward certainty than provisionalism. Also, teachers felt their interaction was more dominated by evaluation of their behavior than toward description of that behavior. All of these behaviors are equated with the defense-inducing behaviors.

At the same time, teachers whose supervisors were seen to operate under Style C (Low Direct/High Indirect) perceived the highest degree of empathy and productivity and the least degree of defense-producing behaviors. Thus, said Blumberg (1980), "Our spoken expectations that Style C would result in communicative freedom and high productivity while Style B would reflect defensiveness and low productivity were met" (p. 69).

Other similar findings by Blumberg and Cusick (1970) present support for the use of both direct and indirect behaviors, together with the first definitive discussion of behaviors and data to dispute the value of the direct style. Their findings support the need to look carefully at the effects of the direct and indirect styles and the probable need to analyze one's supervisory behavior on the basis of these styles. Despite methodological problems in the studies, they provide an interesting parallel to some of the management literature and pose many questions about supervisory style. They have been discussed here in depth because of the significance for the proposal to be made later about supervision in speech-language pathology and audiology.

Interpersonal Approach

Meanwhile, at Teacher's College, Columbia University, Dussault (1970) proposed a middle-range theory of supervision in the education of student teachers that was based on Carl Rogers's theory of therapy and personality change. Dussault discussed the relationships that exist between therapy and the teaching function of supervision and developed a theory that parallels Rogers's writings and, in brief, states that if facilitative interpersonal conditions exist during the supervisory conference, then certain changes will be observed in the supervisee.

Dussault differentiated clearly between the **evaluative** function of supervision and the **teaching** function. Evaluation, he said, is the process of assessment or judgment about the person's readiness to assume professional responsibilities. The teaching function, on the other hand, is the process of helping the student acquire the competencies necessary to fulfill those professional responsibilities. Thus, he made a distinction between evaluation as feedback and guide and evaluation as judgmental assessment. This concept departs from the negative perception of supervisors verbalized by Cogan (1973) as "someone paid to ferret out weaknesses" (p. 78) or specialists "charged with filling cavities" (p. 78).

More discussion of the interpersonal aspects of supervision was presented by Mosher and Purpel (1972), who attended to the psychological factors experienced by students/supervisees during the student teaching experience. They suggested a method of supervision, based on ego-counseling, that focuses on the personal condition with regard to certain roles or situations. Ego-counseling "does not deal with unconscious material" but with the "full range of conscious personal response(s) to teaching—both intellectual and emotional" (p. 128–129). This type of supervision requires specific preparation of the supervisor in order to implement it well, but Mosher and Purpel maintain that preparation is necessary for any type of supervision.

Clinical Supervision

Two other authors at about the same time began advocating a style of supervision called **clinical supervision** (Cogan, 1973; Goldhammer, 1969). Their approach to supervision, although not supported with data, was decidedly more specific and more related to the analysis of actual supervisor behavior than any previous writers. The methodology employs shared interaction between supervisor and supervisee, based on objective data collected and analyzed by both supervisor and supervisee. **Clinical,** a term rarely found in the education literature up to this time, was used by both writers to describe supervision as not referring to the pathological, but to describe "supervision up close" (Goldhammer, 1969, p. 54)—the one-to-one relationships between supervisor and teacher. There is a strong emphasis on the desirability of teachers and supervisors to

> be supportive and empathetic; to perfect technical behaviors and the concepts from which they

are generated; to increase efficiencies and pleasure of learning and becoming; to treat one another decently and responsibly and with affection; to engage with one another, honestly. (Goldhammer, 1969, pp. 55–56)

Cogan (1973) described the genesis of the clinical supervision methodology with students in the Master of Arts in Teaching program at Harvard in the late 1950s and indicated that it grew out of the dissatisfaction of many students about the supervision of their student teaching internship. Cogan also defended the use of the word **clinical** and said, "It was selected precisely to draw attention to the emphasis placed on classroom observation, analysis of the in-class events, and the focus on teachers' and students' in-class behavior" (pp. 8–9). Cogan formulated eight phases in his cycle of supervision.

- Phase 1: Establishing the teacher–supervisor relationship
- Phase 2: Planning with the teacher
- Phase 3: Planning the strategy of the observation
- Phase 4: Observing interaction
- Phase 5: Analyzing the teaching–learning processes
- Phase 6: Planning the strategy of the conference
- Phase 7: The conference
- Phase 8: Renewed planning

Goldhammer (1969) proposed five similar stages for the clinical supervisory process:

- Phase 1: Pre-observation conference
- Phase 2: Observation
- Phase 3: Analysis and strategy
- Phase 4: Supervision conference
- Phase 5: Post-conference (nicknamed the "post-mortem")

Both Cogan's and Goldhammer's methodologies definitely mandate recognition of the contributions of supervisor and supervisee to the supervisory process.

In a revision of Goldhammer's earlier work, Goldhammer, Anderson, and Krajewski (1980) called supervision "that place of instructional supervision which draws its data from first-hand observation of actual teaching events, and involves face-to-face (and other associated) interaction between the supervisor and teacher in the analysis of teaching behaviors and activities for instructional improvement" (pp. 19–20).

Cognitive Coaching

Costa and Garmston (1985a) posited an approach to supervision that they called **cognitive coaching.** It is an approach that supports informed teacher decision making that finds its roots in the ideas of Cogan and Goldhammer about clinical supervision (a relationship to foster the teacher's freedom to act self-sufficiently) rather than an approach to supervision that actually is teacher evaluation in disguise. The rationale for this approach is their belief that the teaching act can best be described as a constant stream of decisions and any teacher behavior used is the result of a decision, either conscious or unconscious. Teachers make many decisions each day about students, curriculum, and teaching strategy. "A supervisory process, therefore, should help teachers make better decisions about instruction. Cognitive Coaching is intended to enhance those intellectual skills which contribute to educationally sound decision making" (p. i).

In Costa and Garmston's (1985b) thinking, the supervisor is seen as a mediator of teachers' intelligent behavior. To stimulate the teacher's intellectual skills, the supervisor must call attention to discrepancies between intended and actual learning outcomes and pose problems designed to invite more than a response based on a memory-type response (Fishler, 1971). For example, Cognitive Coaches ask questions such as the following to facilitate teacher thinking, inference building, self-evaluation, and self-prescription: How do you think the students did in meeting the objective? What data seem to support your line of thinking? What do you think the problem is? "The supervisor's questions and statements can

be designed to elicit specific cognitive functions that produce data, relationships, and generalizations to help resolve the problem (pp. 72–73). They suggest a supervisory process that consists of four phases:

- Auditing (planning/clarification of goals, objectives, strategies)
- Monitoring (gathering data about student and teacher performance)
- Validating (analysis and reflection on student and teacher performance in which cause and effect relationships between teacher performance and student achievement are considered)
- Consulting (evaluating appropriateness of goals/teaching strategies, proscribing alternative strategies, and developing insight into the supervisory process)

The writings of Blumberg (1974), Cogan (1973), Goldhammer (1969), Goldhammer, Anderson, and Krajewski (1980), and Costa and Garmston (1985a, 1985b) have exerted significant influence on the writers of this book as well as on the author of its original edition. Although the proposal for supervision that will be presented in this book is different from that proposed by them, it draws heavily from their writings for illustration and support. Readers are invited to read their original works carefully.

SUPERVISORY APPROACHES IN SPEECH-LANGUAGE PATHOLOGY AND AUDIOLOGY

The literature in the professions of speech-language pathology and audiology has descriptive research findings and theoretical approaches to define the practice of supervision in both disciplines.

Descriptive Findings

There is a fairly large body of information about supervisory conferences in speech-language pathology from many sources. These studies have identified a definite pattern found in the dynamics of the conferences in these studies. The details of the studies will be provided later as appropriate; but if the data from these conferences are combined and the reader conjectures about a typical supervisory conference in speech-language pathology (there are no specific data about audiology conferences), the description of a typical conference would be something like this:

The conference is brief—probably less than thirty minutes. The supervisor assumes a dominant role, doing most of the talking, initiating, and structuring of the discussion, thereby setting the tone for the entire conference. Topics change frequently. Much of the content of the conference consists of the supervisee providing information about what happened in the therapy session and the supervisor making suggestions about strategies to be used in the future. It is not clear how much of this information is data based or analyzed, but it appears to be a "rehash" or recounting of what happened in the therapy session. Supervisors give a great deal of information, make a great many suggestions, and do not spend much time asking the supervisee for suggestions about future action. Supervisors use praise or other supportive behaviors to create a positive social-emotional climate, which probably is perceived by supervisees as reinforcement of certain behaviors. Very little explanation, justification, clarification, elaboration, or summaries of statements (all behaviors that enhance communication) are given by either supervisor or supervisee. Discussion probably deals with maintenance or procedural topics, with discussion of anxieties, defensiveness, or other affective issues being avoided. Supervisors in different settings (university, off-campus practicum, or service delivery settings) may operate differently in some aspects of supervision, although there are not really enough data to substantiate this. Emphasis in discussion is on the teaching-therapy process or the client, not on the supervisee or supervisor. The supervisory process is seldom discussed. Very few evaluative statements are made about the supervisee, perhaps because supervisors assume that supervisees can utilize the discussion of the client to learn about their own behavior. Supervisor style will be much the same from one conference to another, regardless of the supervisee's experience, expertise, or expectations. In general, the discussion is cognitive, not affective.

Supervisees are usually passive participants in the conference and seldom ask questions, initiate a topic, or ask for justification. Instead, they react and respond to the supervisors. Their responses tend to be short, most likely agreeing with the supervisor. Supervisees' needs for indirect behavior from the supervisor and for their own participation are probably not met. As with supervisors, supervisees utilize simple utterances without justification or rationalization and they do not provide reinforcement for the supervisor. (Blumberg, 1980; Culatta & Seltzer, 1976, 1977; Culatta et al., 1975; Dowling & Shank, 1981; Hatten, 1966; Irwin, 1975, 1976, 1981b; McCrea, 1980; Pickering, 1979, 1982, 1984; Roberts & Smith, 1982; Russell, 1976; Schubert & Nelson, 1976; Shapiro, 1985a; Smith, 1978; Smith & Anderson, 1982b; Tufts, 1984; Underwood, 1973; Weller, 1971)

Because there is such overwhelming evidence that this is what happens in conferences, this type of interaction will be referred to as *traditional* supervision.

Theoretical Positions

Although less extensive and covering a shorter period of history than supervision in the disciplines just reviewed, the fields of speech-language pathology and audiology have produced a number of suggested approaches to the supervisory process. Most will reveal influence of work from the other disciplines.

Probably the first in-depth look at the complexities of preparing clinical personnel came almost four decades ago in two thoughtful articles by Ward and Webster (1965a, 1965b). Perhaps not so well known except to those specifically interested in the study of supervision and the preparation of speech-language pathologists and audiologists, these articles should be required reading for everyone in the profession because they raised issues that have not yet been thoroughly resolved. Ward and Webster probed "the nature of human encounter" (1965a, p. 39) and stressed the importance of providing proper conditions for growth and change for students as is done for clients, and for developing "concepts of training in which students may gain repeated experience in exploring and exercising their own humanness" (1965a, p. 39). They defined clinical supervision as "an interactive process between student and supervisor in which both are working together to find the most productive ways of effecting the diagnostic or therapeutic relationship" (1965b, p. 104). Supervisors, they believe, must be willing to examine their own attitudes and relationships—the first mention in the literature that both supervisor and clinician behaviors need the same kind of focus given to client behaviors.

A Rogerian orientation to the relationship between supervisor and supervisee was proposed by Caracciolo and colleagues (1978a). Based on Carl Rogers's (1961, 1962) work on client-centered therapy and Dussault's (1970) theory of supervision, the authors suggested that the same facilitating interpersonal conditions that most speech-language pathologists or audiologists would agree are important to facilitate change in client behavior are also relevant to the supervisory process. These facilitating behaviors, if offered to the supervisee by the supervisor, will "provide a psychosocial environment which enables the student to develop into a competent, secure, and independent professional clinician" (p. 286). Further discussion of this approach by Caracciolo and colleagues suggests that the supervisor, while needing to utilize the nondirective, facilitative orientation to establish a relationship conducive to growth, must also play another role. This role is a more directive one, "when the supervisor must be more directive with respect to giving information to the student, making judgments of the student's behaviors, and establishing requirements and standards for lesson planning, report writing, and so on" (p. 288).

At the same time that interest in the supervisory process in speech-language pathology was growing, a parallel interest was developing in audiology. An approach to supervision by Rassi (1978) utilizes a framework of competency-based instruction that includes skills in testing, writing, and interpersonal and decision-making areas. Her definition of supervision is clinical teaching in which the student is taught "in a one-to-one situation how to apply his academic knowledge in a practical clinical setting as he functions in that setting. The ultimate goal is to transform the student into an independent clinician" (p. 9).

Later, Rassi (1985, 1987) provided arguments for differences between supervision of audiology and speech-language pathology. The preponderant diagnostic nature of work inherent in the practice of audiology dictates a different approach to supervision, according to her. This approach, she said, requires competency-based instruction.

Schubert (1978) suggested an approach to supervision based on the use of an interaction analysis system, the "Analysis of Behavior of Clinicians." This system will be discussed in Chapters 6 and 7. The Integrative Task Maturity Model of Supervision (ITMMS), discussed by Mawdsley (1985a) at an ASHA convention, is an ingenious combination of the Hersey and Blanchard Situational Leadership Model (1982), the Wisconsin Procedure for Appraisal of Clinical Competence (Shriberg et al., 1975), and the clinical supervision model of Cogan (1973). It includes a system for analyzing appropriate supervisory styles and specific techniques to be utilized at different levels of maturity. Crago and Pickering (1987) published a book that discussed several facets of the supervisory process with a major emphasis on its interpersonal aspects.

Farmer and Farmer (1989) promote a Trigonal Model of Communication Disorders supervision, which identified three components of the supervisory process. In addition to positing the model itself, they proposed specific activities to implement it which were consistent with its theoretical constructs.

Gillam and Pena (1995) and Gillam (1999) suggested that clinical education can best be thought of as a socialization process in which supervisors demonstrate and mediate the ideals and practices that are valued by the profession. In this model, which is based on Vygotsky's (1978) social constructivist theory of learning, supervisors are seen as socialization agents who mediate the values, ideals, and practices that are valued by the professions. In the initial stages of their training, student clinicians are assigned to supervisors who function as master clinicians and who model and interpret clinical behavior for students during an initial period of highly structured, specific observation. Gradually, supervisors should encourage student participation at a comfortable, yet challenging level and should provide a bridge for generalizing skills and approaches from familiar to novel situations. As students become more responsible for the provision of direct clinical service, the clinical education experience might develop into a coaching relationship between supervisor and student. This approach is perhaps best described as an apprenticeship model of supervision and may have real utility as a downward extension of the model of supervision proposed by this book within the dynamics of certain situations: undergraduate practicum; graduate practicum under Medicare Part B regulations; concurrent observation under the new ASHA standards (ASHA 2000a) which are scheduled to begin implementation in 2003; and the utilization of assistants who will provide direct service to patients/clients.

Subsequent to the publication of the original edition of this book, Dowling (1992, 2001) authored two books that also enhanced the literature base in the supervisory process in speech-language pathology. They both were predicated on a broad, interdisciplinary compilation of theory and research in leadership and supervision with a expanded focus on the application of this information to clinical supervision in speech-language pathology and audiology (ASHA, 1985a) and the continuum model of supervision developed by Anderson (1988).

It is Anderson's model that forms the foundation of this book. In writing about her original motivation for this model, Anderson (1981) wrote:

The pervading belief underlying the program is that supervision at any level is teaching—a very special kind of teaching—and that, like all teaching, it requires the involvement of the learner.

Therefore, the supervisee is not an apprentice to be molded into a model of the supervisor, is not "slave labor," and, although often but not always "less knowing," is not *subordinate* to the supervisor. The model that is developing and being tested through self-study and research is one of joint problem solving by supervisor and supervisee related to client or program needs. It includes maximal use of objective data collection and self-analysis techniques by both supervisor and supervisee. It assumes a dual role for the clinician—that of clinician to the client, and supervisee to the supervisor. Each of these roles demands a different set of behaviors that can and must be identified, observed, quantified, analyzed, and if necessary, modified. The model utilizes an analytical approach to behavior in the supervisory conference and assumes that interaction between supervisor and supervisee is as important to the total learning process and as measurable as the interaction between clinician and client. It also assumes that supervisors, as well as supervisees, can and must grow and develop and improve their own skills as they participate in the supervisory process. (p. 79)

THE CONTINUUM OF SUPERVISION IN SPEECH-LANGUAGE PATHOLOGY AND AUDIOLOGY

The definition and description of the supervisory process given in Chapter One is the professional growth of both supervisor and supervisee. Expansion of that idea leads to the concept of the supervisor's role as assisting the supervisee in reaching a level of independence in which their relationship is one of peer-consultation rather than dependency. To create a situation where supervisees can say, "We did it ourselves" (as they provide quality service) seems the ultimate in the supervisory relationship. This conceptualization of the supervisory relationship is in contrast to the descriptive data that identified the *traditional* approach to supervision detailed earlier in this chapter. It is, however, a process that is consistent with those described by Blumberg (1980), Cogan (1973), Goldhammer (1969), Goldhammer, Andersen, and Krajewski

(1980), Costa and Garmston (1985a, 1985b), and the clinical education process identified by McAllister (2000). Indeed, it is the process implied by the current standards for accreditation of academic training programs in the communication sciences and disorders (ASHA, 2000a).

The remainder of this chapter will discuss a continuum of supervision in which the goal is the type of supervisory practice that is appropriate to the "student's level of knowledge, experience, and competence" (ASHA, 2000a) and that will help develop a speech-language pathologist or audiologist who is able to think critically, make decisions, and solve problems (ASHA, 2000a). Further, this continuum is applicable to the professional whose continued growth is necessary to meet the demands of the profession's scope of practice and the ethical commitment to quality (and continuous quality improvement) in order "to hold paramount the welfare of the clients served" (ASHA, 1997).

It will become immediately clear that the continuum model recognizes that there is not just one way to supervise. In fact the model is predicated on the belief that supervision exists on a continuum and employs different strategies and styles that are appropriate at different points in time. These styles are determined by the variables inherent in the process—that is, the needs, competencies, expectations, and philosophies of both supervisor and supervisee as well as variables associated with the setting (task, client, organizational structure, etc). The model offers a structure for supervisors and supervisees to examine their own philosophies about supervision, identify their own behaviors, and determine what changes they want to make, if any. As a result, it suggests an approach of continuous improvement that can span a career from preprofessional training and the CF as a supervisee through experienced supervisory and clinical practice.

Stages of the Continuum

The continuum of supervision is based on the assumption that professionals will be involved in some supervisory or consultative experience for the duration of their professional lives and that the expectations and needs of supervisees change throughout this period of time. The continuum is comprised of three stages:

- Evaluation-Feedback Stage
- Transitional Stage
- Self-Supervision Stage

The continuum mandates a change over time in the amount and type of involvement of both supervisor and supervisee in the supervisory process. As the degree of dominance of the supervisor decreases, participation by the supervisee increases across the continuum. As they move into the Self-Supervision Stage, the balance changes to an equal interaction of peers. Each stage and its appropriate style will be discussed briefly here with more detailed discussion to follow in succeeding chapters.

Perhaps the most significant feature of the continuum that must be fully appreciated is that **none of the stages are time-bound.** Individual supervisees may be found at any point on the continuum throughout their career, depending on personal and professional situational variables. Some may never reach the Self-Supervision Stage and others may begin well beyond the Evaluation-Feedback Stage.

It is assumed that this continuum applies to both speech-language pathology and audiology. In fact, Rassi (1978), in discussing supervision in audiology, presented a similar continuum that identified eight possible levels of supervision beginning with detailed explanation accompanied by demonstration to a final level where the student is working independently with monitoring and suggestions provided by the supervisor only when necessary. Rassi stated, "Each succeeding level requires less active participation by the supervisor, while at the same time, the student's direct involvement and attendant responsibilities increase" (p. 15). Indeed, it may also be assumed that within each level there will be shifts in the supervisor-supervisee balance over time.

Evaluation-Feedback Stage.   In the evaluation feedback stage, the supervisor is dominant. This is where the beginning supervisee may be found, or the supervisee who is working with a new type of client, or one who has just entered a new setting. The supervisee who is unknowledgeable or has difficulty applying academic information to the clinical process, often called the "marginal student," may perseverate at this stage. Unprepared for clinical interaction for whatever reason, unable to problem-solve, overwhelmed by the dynamics of a given situation, or accustomed to being told what to do, the supervisee at this stage assumes a very passive role. Additionally, supervisees may also be placed at this stage by supervisors who perceive their role to be strictly that of instructor or evaluator.

Whatever the reason for dynamics of the Evaluation-Feedback Stage, the goal for both supervisor and supervisee is to work together to move quickly from this point. Hersey and Blanchard (1982) identified eight variables that influence the amount and degree of supervisor involvement:

- Supervisee's clinical competence (i.e., ability, technical knowledge, and practical skills)
- Supervisee's psychological maturity and commitment (i.e., degree of self-confidence, motivation, and self-respect)
- Supervisee's perception of supervisor's expertise
- Supervisee's expectations of what the supervisor should or should not be able to do and provide
- The styles and expectations of the supervisor's superior/boss
- The colleagues with whom a supervisor interacts on a regular basis
- Organizational/institutional expectations, goals, policy, and philosophy
- Amount of time

Transitional Stage. The Transitional Stage follows the Evaluation-Feedback Stage. It is perceived as the place where the supervisee has reached a level of competency, that is, knowledge and skill, and the supervisor has achieved an attitude that results in participation by both in joint problem solving and peer interaction. Supervision

in this stage is a shared process. The supervisee is not able to operate independently but is moving along the continuum in that direction.

At this stage, supervisees are able to participate in varying degrees in decision making. They are learning to analyze their clinical behavior and action and plan future strategies on the basis of that analysis; to make modifications during their clinical sessions; to problem-solve; and to collaborate within the supervisory conference. Moreover, the supervisor is able to allow the supervisee to assume these responsibilities. As the supervisory dyad moves along the continuum, the interaction becomes increasingly closer to peer interaction or colleagueship (Cogan, 1973) with the ever-present goal of independence or self-supervision. Supervisees may move back and forth within the Transitional Stage depending on many variables, but most especially those of experience, task, and setting. Some supervisees may have skills that enable them to begin their supervisory experience at any point in the Transitional Stage. Some may have had many hours of experience with language delayed children and be able to work independently with them, but when they are assigned to their first traumatic brain injury client may find it necessary to move back to the Evaluation-Feedback Stage and receive more direct and structured input from their supervisor. Such situations may occur in either the educational setting or the service delivery setting but the key is that when they do, supervisees are able to "recover" their positions in the Transitional Stage sooner rather than later because of their previous experience within the clinical process and their growing understanding of themselves as clinicians.

Self-Supervision Stage. Self-Supervision is defined as a stage in which supervisees have the ability to accurately analyze their clinical behavior and its outcomes and to alter it based on that analysis. It denotes a level of independence in problem solving in which supervisees are no longer dependent on supervisors for observation, analysis, and feedback about their clinical work. It is the stage in which supervisees become responsible for their own professional growth. It is also a stage in which, despite their independence, supervisees still desire peer interaction and consultation. Indeed, as rapidly as research and regulation are changing the dynamics of clinical service delivery, the consultation process is becoming an increasingly important professional dynamic. Some professionals may never reach a total level of independence.

Implications of the Continuum

This continuum has important implications in terms of expectations for professionals during their educational program and after they leave it. Some supervisees may not reach the independence of the Self-Supervision Stage across the spectrum of age and disorders for which they must be trained to provide service or they may not reach independence in relation to certain aspects of it despite the efforts of the educational training program. This then becomes a question of accountability for the educational program, particularly in light of the new standards for training programs (ASHA, 2000a), which will be discussed in later chapters. If the supervisee enters an externship, the Clinical Fellowship (CF), or the work force at a point on the continuum below the Self-Supervision Stage, the supervisor in this situation must then implement a style relevant to that point. In other words, supervisors in all situations must be aware of the continuum as they determine the appropriate style for each supervisee. Additionally, they must possess the flexibility that will enable them to adjust their behaviors as they move back and forth on the continuum with their supervisees. The task of identifying the place at which the supervisor and supervisee should be operating and the behaviors that make up the appropriate style will be the focus of much of the remainder of this book.

Appropriate Styles for Each Stage

The appropriate supervisory style for each stage of the continuum is determined by the skill level of the supervisee and the nature of the task as related to the client. The supervisor's flexibility in adapting to these variables also affects the appropriateness of the interaction.

Direct-Active Style. The Direct-Active Style of supervisor interaction is most appropriate for the Evaluation-Feedback Stage of the continuum. It embodies what might be thought of as stereotypical supervisor behavior: telling, criticizing, evaluating. In this style, the supervisor is in a controlling, superior position; the supervisee is in a passive, at best respondent, and subordinate position.

This style at its extreme embodies maximum control and responsibility in the supervisor's role; dependence and minimal participation in the supervisee's role. It is the High Direct-Low Indirect style of Blumberg (1980), the Domination Style of Farris (1974), and the style of choice of many supervisors. According to the literature, it is comparable to the High Task/Low Relationship Stage of the Hersey and Blanchard (1982) model. It may be appropriate, depending on the needs of the supervisee in relation to the client or specific setting. The frequency with which it is used may depend on the perceptions that both supervisor and supervisee have of their role in the supervisory process. Some supervisors may hold a firm conviction that direct behavior produces greater change in supervisees and, therefore, prefer this style.

Available time is perceived by some as the variable that influences the use of this style by the supervisor more than any other (Irwin, 1976). Those who use this reasoning say that joint problem-solving, which is a characteristic of the Collaborative or Consultant Style, takes time that most supervisors do not have, especially today in settings where billable hour productivity is an important dynamic. Supervisors may feel that it is necessary to be more directive with supervisees in the interest of the client and the bottom line when time is limited. This assumption has not been empirically tested, however, and the ramifications of time in the supervisory process are unknown.

Although it seems clear that there are situations in which the supervisee is in the Evaluation-Feedback Stage and the direct style is appropriate, especially with the inexperienced or unskilled student, the decision to use this Direct-Active Style must be made carefully. A number of questions need be to asked and answered to help determine if this style is indeed appropriate:

- By whose judgment is the supervisee determined to be inexperienced or unskilled?
- On what basis has the judgment been made that the supervisee is at the Evaluation-Feedback Stage?
- Has the judgment been made on the basis of objective data?
- Is the judgment merely the result of the subjective appraisal of the supervisor, biased by his or her own experiences and preferences?
- Is it the supervisor's style with all supervisees?

This style used exclusively has certain hazards. Theoretical writings and research on leadership and human interaction clearly negate the use of any single style for all situations because of differences in supervisee, supervisor, and situation (Gouran, 1980). One outcome of the exclusive use of this style is the phenomenon of modeling (see Figure 2.1). Although a certain amount of directing, suggesting, and modeling by supervisors may be necessary, appropriate, and desirable at some times, it may also be a deterrent to growth and development of the supervisee. The constant shaping of the supervisee's behavior to match that of the supervisor based on what his or her performance would probably have been in a similar situation, has the potential for the outcome of the supervisory process to be the creation of a mirror image of the supervisor.

This outcome is not consonant with the supervisory process implied by current ASHA (2000a) standards and possibly will create problems for the professions. If each new generation of professionals does no more than model the behaviors of its supervisors, it does not bode well for the development of critical-thinking and problem-solving professionals who are able to develop efficacious systems for delivering services, nor for the welfare of clients. **The purpose of supervision is not cloning.**

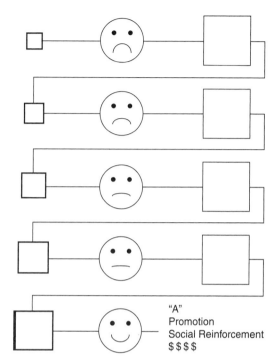

FIGURE 2.1 Social Promotion

Although supervisors do have experiential and academic information to share with their supervisees (if they didn't, they should not be supervising), no supervisor can possibly have all the definitive answers to every clinician-client transaction. Certainly with the proliferation of knowledge from which speech-language pathologists and audiologists draw, each generation of professionals should proceed beyond the level of the last. The objective of supervisors should be not only to impart their own experience but also to encourage their supervisees to go beyond them. The pervasive use of the Direct-Active style would seem not to accomplish this.

Confusion about Direct-Indirect. Those who have studied the supervisory process in recent years have been introduced to the Direct-Indirect concept and certain misconceptions have grown up around it. Its characteristics have often been distorted from the original description by Blumberg (1974) and its use has been subject to a variety of interpretations. Additionally, a value judgment has been placed on the two styles in some instances—direct supervisory behavior is wrong, indirect is right—which is not at all consistent with the results of early research.

It is simplistic to discuss any style of human behavior restrictively. Blumberg (1974) himself made it clear that he and his associates perceived at least four combinations of direct and indirect supervisory behavior and that teachers perceived a combination of both types of behavior to be more effective than either one alone. In reality, what becomes important in terms of the continuum is the balance of these behaviors and the appropriateness of that balance to the situation.

Some supervisors have not interpreted the behavioral components of these styles accurately. Some assume that the mere asking of questions makes an interaction indirect, ostensibly because the supervisor is not telling the supervisee to do something; however, there are many ways of framing questions. "Do you think the client would benefit from…?" may appear just as direct as "Have him do this next time."

Perhaps it would be more productive to describe these behaviors as active and passive rather than direct and indirect to more accurately and precisely capture the behavior of both supervisors and supervisees. Accordingly, a supervisor's behavior may be direct-active, characterized by the descriptors for direct behavior; indirect-active, characterized by purposeful behaviors that encourage problem solving, such as asking for opinions and suggestions, accepting and expanding supervisee's ideas, or asking for rationale and justification of supervisee statements; indirect-passive, characterized by listening and waiting for supervisees to process ideas and problem solve; or passive, characterized by not listening, providing little or no input, or not responding to supervisee input or requests. Similarly, an active supervisee would participate by collecting and analyzing data, initiating discussion, problem solving, questioning, giving opinions, and requesting rationale and justification for supervisor statements. A passive supervisee

would be listening, accepting, asking for suggestions and guidance, seeking strategies, and waiting for information from the supervisor.

The clinical supervision approach (Cogan, 1973; Goldhammer, 1969), which has influenced much of the thinking about supervision in recent years, makes no allowances for a direct style. Cogan rejected the superior/subordinate relationship between supervisors and supervisees as incompatible with his approach; Goldhammer insisted on cooperative, shared interactions. However, they were writing about the professionally employed teacher. It is the opinion of the writers that, particularly in an educational program, supervisors must allow for the fact that some supervisees will need varying amounts of direct assistance in learning how to begin their work as professionals, and that there are times when supervisors will legitimately need to provide specific directions or demonstrate techniques. Certainly, Gillam and Pena (1995) would advocate for this position. It is only when direct behavior persists throughout the interaction or with all supervisees and inhibits their opportunities for problem solving that it should be viewed as inappropriate.

Collaborative Style. The Collaborative Style is the appropriate style for moving away from the Evaluation-Feedback Stage through the Transitional Stage to Self-Supervision. This style is a dynamic, problem-solving process wherein supervisor and supervisee work together to achieve optimum service for clients as well as for the professional growth and development of both participants. The supervisor's role is less direct but not inactive. Both participants assume responsibility and provide input in varying degrees at different times about both the clinical and the supervisory process. Objectives are established jointly. The supervisor provides feedback but also encourages input from the supervisee, accepts the supervisee's ideas, problem solves with the supervisee, analyzes clinical behavior, encourages self-analysis and further planning by the supervisee, and recognizes and respects the worth of the supervisee as a professional and as a person. The supervisee, in turn, accepts responsibility for participation in the clinical and supervisory process, provides input, accepts suggestions, questions the supervisor, requests rationale and justification for supervisor statements, engages in self-analysis and problem solving, and works toward independence. The supervisor, though responsible for structuring and facilitating interaction, is *not* the only responsible individual within the interaction and does not make all the decisions or provide all the information. Rather, supervision is seen as a joint process in which the supervisor and supervisee share responsibilities and interact as professionals to meet common objectives. As progression continues along the continuum, the amount of participation from each is altered as shown in Figure 2.2. This becomes what Kurpius and colleagues (1977) termed *increased ownership* by the trainee in the joint experience of supervision. Furthermore, the interactions between supervisor and supervisee are subject to study to increase the learning that results from participation in the supervisory process. Based on clinical supervision as presented by Cogan (1973) and Goldhammer (1969), this style is seen as necessary to move from the Evaluation-Feedback Stage to the ultimate objective of Self-Supervision.

Some supervisors resist the Collaborative Style because they assume it means a compromising of the supervisor's position or that it is impossible to obtain appropriate input from the supervisees. Some do not realize that it employs a mix of behaviors. This is definitely a misunderstanding of the style. The supervisor who uses the Collaborative Style may employ both direct, indirect, active, or passive behaviors in any combination, depending on the situation. None of these styles will be seen in a pure form. Only in the Evaluation-Feedback Stage does the supervisor come close to totality of direct behavior, and even then there will be a mix of behaviors. **The aim of the Collaborative Style is to move away from the direct supervisor and passive supervisee behavior as rapidly as possible to involve the supervisee in decision making.** Supervisors should continue to have input, however. They must share their experience and expertise, but not to the exclusion of meaningful participation by the supervisee.

Munson (1983) described supervision in social work in terms that are similar to the Collaborative Style proposed here:

> If we enter supervision viewing it as the place where supervisors give answers, check up on the practitioner's work, and find solutions for the therapist, we will have started off on the wrong foot and will stumble. Supervision should be a mutual sharing of questions, concerns, observations, speculations, and selection of alternative techniques to apply in practice. I call this process the *congruence of perceptions* in supervision. Practitioners should, and want to, participate in supervision rather than be recipients in it. (p. 4)

Caracciolo and colleagues (1978b) described this mix of behaviors when they said that the supervisor plays two roles—a nondirective one that enables the student to express ideas without fearing judgment or penalty, and a directive one that gives information when appropriate, establishes standards and guidelines, and judges when appropriate.

> The speech-language pathology supervisor must, therefore, be sensitive to the continuously changing needs of the student clinician within any given moment of the supervisory conference period and must be able to match the supervisory behavior to the student clinician's needs and expectations. (p. 288)

In certain instances, a supervisor and supervisee may change roles at some points in the

Collaborative Style for the Transition Stage

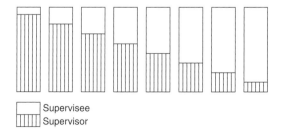

☐ Supervisee
▥ Supervisor

FIGURE 2.2   Collaborative Style

Transitional Stage. For example, a student clinician, well-trained and with extensive experience in the clinical process within a specific disorder area, might work with a supervisor whose background in this area is different, limited, or not current. The supervisee might then assume a more active role in the collaboration, with the supervisor being the beneficiary of input about certain techniques, new research, or a differing philosophy. This requires openness on the part of the supervisor, and confidence, if not courage, on the part of the supervisee.

As in the Evaluation-Feedback Stage, there may be hazards. If the proper place on the continuum is not identified, supervisors may expect supervisees to operate beyond their level, resulting in frustration for both. The Collaborative Style could easily become more of an *abdication style* if supervisors do not provide the correct amount of input. However, the benefits of the Collaborative Style are worth the risks associated with it. Collaborative behaviors on the part of supervisors can begin the process of empowerment and acceptance of responsibility for their behavior on the part of supervisees. It facilitates the process of independent critical thinking and problem solving that is requisite to practice in the professions.

Consultative Style. Following the continuum through to its conclusion of Self-Supervision, the burden of responsibility now shifts to the supervisee. Self-supervision requires a continuing search for professional growth through self-analysis. It suggests a peer relationship between supervisor and supervisee, which is represented in Figure 2.3 by the horizontal lines, which signify the ultimate cooperative interaction between supervisor and supervisee. This interaction has been developing throughout the previous stages of the continuum and the supervisee is now empowered to make decisions about his or her own needs, and can proceed to find solutions.

The preprofessional or professional who reaches this stage will be able to self-identify strengths or weaknesses, make appropriate behavioral modifications, and seek assistance or further knowledge when appropriate. Although this knowledge may come from other sources—peers,

Consultative Style

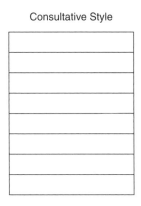

FIGURE 2.3   Consultative Style for the Self-Supervision Stage

in-service or course offerings, readings, or creative problem solving—the supervisory relationship remains important, even though supervisees now have the major responsibility for initiating consultation, even if it is not automatically made available to them.

By definition, *consult* means "to seek advice or information" as in "consult a specialist," "to exchange views," or "to give professional advice" (*Webster's,* 1984, p. 303). This is exactly the concept intended in the use of this term as the appropriate style for Self-Supervision, a style that involves a more voluntary nature of interaction between peers than the previous styles.

> *Consultation* is a helping process which emerges out of a need to solve a problem. The consultant and consultee engage in a voluntary relationship which focuses on change (i.e., behaviors, structures, system and/or situations). In the work-related process of consultation, the consultant helps the consultee use his/her knowledge, skills, and expertise to solve a problem. (Brasseur, 1978, p. 2)

As with the other stages, Self-Supervision is **not time bound,** and therefore, the Consultative Style may be utilized at appropriate times in the educational program, the off-campus or CF experience, or the employment setting. The supervisor may serve in this capacity when the supervisee no longer needs continuous monitoring. This style may be used when supervisees are working with certain types of clients with which they have developed expertise while, at the same time, the supervisor may be utilizing a Direct-Active Style with the same supervisee while working with another client. In the employment setting where supervisors are often less available, supervisees may find it necessary to be specific in their requests for help. If a true consultative style is to be a reality here, both participants must enter the interaction with a clear concept of their roles, the problems to be solved, and the procedures to be followed. As with other stages, differences in perceptions and unmet expectations can create negative reactions, leading to a variety of negative results.

Supervisor behaviors used in the Consultative Style will be mainly listening, supporting, problem solving, and, where appropriate, giving direct suggestions. If a true peer relationship exists, these suggestions may be accepted, rejected, or built on by the supervisee. The two will be relating as peers in a productive interaction. It is critical, therefore, that the supervisor recognizes and accepts the supervisee's options, especially that of rejecting suggestions.

Striving to reach the Self-Supervision Stage is important in speech-language pathology and audiology because so many professionals work alone or without supervision or consultation from persons trained in their own profession. Working alone is not necessarily synonymous with self-supervision. When working in such situations, the responsibility for professional growth lies with the individual. Some professionals are able to continue their self-analysis and professional growth to a greater extent than others. Supervision in the service delivery setting will be discussed in greater depth in Chapter 11, but it should be said here that the lack of supervision or consultation in the employment setting by trained people is a serious issue in terms of continuing professional growth. This lack increases the need for educational programs to produce self-analytical students. The continuum model of supervision presented in this book offers a process as well as strategies for accomplishing this important goal.

Place on the Continuum

A composite of the stages of the continuum and their appropriate styles is seen in Figure 2.4. Determining the level at which the supervisor and

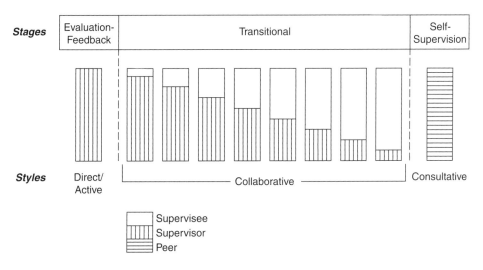

FIGURE 2.4 Full Continuum

supervisee are functioning and, therefore, the appropriate style to use, is a decision that requires insight and analysis on the part of both participants. It is somewhat analogous to the diagnostic process used to determine the needs of clients. This process will be discussed in Chapter 5. Samples of the three styles in hypothetical conferences are shown in Appendix 2A.

Attitudes toward the Continuum

Most supervisors would probably say that this continuum *is* what they actually are following, that they *do* treat supervisees differently, that they *do* change their style depending upon the level of expertise of the supervisee, and that their style *is* a collaborative one. In reality, as has been seen, data on the supervisory conference indicate that not only is the Direct-Active Style the most frequently used style, but that supervisors *do not* change their styles over time, even when they perceive that they do (Blumberg, 1980; Culatta & Seltzer, 1976, 1977; Culatta et al., 1975; Dowling & Shank, 1981; Hatten, 1966; Irwin, 1975,1976, 1981b; McCrea, 1980; Pickering, 1979, 1981a, 1981b, 1982, 1984; Roberts & Smith, 1982; Russell, 1976; Schubert & Nelson, 1976; Shapiro, 1985a; Smith, 1978; Smith & Anderson, 1982b; Tufts, 1984, Underwood, 1973; Weller, 1971). Despite the fact that these data are historical, very little training of supervisors has occurred since they were first collected and so it is highly likely that supervisors continue to demonstrate a single supervisory style over a period of time, even when they perceive that they do not. In sum, supervisors appear to have one style that they use consistently with all supervisees. Some supervisors, accustomed to the Direct-Active Style, may be unwilling to change their style; some supervisees may prefer to remain dependent and passive. Nonetheless, the continuum is presented as a vehicle for helping to develop supervisees who are able to think independently, critically, and solve their own professional problems as well as for a vehicle for lifelong professional learning and development.

SUMMARY

Philosophy and procedures in supervision in speech-language pathology and audiology have their historical foundation in the literature from other disciplines as well as from the experiences of people in the professions themselves. It is important for students of the supervisory process to have a broad view of the accumulated knowledge about supervision so that they can build on rather than repeat the events of the past.

Supervision exists on a continuum along which supervisors and supervisees progress during individual supervisory interactions as well as throughout their professional career. Although individuals may enter the continuum at any point or may move back and forth along it, depending upon situational variables, it is the continuous **movement** along the continuum toward the ultimate objective of independence that is critical. The Collaborative Style is seen as a means to facilitate this movement.

Sample Scripts of a Direct, Direct-Indirect, and Indirect Supervisory Conference

In all three scripts, the clinical problem, therapy strategies, and outcomes of the conference are the same. The scripts differ only in the proportions of direct and indirect behaviors (validated by panel of five experts, using Blumberg's 1970 Interaction Analysis System to code behaviors every three seconds).

Key:
SR—Supervisor
SE—Supervisee

DIRECT/ACTIVE SUPERVISORY STYLE

SR: Hi Ann.... How are you today?

SE: Fine. Were you able to watch my session with Johnny yesterday?

SR: Um hmm.

SE: What did you think about it?

SR: Well, I noticed that he still isn't able to produce /s/ in final position words. Let's see…if I'm right, he is able to produce syllables—different vowels plus /s/—without a model from you with 90% accuracy. Is that right?

SE: Um hmm. But I'm getting frustrated…I'm not quite sure what to do because as soon as I give him a word, he goes back to his error…he omits the sound. And I thought I had a pretty good program planned…I mean he *is* 7 years old and he omits /s/, /z/, sh, ch, zh, and j. And so after you suggested working on /s/ and checking for generalization to untrained /s/ words and the other sibilants—and helped me figure out where to start training with him—I thought I'd be on my way. But right now, I doubt if he'll ever learn to say the 10 final position /s/ words that I'm trying to train…much less generalize to untrained items.

SR: Well, maybe I can give you some help. I'm sure that I can think of some strategies that would work with Johnny.... After all, that's part of my job…to help you so you can be more effective with Johnny.

SE: Oh good. It's kinda hard for me because all this is so new to me. And of course, you've had a lot more experience, so you know what works and what doesn't work.

SR: Okay, first tell me what you've tried, Ann.

SE: Okay. Well, I've shown him some pictures that have a final /s/ like *bus, goose, base, race*… and here are my pictures (SE shows cards to SR). See, *bus, base, piece, mice, moose, case, geese, goose, rice, race,* and *house.*

SR: Um hmm.

SE: Um, I've shown him these pictures and asked him to say the words.... But when I do that, he omits the final sound.

SR: Um hmm. But Ann, you've, um, you've missed an important point. You went from training in syllables where first you modeled the syllable, had him make an attempt, and then gave him feedback. Once he reached criteria for this step, you stopped modeling, but continued to provide feedback—which acted as a reinforcer—and you did that until he reached criteria. Then, in making the transition from production in syllables to production in words, you left out a few very important details. Um, you gave him one model—asked him to make five attempts—then after all of his attempts, you gave him feedback. (SR looks at clipboard). In my notes from observing your therapy session yesterday, I wrote down that I needed to talk to you about learning theories, because obviously you've forgotten some things…or you're having trouble applying what you've had in classes to what you're doing in therapy. So that's one of the things I want to discuss with you today. Is that all right with you?

SE: Yes, that's fine.

SR: Okay, first let me review operant conditioning with you. Remember that behaviorists maintain that a behavior is influenced by its consequences. In trying to establish a new behavior, you devise small steps that lead to that goal behavior. You decide what stimuli you will provide…and what the desired response is…and what the consequences of a response will be. Any consequence that increases a behavior is a reinforcement and any consequence that decreases a behavior is a punishment. So you're working with this, um, Stimulus—Response—Reinforcement paradigm (SR writes and shows to SE).

Consequences must be provided consistently, if you expect to change a behavior. Um, I think consistency may have been part of the reason why Johnny didn't do well in your last session. I think the stimuli that you provided may be the other part of the reason he couldn't successfully produce those final position /s/ words. I would suggest that in your sessions next week, you do two things.

First, give him feedback after *every* response…that is, provide consistent consequences. When he's right, let him know. When he's wrong, let him know that too. It might also be helpful to let him know *why* he's wrong when he has incorrect responses. That is, you give him informative feedback…like, "Johnny, you forgot to say /s/ at the end of the word. Watch me, say *mice*." Emphasize the final sound.

Second…change the way you are providing the stimulus…give him a verbal model *every* time. Show him the picture, then you say the word, then ask him to say it.

Do you understand what I mean? Is that clear to you?

SE: Um hmm. I remember talking about that stuff in classes. Now I think I have a better

idea about how to use it in therapy. Um…I mean, your suggestions really were helpful.

SR: Good, good. Also, you want to be sure that you tabulate each one of his responses during your sessions…. That way we can tell if the feedback is acting as a positive reinforcement. Why don't you take a minute and write all of this stuff down, so you don't forget. Um, do you have any questions so far?

SE: No, not right now.

[SE writes:

1. Give feedback to client after each response. Give informative feedback for incorrect responses.
2. Provide a model with each presentation of stim card. Also, provide model before requesting subsequent attempt.
3. Tally responses]

[SE looks at notes.] It looks like my sessions next week should be pretty good. Um…in my lesson plan, my overall objective is to have him say 9 out of 10 words correctly on his first attempt…this is in four consecutive sets.

So, on Tuesday, I'm not sure if he'll be able to reach that criteria…it might be a little bit too high.

SR: I think you're probably right. I think 90% is probably a little too high…. I think that you should leave the 90% on four consecutive sets as your overall goal…but on Tuesday, set your objective at 70%. See if he can reach a 70% level of proficiency when you provide a model each time, and when you are providing consistent feedback. That seems like a pretty reasonable expectation for the session.

SE: Yeah, it does. Um [silence; SE thinking]… Suppose he doesn't reach criteria…say after 10 sets, or 100 trials, he still can't get that 70% correct…. What do you think I should do?

SR: What do you think you should do?

SE: I probably should have some alternative strategies planned.

SR: I think that's a good idea. Do you have some strategies in mind?

SE: Um, not anything specific.... I just know that I ought to be able to modify my plan so that I can increase the probability of getting correct responses.

SR: Good point. That leads to another thing that I wanted to review with you today.... I wanted to talk about operant conditioning *and* social learning theory. I'd like to show you how you can apply some of the principles of social learning theory to what you're doing in therapy...just like I did with operant conditioning. Then we can talk about some strategies that are based on social learning theory.... Okay, according to social learning theory, what are the factors that facilitate learning?

SE: Um, feedback...cognitions, modeling, and reinforcement.

SR: Um hmm.... Of these factors, which ones have already been incorporated into the strategies that we've discussed today?

SE: Umm...modeling, feedback, and reinforcement.

SR: Right.... That's good. So, lets focus on cognitions now....

DIRECT-INDIRECT/ COLLABORATIVE STYLE

SR: Hi Ann.... How are you today?

SE: Fine. Were you able to watch my session with Johnny yesterday?

SR: Um hmm.

SE: What did you think about it?

SR: Well, why don't you tell me what *you* thought about it.

SE: Well, he still isn't getting those /s/s in words...even though he can do them when they're in a vowel–consonant unit.... I'm getting frustrated...I'm not quite sure what to do because he can produce a vowel plus /s/ without a model from me, and he does it right 90%

of the time. But as soon as I give him a word, he goes back to his error and he omits the sound. He *is* 7 years old and he omits /s/, /z/, sh, ch, zh, and j. So after we decided to work on /s/ and you told me about checking for generalization—and helped me figure out where to start training with him—I thought I'd be on my way. With the way he is now, though I doubt if he'll ever be able to learn /s/ with 10 final /s/ words...much less generalize to untrained /s/ words and other sibilants!

SR: I can tell you're frustrated...and it *is* frustrating when you think you've got a super plan and then for some reason, um, things don't quite work out the way you planned.... Let's see if we can figure out some things that might help Johnny produce /s/ correctly in final position words.

SE: Okay.

SR: Okay. What kinds of strategies do you think might facilitate correct production of /s/ in final position words?

SE: I don't know...I've tried everything that I can think of. Do you have any ideas?

SR: First, tell me what you've tried, Ann.

SE: Okay. Well, I've shown him pictures that have a final /s/ like *bus, goose, base, race*... well, wait, here are my pictures [SE shows pictures to SR]. There's *bus, base, piece, mice, moose, case, geese, goose, rice, race,* and *house.* I've shown him these pictures and asked him to say the words.... But when I do that, he omits the final sound.

SR: Ann, in changing from production in syllables to production in words, you left out a few very important details. There are some questions you should ask. What were your procedures for production in syllables? And what were the procedures that you used when you made the transition to production in words? How are the two sets of procedures different?

SE: Um well, obviously I used syllables first... then I used words. But I don't think that's what you're getting at.

SR: No, it isn't. Let's back up a little bit. Tell me exactly what you did when you started production in words.

SE: When he wasn't able to say /s/ when I showed him the pictures, I changed my strategy. I said the name of the picture and asked him to say it five times…then I told him how many he had right and how many he had wrong. But that didn't help either…he still omitted /s/.

SR: All right. So you know that providing one model, having Johnny make five attempts, and then giving him feedback doesn't result in correct production right now. Think about what you know about how people learn. How can you apply what you know about that to your therapy with Johnny?

SE: Hmm…[silence; SE thinking].
    Well, I know about operant conditioning and I know about Bandura's social learning theory.

SR: Let's talk about one at time. Let's talk about operant conditioning first. What can you tell me about it?

SE: Well, I know that a behavior is influenced by its consequences.… And when you're trying to get someone to learn a new behavior, you devise small steps that lead to the goal behavior.

SR: Um hmm. What else?

SE: Um, you decide what stimuli you will provide…and what the desired response is…and what the consequences of a response will be.… Also, any consequences that increase a behavior is a reinforcement and any consequence that decreases a behavior is a punishment.

SR: Right. Also, consistency is a very important factor…Consequences must be provided consistently if you expect to change a behavior. Let's take this framework and analyze the strategies that you've used in your therapy with Johnny.

SE: Okay.

[SR writes:]

STIM	RESPONSE	RF	DESIRED OUTCOME?
1. Present pics	client omits /s/	?	No
2. Clin models 1x	client says 5x omits all /s/s	intermittent	No

SR: Okay, look at this a minute [SR show notes to SE]. When you were training /s/ syllables, what kind of stimuli and consequences did you provide?

SE: I modeled each time…then I had him make an attempt…and then I gave him feedback. And once he reached criteria for that step, I stopped modeling…but continued to provide verbal feedback after each attempt.

SR: Um hmm. And your feedback acted as a reinforcer because Johnny's correct productions increased. How did you change your strategies when you started training words? [SR points to paper.]

SE: Oh…I know—I changed two things. I changed my method of presenting stimuli…I stopped providing a model for each attempt.… Also, I didn't provide consistent feedback after his attempts.

SR: So what do you think you'll want to do in your next session?

SE: Well for one thing, every time I show him a picture, I'll say the word first—before I ask him to say it. Um…second, I'll give him verbal feedback after every response. And if his correct production of /s/ increases, then I can say that my verbal feedback is reinforcing. I'm going to jot this down [SE writes]…I should have figured this out…What a dummy I am!

SR: Ann, you're not a dummy.… You're just new at this game. Sometimes it's hard to take things that you've learned in class and apply them to what you're doing in therapy. Anyway, now you have two strategies for your next session [brief pause]. I think that, in addition to providing consistent feedback, it would also be helpful if you'd give him *informative* feedback when he has incorrect responses. I mean, not only let him know *when* he's wrong…but also let him know *why* he's wrong.

SE: Hmm.

SR: Can you give me an example of informative feedback, so I know that this is clear to you?

SE: If I model the word *mice* and he responds "mi__," I could say, "No, Johnny, you forgot to say /s/ at the end of that word. Watch me, say "mi*ce*"…You know, emphasize the /s/.

SR: Good. You've also described modeling… that is, providing an additional model before asking your client to make a subsequent attempt. Why don't you add those things to your list of strategies?

SE: Okay [SE writes strategies]. It looks like my sessions next week should be pretty good.

SR: Okay. Let's take these ideas and develop some specific objectives for your therapy sessions. What will your objectives be for your session on Tuesday?

SE: In my lesson plan, my overall objective is to have him say 9 out of 10 words correctly on his first attempt in four consecutive sets.… That criteria might be a little too high to expect on Tuesday.

SR: I think you're probably right. Um, what do you think would be an appropriate criteria?

SE: If I could get him to say the words correctly 70% of the time…producing them right, after I give him a verbal model—I'd say that would be pretty good. Don't you think?

SR: A 70% proficiency level sounds reasonable to me.

SE: Okay [silence; SE thinking]. Um, suppose he doesn't reach the criteria? Say that after 10 sets, or 100 trials, he still can't get 70% correct.… What do you think I should do then?

SR: What do you think you should do?

SE: Hmm.… I suppose I should have some alternative strategies planned.

SR: I think that's a good idea. Do you have any alternatives in mind?

SE: Not anything specific.… I just know that I ought to be able to modify my plan so that I can increase the probability of getting correct responses.

SR: Um, good point. Why don't we back up a bit…you mentioned earlier, when we were talking about how people learn, that you know about operant conditioning and Bandura's social learning theory. We've developed some strategies based on operant conditioning. Let's see if we can develop some based on social learning theory.… First, what can you tell me about social learning theory?

SE: Well, I know that cognitions, modeling, feedback, and reinforcement are the primary things that facilitate learning.… And I know that modeling is the most powerful of all of these.

SR: Um hmm.… And modeling, feedback, and reinforcement have already been incorporated into the strategies that you'll be using next week. So it looks like we need to focus on cognitions.

INDIRECT/CONSULTATIVE SUPERVISORY STYLE

SR: Hi Ann.… How are you today?

SE: Fine. Were you able to watch my session with Johnny yesterday?

SR: Um hmm.

SE: What did you think about it?

SR: Well, why don't you tell me what *you* thought about it.

SE: Well, he still isn't getting those /s/s in words…even though he can do them when they're in a vowel–consonant unit.… I'm getting frustrated...I'm not quite sure what to do because he can produce a vowel plus /s/ without a model from me, and he does it right 90% of the time. But as soon as I give him a word, he goes back to his error and he omits the sound.

I thought I had a pretty good program planned...I mean he *is* 7 years old and he omits /s/, /z/, sh, ch, zh, and j. So after I decided to work on /s/ and you told me about checking for generalization—and helped me figure out where to start training with him—I thought I'd be on my way.

With the way he is now, though, I doubt if he'll ever be able to master 10 final /s/ words... much less generalize to untrained /s/ words and other sibilants that he omits!

SR: I can tell you're frustrated...and it *is* frustrating when you think you've got a super plan, and then for some reason things don't quite work out the way you planned. Let's see if we can figure out some things that might help Johnny produce /s/ correctly in final position words.

SE: Okay.

SR: What kinds of strategies do you think might facilitate correct production of /s/ in final position words?

SE: I don't know...I've tried everything that I can think of. Do you have any ideas?

SR: Well, let's take a look at what you've tried.

SE: Okay. I've shown him pictures that have a final /s/...like *bus, goose, base, race*...well, here are my pictures [SE shows cards to SR].... Um, *bus, base, piece, mice, moose, case, geese, goose, rice, race*, and *house.*

SR: Um hmm. Okay, can you tell me *how* you've used these pictures?

SE: Well, I've shown him these and asked him to say the words. Um...but when I do that, he omits the final sound.

SR: Okay...so you know one thing about Johnny.... You know that showing him a picture card and asking him to say the name doesn't work at this point.

SE: Yeah.

[SR writes on paper:]

STIM	RESPONSE	RF	DESIRED RESULT?
1. present pics	client omits /s/	?	No

SR: Have you tried any other strategies?

SE: Yeah. I said the name of the picture and asked him to repeat it five times.... Doing that didn't work either...he still omitted /s/.

SR: Okay.

[SR writes:]

STIM	RESPONSE	RF	DESIRED RESULT?
clin models 1x omits all /s/	client says 5x	interm	No

All right.... So you know something else about Johnny. You know that providing one model, having him make five attempts, and then giving him feedback doesn't result in correct productions right now. Think about what you know about how people learn. How can you apply what you know about that to your therapy with Johnny?

SE: Hmm...[silence; SE thinking].

Well, I know about operant conditioning and I know about Bandura's social learning theory.

SR: Okay, let's take one at a time. Umm...tell me what you know about operant conditioning.

SE: Well, I know that it involves Stimulus—Response—Reinforcement.

SR: Um hmm.... What else?

SE: I know that reinforcement increases a behavior and punishment decreases it.

SR: Um hmm. Can you tell me more about that?

SE: I guess I'm not sure what you're getting at.

SR: What do you know about schedules of rein-forcement? How important are the schedules of reinforcement in establishing a new behavior?

SE: Oh!... I know.... um...uh oh...maybe that's why Johnny didn't get any correct responses in words last time. At first, I should give him feed-back after every response. And if his correct production of /s/ increases, then I can say that my verbal feedback is reinforcing.

Oh boy, what a dummy I am. Why didn't I think of that before?

SR: Ann, you're not a dummy.... You're just new at this game. Sometimes it's hard to take things that you've learned in class and apply them to what you're doing in therapy. Let's take your rediscovery and write it down as a possible solution for next time.

SE: Okay.

SR: [SR writes] All right, so one possible strat-egy is that you will give him feedback after each response and see if that increases his cor-rect production of /s/. What kind of feedback do you think you'll have to give him?

SE: Well...I could say "yes" and "no"...or "right" and "wrong." I don't want him to get discouraged though...I mean if I always say "no" or "wrong," he might feel bad.

SR: Um hmm. I think that's a valid concern. How do you think you want to handle that?

SE: Hmm [SE thinks]. Maybe I could say things like, "No, Johnny...you forgot to say /s/ at the end of that word. Watch me, say m*ice*"...You know, emphasize the sound.

SR: Yeah...emphasize the target, and what you've described also includes giving informa-tive feedback...telling him *why* a production is incorrect. You've also described modeling.... Um...you're going to provide a model before asking him to give it another try.

SE: Yeah! [Smiles] You know, I might even try giving him a model every time...I mean before I ask him to say a word, I'll name the picture first, and then have him say it. That might work better right now...I mean better

than me saying the word once and having him say it five times.

SR: Okay. Let me write all of this down, so we don't forget.

[SR writes and talks while writing]. Let's see...(a) clinician will give informative feedback for client's incorrect productions, (b) clinician will provide a model before asking the client to make a subsequent at-tempt, and (c) clinician will provide a model for each presentation of a stim card.

Well, Ann, it looks like you're on your way! Let's take your ideas and develop some specific objectives for your next therapy ses-sion. Given these methods, what will your ob-jectives be for your next session on Tuesday?

SE: Hmm. [Looks at paper]...I'm thinking [pause]. Well, my overall objective is to have him say 9 out of 10 words correctly on his first attempt in four consecutive sets.... That's on my lesson plan, you know.

SR: Um hmm [nods head].

SE: So on Tuesday, if I could get him to say the words correctly 70% of the time...producing them right, after I give him a verbal model... I'd say that would be pretty good. Do you think so?

SR: Yes I think correct production after a model at 70% proficiency level sounds reason-able to me. Um, suppose that after you've completed 10 sets...which would be 100 trials or productions...that he hasn't met your crite-ria. What would you think?

SE: Oh no...I hope that doesn't happen!

SR: Suppose it does.... What would you think?

SE: I think I'd be ready to commit suicide [Laughs]. I think I should have some aces up my sleeve. I mean I ought to have some other alternative strategies.

SR: Um hmm [smiles].

SE: I'm not sure I know what else I could do. Do you have any suggestions?

SR: Well, you mentioned earlier...when we were talking about how people learn...that you know about operant conditioning and social learning theory. Um…you've come up with some strategies based on operant conditioning. Let's see if we can develop some strategies based on what you know about social learning theory…. What do you know about social learning theory?

SE: Well, I know that cognitions, modeling, reinforcement, and feedback are the primary thing that facilitate learning…and I know that modeling is the most powerful.

SR: Um hmm.

SE: I've already incorporated modeling, feedback, and reinforcement into the strategies that I'm planning to use…so I guess I need to think about cognitions.

Adapted from Brasseur, J. (1980). The observed differences between direct, indirect, and direct/indirect video-taped supervisory conferences by speech-language pathology supervisors, graduate students, and undergraduate students (Doctoral dissertation, Indiana University, 1980). *Dissertation Abstracts International, 41,* 2131B. (University Microfilms No. 80-29, 212)

CHAPTER THREE

COMPONENTS OF THE SUPERVISORY PROCESS

Supervision, as a field of study, is filled with myths, unclear definitions and distinctions, and untrained supervisors who operate with good intentions as their main resource.
—Hart (1982, p. 5)

What are supervisors and supervisees talking about when they talk about supervision? Where do they begin in studying such a complex process? What do they mean when they say they are supervising? What is involved in carrying out the task they assume as supervisors? The Position Statement on Clinical Supervision in Speech-Language Pathology and Audiology (Appendix 3A) (ASHA, 1985b) legitimized supervision as a distinct area of expertise and practice and stipulated that special skills need to be developed to be a competent and effective supervisor. These special skills were defined as 13 tasks:

1. Establishing and maintaining an effective working relationship with the supervisee
2. Assisting the supervisee in developing clinical goals and objectives
3. Assisting the supervisee in developing and refining assessment skills
4. Assisting the supervisee in developing and refining management skills
5. Demonstrating for and participating with the supervisee in the clinical process
6. Assisting the supervisee in observing and analyzing assessment and treatment sessions.
7. Assisting the supervisee in development and maintenance of clinical and supervisory records.
8. Interacting with the supervisee in planning, executing, and analyzing supervisory conferences.
9. Assisting the supervisee in evaluation of clinical performance.
10. Assisting the supervisee in developing skills of verbal reporting, writing, and editing.
11. Sharing information regarding ethical, legal, regulatory, and reimbursement aspects of the profession.
12. Modeling and facilitating professional conduct.
13. Demonstrating research skills in the clinical or supervisory processes.

Now that we know **what** we need to do, we need to know **how** to do these tasks. We need to understand the components of the supervisory process and how we use the components to effect the professional growth and development of supervisees and supervisors.

Although the clinical process is at times puzzling and challenging, it is conceptually well known to speech-language pathologists and audiologists. A great deal of attention has been given to studying the clinical process. Student clinicians have been carefully prepared in observation and analysis of the clinical process. They have been taught to isolate the components of the clinical process with informal supervisor-developed methodologies or by the use of highly structured behavior recording systems such as those described by Boone and Prescott (1972) and Schubert, Miner and Till (1973). They have come to understand the importance of principles of learning such as modeling, reinforcement, and sequencing in discussions with their supervisors and in reading texts targeted at clinical practice (e.g., Goldberg, 1997; Hegde & Davis, 1995; Moon Meyer, 1998). If supervisors and supervisees are to understand the supervisory process in the same way they understand the clinical process, they need to attend to its various parts. They need to be able to dissect and examine the components that make up the total process. The supervisory process deserves at least the same degree of systematic attention that has been given to the clinical process.

The continuum introduced in the previous chapter consists of three stages: Evaluation-Feedback, Transitional, and Self-Supervision. A Collaborative Style is seen as the appropriate supervisory style to facilitate movement of supervisees along the continuum. This style consists of certain components: (I) Understanding the Supervisory Process, (II) Planning, (III) Observing, (IV) Analyzing, (V) Integrating. The point on the continuum at which supervisor and supervisee are operating will dictate the quantity of time spent on each component, the amount of input from supervisor and supervisee in each component, and the operational specifics of each supervisory interaction.

Each component will be treated in a separate chapter. A brief overview of all the components is presented here.

COMPONENT I—UNDERSTANDING THE SUPERVISORY PROCESS

One of the premises of this book is that supervisors need to be prepared for their roles. Another premise is the need for collaboration between supervisor and supervisee in the process. Given that both are valid assumptions, it follows that supervisees need preparation for their role. For some supervisees, formal preparation is nonexistent. For others, it may consist of a brief discussion or unit of study in a pre-practicum course. Whatever previous information has been accrued, it is proposed here that the supervisory process should be a topic of discussion between supervisors and supervisees at the beginning of every new supervisory experience and throughout the relationship.

Each person brings to the total supervisory experience his or her own needs, expectations, concerns, and objectives. Because of the variety of stereotypes brought into the supervisory experience and because supervisors and supervisees have different perceptions of the same supervisory interaction (Blumberg, 1980; Culatta et al., 1975; Smith & Anderson, 1982b), it is important for the two to discuss the supervisory process throughout the entire interaction. If there is a lack of congruency about objectives and procedures at this point, attempts can be made to resolve it. If not resolved, differences can at least be raised to a level of consciousness or compromise.

For example, supervisors who believe that the "best" supervisory style is the Collaborative Style may incorporate into their behavior such activities as broad questioning, listening, using supervisee's ideas, and supportive responses to supervisee's ideas with strong attention to encouraging problem solving by the supervisee. If supervisees, however, perceive that the supervisor's role is to evaluate, tell them what they did right or wrong, and help them to "do better," there will be an incongruency which may disrupt the supervisory relationship and the learning that should take place (Larson, 1982). A period of discussion about the process into which the supervisor and supervisee are about to embark, preparation of the supervisee for his or her part in the experience, and sharing expectations and objectives that should alleviate problems that might arise from such differences in perceptions.

This activity should be more than just an introductory phase, however. It is important that such discussions of the supervisory process be **ongoing** as needs and objectives are altered, levels of expertise change, and new insights or problems arise.

COMPONENT II—PLANNING

Speech-language pathologists and audiologists have spent a great deal of time planning for the client, and supervisors have spent time educating their students in the planning process. This client-centered approach is certainly necessary and important, but other planning is needed. Following the continuum requires **joint** planning as follows:

- Planning for the Clinical Process
  A. Planning for the client
  B. Planning for the clinician
- Planning for the Supervisory Process
  A. Planning for the supervisee
  B. Planning for the supervisor

Planning for the client is not new. Planning for the clinician may not be new for many; planning for the supervisory process itself may be a novel task for most supervisors and supervisees.

COMPONENT III—OBSERVING

Traditionally, the script for observation has often been as follows: Supervisor enters observation room, pencil in hand. Observes clinician at work. Takes notes continuously or intermittently. Notes consist primarily of evaluations of the clinician's behavior. Supervisor leaves observation room. Evaluations are communicated to the clinician in a variety of ways (verbally immediately after the session, written notes or checklists given to clinician, etc.).

Observation should not be the time when evaluation takes place. It is no mistake that observation (Task 6) and evaluation (Task 9) are two separate entities for effective supervision. Observation is the place where real objectivity begins in the supervisory process. During observation, data are collected and recorded by both the supervisor and supervisee for subsequent analysis and interpretation, which then lead to evaluation. A good operational definition of observation is obtained by editing Cogan's (1973) definition: those operations by which individuals make careful, systematic scrutiny of the events and interactions occurring during clinical or supervisory sessions. The term also applies to the records made of these events and interactions (p. 134).

COMPONENT IV—ANALYZING

The analysis stage of the supervisory process is a bridge between observation and evaluation. The objective data collected during the observation mean little by themselves. It is in the analysis component that the supervisor and supervisee begin to make sense of the data (Cogan, 1973; Goldhammer, 1969). The data are examined, categorized, and interpreted in relation to the change, or lack of change, in the client or clinician. Analysis comes naturally from the planning and observation stages because if planning is well done, both supervisor and supervisee will have determined exactly what data will be collected and what will be done with them.

An important facet of the analysis stage is the joint responsibility for analysis or interpretation of the data. This is where supervisees, to whatever extent possible, begin to self-analyze, to problem-solve about their own behavior, and to look for the relationship between their behaviors and those of the client.

COMPONENT V—INTEGRATING

At various points throughout each supervisory experience the contents of the components must be integrated. This is ordinarily done in a conference between supervisor and supervisee, individually or in groups, although there are other procedures that contribute to integration.

PRACTICAL RESEARCH IN SUPERVISION

Task 13: Demonstrating research skills in the clinical or supervisory processes. Competencies required:

13.1   Ability to read, interpret, and apply clinical and supervisory research

13.2   Ability to formulate clinical or supervisory research questions

13.3   Ability to investigate clinical or supervisory research questions

13.4   Ability to support and refute clinical or supervisory research findings

13.5   Ability to report results of clinical or supervisory research and disseminate as appropriate (e.g., in-service, conferences, publications)

As Ulrich (1990) stated, "The degree to which we are able to carry out this task is very likely to determine our future as an area of specialized expertise and practice" (p. 15). In the course of reading this text, it will become apparent that there is a significant body of research in supervision. And, there remains a great need for continued research in the supervisory process. Significant questions emerge from actual practice and it is essential that our practices be based on the theories and findings that come from rigorous research. This is true for both the supervisory and clinical processes and is mandated in the new standards for CCC, which stipulate that applicants "must demonstrate knowledge of processes used in research and the integration of research principles into evidence-based clinical practice" (ASHA, 2000a).

"Practical research" is essential for supervisors who want to know what they can do to improve the interaction between themselves and their individual supervisees (Strike & Gillam, 1988).

Likewise, it is essential for professionals who want to answer questions about the clinical process (Rassi & McElroy, 1992; Richardson & Gillam, 1994). Practical supervision research seeks to answer questions about supervisory procedures. It explores such matters as the relationships between particular supervision procedures and various clinician variables (e.g., experience, motivation) or techniques for solving difficulties inherent in the supervisory process. It identifies which of the 81 competencies (ASHA, 1985b) are most effective at different stages on the continuum. Practical clinical research seeks to answer questions about treatment efficiency and effectiveness.

Generating practical research requires that those involved in the supervisory process also be actively involved in the research process. This is a bit difficult for a couple of reasons. "Time and knowledge of research principles are the two most frequent factors that interfere with ongoing supervision research" (Strike & Gillam, 1988, p. 274). Supervisors may be inclined to believe that research can only be done by academics who have formal preparation in research methods and the time to devote to the endeavor. Some of this perception may be accurate or valid. Although Ph.D.'s in academic settings have the skills needed to design and conduct research, many are not familiar with supervisory issues. Likewise, supervisors who have a pulse on the important issues and daily opportunities to collect relevant data are not often seasoned researchers. This poses a dilemma.

Rassi, Dodd, and Baer (1993) stated that the dichotomy between clinical practice and research is perpetuated by university programs and in various ways. For example: (a) the researcher/teacher who investigates and professes to know clinical matters, but does not engage in clinical practice; (b) the clinical educator who supervises students without discussing or applying cutting-edge techniques—or without using research to substantiate or refute practices they advocate. Programs that almost exclusively have master's level preparation grounded in a clinical orientation and doctoral degrees with a research-only focus also perpetuate this dichotomy (Rassi, Dodd, & Baer, 1993). Ulrich (1990) stated that clinicians and supervisors do indeed have the skills needed to carry out most of the competencies associated with Task 13. Every time we assess, plan, and implement treatment programs, we employ the scientific methodology of research (Ulrich, 1990). Numerous experts have suggested collaboration between students, supervisors, professors, and/or clinicians in different work settings (Dowling, 2001; Rassi, Dodd, & Baer, 1993; Richardson & Gillam, 1994; Schiavetti & Metz, 1997; Strike & Gillam, 1988) as a viable solution. Such collaboration would entail joint research in which each professional contributes his or her expertise to developing research questions, planning the appropriate design for answering the questions, and conducting the investigation.

In recent years leaders of both ASHA and the Council of Academic Programs in Communication Sciences and Disorders (CAPCSD) have voiced concerns about the erosion of the scientific bases of our professions and the need to invigorate research efforts in our professions. Numerous research initiatives evolved, and it has become increasingly apparent that colleges and universities need to revamp curricula to close the gap between academic and clinical education, as well as the gap between research and practice. Miller (1996) suggested that we need to promote interest among neophyte professionals, noting the importance of increasing research opportunities for *undergraduate* students in our programs. He offered several reasons for expanding research opportunities for undergraduate students:

1. Appreciate the role science plays in the field, that of contributing new knowledge about specific disorders, new and improved measurement systems, and the documentation of treatment efficacy
2. Learn the scientific method as the foundation of clinical work
3. Be better consumers by learning how to read and evaluate research
4. Bring life and reality to the research studies read in class
5. Empower students to create new knowledge in the field
6. Recruit students into research careers (Miller, 1996, p. 56)

Scott (1996) suggested, "We should encourage faculty to develop programmatic research and invite students interested in those topics to join the effort on pieces of that research" (p. 64). Modeling for and involving students in research seem to be important first steps in changing the attitudes about clinicians versus researchers and facilitating the evolution of the clinician-researcher practitioner.

Richardson and Gillam (1994) provide an innovative example of merging clinical research with clinical teaching. They discussed the "sometimes discordant nature of our dual roles as supervisors and researchers that served as frequent sources of tension throughout the study" (Richardson & Gillam, 1994, p. 204). Combining practicum and research adds a layer of issues to both the clinical and supervisory processes. But the kind of efficacy research that Richardson and Gillam completed with three graduate students and clients is precisely the type of collaboration that answers important clinical questions and has the potential to instill the interest in and passion for research that students need to develop if we are to invigorate research efforts.

Pickering (2001) offered a thought-provoking perspective on the nature of joint research and collaborative scholarly work. Citing the work of Boyer (1990) at the Carnegie Foundation for the Advancement of Teaching, she stressed that professionals need to go beyond what is traditionally perceived of as research and broaden their perspective of scholarship. Boyer's four-part model of scholarship includes scholarship of discovery, integration, application, and teaching. The scholarship of discovery involves the quest for new knowledge. The scholarship of integration provides the way to give meaning to isolated facts and to make connections within and across disciplines. The scholarship of application puts the knowledge gained from discovery and integration into practice. The scholarship of teaching involves not merely transmitting knowledge but "transforming and extending it as well" (Boyer, 1990, p. 24). Pickering (2001) illustrated how clinical educators have used all four kinds of scholarship to expand our knowledge base about supervision and added that viewing scholarship from this larger perspective demonstrates how *all* professionals can be involved in research and scholarly endeavors.

In subsequent chapters, "Research Issues and Questions" will be presented. The purpose of these research sections is not to provide an exhaustive review of the studies for a particular topic area that have been completed to date. Rather, it is an attempt to highlight some of what we currently know from the research on a particular aspect of the process and to suggest some directions for future research. Our hope is that it will stimulate interest and collaboration among academicians, supervisors, and supervisees in universities, schools, and medical settings and lead to the publication of new investigations that demonstrate the effectiveness of clinical supervision.

IMPORTANT FACTORS TO CONSIDER IN DESIGNING FUTURE STUDIES

Naremore (1984) emphasized that because supervision is a *process,* exploring it demands a multiple focus. Researchers cannot afford to focus on single variable. She stated, "We are dancing around the process with 'it' questions." We need to be cognizant of the multilayered complex process that is supervision when selecting dependent variables but also realize we can't study everything at once. Thus, we have to select a piece of the process to investigate.

Numerous *descriptive* studies have provided important information about the supervisory process and a foundation for experimental investigations. We need to identify what things we do as supervisors that make a difference in the professional growth and development of our supervisees. What is effective practice? What are best practices? What should supervisors be prepared to do? Is one methodology better than another? What changes do supervisees make as a result of

their supervisory experiences? What supervisor variables enhance efficiency?

In designing experimental studies to help in the discovery of new knowledge and in making connections between theory and practice, one kind of design is particularly appealing because the methods closely parallel what good clinicians do in their daily practice. Single-subject designs require establishing a stable baseline, applying a treatment, and systematically collecting objective data relative to the treatment. Given the flexibility and relative ease in using single-subject experimental research designs (Connell & Thompson, 1986; Herson & Barlow, 1976; Kearns, 1986; McReynolds & Thompson, 1986; McReynolds & Kearns, 1983) they would be "user-friendly" for all members of a research team. Furthermore, these designs are appropriate for answering the kinds of practical research questions advocated in this text. These functional analysis designs clearly allow cause–effect relationships to be demonstrated, while avoiding the multitude of problems inherent in group experimental designs.

SUMMARY

The complexities of the supervisory process will be better understood if they can be isolated into specific components for discussion and study. Thus, this chapter has presented five components: understanding, planning, observing, analyzing, and integrating, which make up the content of supervision. Each will be discussed thoroughly in subsequent chapters. Furthermore, questions relative to each of the cases are posed so that readers may attempt to apply the text to a specific problem. Finally, chapters also contain some research issues and questions that are intended to spark interest in collaborative investigations to study the supervisory process.

Clinical Supervision in Speech-Language Pathology and Audiology: A Position Statement

INTRODUCTION

Clinical supervision is a part of the earliest history of the American Speech-Language-Hearing Association (ASHA). It is an integral part of the initial training of speech-language pathologists and audiologists, as well as their continued professional development at all levels in all work settings.

ASHA has recognized the importance of supervision by specifying certain aspects of supervision in its requirements for the Certificates of Clinical Competence (CCC) and the Clinical Fellowship Year (CFY) (ASHA, 1982). Further, supervisory requirements are specified by the Council on Professional Standards in its standards and guidelines for both educational and professional services programs (Educational Standards Board, ASHA, 1983). State laws for licensing and school certification consistently include requirements for supervision of practicum experiences and initial work performance. In addition, other regulatory and accrediting bodies (e.g., Joint Commission on Accreditation of Rehabilitation Facilities) require a mechanism for ongoing supervision throughout professional careers.

It is important to note that the term **clinical supervision,** as used in this document, refers to the tasks and skills of clinical teaching related to the interaction between a clinician and client. In its 1978 report, the Committee on Supervision in Speech-Language Pathology and Audiology differentiated between the two major roles of persons identified as supervisors: clinical teaching aspects and program management tasks. The Committee emphasized that although program management tasks relating to administration or coordination of programs may be a part of the person's job duties, the term **supervisor** referred to "individuals who engaged in clinical teaching through observation, conferences, review of records, and other proce-

dures, and which is related to the interaction between a clinician and a client and the evaluation or management of communication skills" (ASHA, 1978, p. 479). The Committee continues to recognize this distinction between tasks of administration or program management and those of clinical teaching, which is its central concern.

The importance of supervision to preparation of students and to assurance of quality clinical service has been assumed for some time. It is only recently, however, that the tasks of supervision have been well-defined, and that the special skills and competencies judged to be necessary for their effective application have been identified. This Position Paper addresses the following areas:

- tasks of supervision
- competencies for effective clinical supervision
- preparations of clinical supervisors

Tasks of Supervision

A central premise of supervision is that effective clinical teaching involves, in a fundamental way, the development of self-analysis, self-evaluation, and problem-solving skills on the part of the individual being supervised. The success of clinical teaching rests largely on the achievement of this goal. Further, the demonstration of quality clinical skills in supervisors is generally accepted as a prerequisite to supervision of students, as well as of those in the Clinical Fellowship Year or employed as certified speech-language pathologists or audiologists.

Outlined in this paper are 13 tasks basic to effective clinical teaching and constituting the distinct area of practice which comprises clinical supervision in communication disorders. The committee stresses that the level of preparation and experience of the supervisee, the particular work setting of the supervisor and supervisee, and client variables will influence the relative emphasis of each task in actual practice.

The tasks and their supporting competencies which follow are judged to have face validity as established by experts in the area of supervision, and by both select and widespread peer review. The committee recognizes the need for further validation and strongly encourages ongoing investigation. Until such time as more rigorous measures of validity are established, it will be particularly important for the tasks and competencies to be reviewed periodically through the quality assurance procedures. Mechanisms such as Patient Care Audit and Child Services Review System appear to offer useful means for quality assurance in the supervisory tasks and competencies. Other procedures appropriate to specific work settings may also be selected.

The tasks of supervision discussed above follow:

1. establishing and maintaining an effective working relationship with the supervisee;
2. assisting the supervisee in developing clinical goals and objectives;
3. assisting the supervisee in developing and refining assessment skills;
4. assisting the supervisee in developing and refining clinical management skills;
5. demonstrating for and participating with the supervisee in the clinical process;
6. assisting the supervisee in observing and analyzing assessment and treatment sessions;
7. assisting the supervisee in the development and maintenance of clinical and supervisory records;
8. interacting with the supervisee in planning, execution, and analyzing supervisory conferences;
9. assisting the supervisee in evaluation of clinical performance;
10. assisting the supervisee in developing skills of verbal reporting, writing, and editing;
11. sharing information regarding ethical, legal, regulatory, and reimbursement aspects of professional practice;
12. modeling and facilitating professional conduct; and
13. demonstrating research skills in the clinical or supervisory processes.

Competencies for Effective Clinical Supervision

Although the competencies are listed separately according to task, each competency may be needed to perform a number of supervisor tasks.

1.0 Task: Establishing and maintaining an effective working relationship with the supervisee

Competencies required:

1.1 Ability to facilitate an understanding of the clinical and supervisory processes.

1.2 Ability to organize and provide information regarding the logical sequences of supervisory interaction, that is, joint setting of goals and objectives, data collection and analysis, evaluation.

1.3 Ability to interact from a contemporary perspective with the supervisee in both the clinical and supervisory process.

1.4 Ability to apply learning principles in the supervisory process.

1.5 Ability to apply skills of interpersonal communication in the supervisory process.

1.6 Ability to facilitate independent thinking and problem solving by the supervisee.

1.7 Ability to maintain a professional and supportive relationship that allows supervisor and supervisee growth.

1.8 Ability to interact with the supervisee objectively.

1.9 Ability to establish joint communications regarding expectations and responsibilities in the clinical and supervisory processes.

1.10 Ability to evaluate, with the supervisee, the effectiveness of the ongoing supervisory relationship.

2.0 Task: Assisting the supervisee in developing clinical goals and objectives.

Competencies required:

2.1 Ability to assist the supervisee in planning effective client goals and objectives.

2.2 Ability to plan, with the supervisee, effective goals and objectives for clinical and professional growth.

2.3 Ability to assist the supervisee in using observation and assessment in preparation of client goals and objectives.

2.4 Ability to assist the supervisee in using self-analysis and previous evaluation in preparation of goals and objectives for professional growth.

2.5 Ability to assist the supervisee in assigning priorities to clinical goals and objectives.

2.6 Ability to assist the supervisee in assigning priorities to goals and objectives for professional growth.

3.0 Task: Assisting the supervisee in developing and refining assessment skills.

Competencies required:

3.1 Ability to share current research findings and evaluation procedures in communication disorders.

3.2 Ability to facilitate an integration of research findings and evaluation procedures in communication disorders.

3.3 Ability to assist the supervisee in providing rationale for assessment procedures.

3.4 Ability to assist supervisee in communicating assessment procedures and rationales.

3.5 Ability to assist the supervisee in integrating findings and observations to make appropriate recommendations.

4.0 Task: Assisting the supervisee in developing and refining management skills.

Competencies required:

4.1 Ability to share current research findings and management procedures in communication disorders.

4.2 Ability to facilitate an integration of research findings in client management.

4.3 Ability to assist the supervisee in providing rationale for treatment procedures.

4.4 Ability to assist the supervisee in identifying appropriate sequences for client change.

4.5 Ability to assist the supervisee in adjusting steps in the progression toward a goal.

4.6 Ability to assist the supervisee in the description and measurement of client and clinician change.

4.7 Ability to assist the supervisee in documenting client and clinician change.

4.8 Ability to assist the supervisee in integrating documented client and clinician change to evaluate progress and specify future recommendations.

5.0 Task: Demonstrating for and participating with the supervisee in the clinical process.

Competencies required:

5.1 Ability to determine jointly when demonstration is appropriate.

5.2 Ability to demonstrate or participate in an effective client-clinician relationship.

5.3   Ability to demonstrate a variety of clinical techniques and participate with the supervisee in clinical management.

5.4   Ability to demonstrate or use jointly the specific materials and equipment of the profession.

5.5   Ability to demonstrate or participate jointly in counseling of clients or family/guardians of clients.

6.0   Task: Assisting the supervisee in observing and analyzing assessment and treatment sessions.

Competencies required:

6.1   Ability to assist the supervisee in learning a variety of data collection procedures.

6.2   Ability to assist the supervisee in selecting and executing data collection procedures.

6.3   Ability to assist the supervisee in accurately recording data.

6.4   Ability to assist the supervisee in analyzing and interpreting data objectively.

6.5   Ability to assist the supervisee in revising plans for client management based on data obtained.

7.0   Task: Assisting the supervisee in development and maintenance of clinical and supervisory records.

Competencies required:

7.1   Ability to assist the supervisee in applying record-keeping systems to supervisory and clinical processes.

7.2   Ability to assist the supervisee in effectively documenting supervisory and clinically related interactions.

7.3   Ability to assist the supervisee in organizing records to facilitate easy retrieval of information concerning clinical and supervisory interactions.

7.4   Ability to assist the supervisee in establishing and following policies and procedures to protect the confidentiality of clinical and supervisory records.

7.5   Ability to share information regarding documentation requirements of various accrediting and regulatory agencies and third-party funding sources.

8.0   Task: Interacting with the supervisee in planning, executing, and analyzing supervisory conferences.

Competencies required:

8.1   Ability to determine with the supervisee when a conference should be scheduled.

8.2   Ability to assist the supervisee in planning a supervisory conference agenda.

8.3   Ability to involve the supervisee in jointly establishing a conference agenda.

8.4   Ability to involve the supervisee in joint discussion of previously identified clinical or supervisory data or issues.

8.5   Ability to interact with the supervisee in a manner that facilitates the supervisee's self-exploration and problem solving.

8.6   Ability to adjust conference content based on the supervisee's level of training and experience.

8.7   Ability to encourage and maintain supervisee motivation for continuing self-growth.

8.8   Ability to assist the supervisee in making commitments for changes in clinical behavior.

8.9 Ability to involve the supervisee in ongoing analysis of supervisory interactions.

9.0 Task: Assisting the supervisee in evaluation of clinical performance.

Competencies required:

9.1 Ability to assist the supervisee in the use of clinical evaluation tools.
9.2 Ability to assist the supervisee in the description and measurement of his/her progress and achievement.
9.3 Ability to assist the supervisee in developing skills of self-evaluation.
9.4 Ability to evaluate clinical skills with the supervisee for purposes of grade assignment, completion of Clinical Fellowship Year, professional advancement, and so on.

10.0 Task: Assisting the supervisee in developing skills of verbal reporting, writing, and editing.

Competencies required:

10.1 Ability to assist the supervisee in identifying appropriate information to be included in a verbal or written report.
10.2 Ability to assist the supervisee in presenting information in a logical, concise, and sequential manner.
10.3 Ability to assist the supervisee in using appropriate professional terminology and style in verbal and written reporting.
10.4 Ability to assist the supervisee in adapting verbal and written reports to the work environment and communication situation.
10.5 Ability to alter and edit a report as appropriate while preserving the supervisee's writing style.

11.0 Task: Sharing information regarding ethical, legal, regulatory, and reimbursement aspects of the profession.

Competencies required:

11.1 Ability to communicate to the supervisee a knowledge of professional codes of ethics (e.g., ASHA, state licensing boards, and so on).
11.2 Ability to communicate to the supervisee an understanding of legal and regulatory documents and their impact on the practice of the profession (licensure, PL 94-142, Medicare, Medicaid, and so on).
11.3 Ability to communicate to the supervisee an understanding of reimbursement policies and procedures of the work setting.
11.4 Ability to communicate a knowledge of supervisee rights and appeal procedures specific to the work setting.

12.0 Task: Modeling and facilitating professional conduct.

Competencies required:

12.1 Ability to assume responsibility.
12.2 Ability to analyze, evaluate, and modify own behavior.
12.3 Ability to demonstrate ethical and legal conduct.
12.4 Ability to meet and respect deadlines
12.5 Ability to maintain professional protocols (respect for confidentiality, etc.).
12.6 Ability to provide current information regarding professional standards (PSB, ESB, licensure, teacher certification, etc.).
12.7 Ability to communicate information regarding fees, billing procedures, and third-party reimbursement.

12.8 Ability to demonstrate familiarity with professional issues.

12.9 Ability to demonstrate continued professional growth.

13.0 Task: Demonstrating research skills in the clinical or supervisory processes.

Competencies required:

13.1 Ability to read, interpret, and apply clinical and supervisory research.

13.2 Ability to formulate clinical or supervisory research questions.

13.3 Ability to investigate clinical or supervisory research questions.

13.4 Ability to support and refute clinical or supervisory research findings.

13.5 Ability to report results of clinical or supervisory research and disseminate as appropriate (e.g., in-service, conferences, publications).

Preparation of Supervisors

The special skills and competencies for effective clinical supervision may be acquired through special training which may include, but is not limited to, the following:

1. Specific curricular offerings from graduate programs: examples include doctoral programs emphasizing supervision, other postgraduate preparation, and specified graduate courses.
2. Continuing educational experiences specific to the supervisory process (e.g., conferences, workshops, self-study).
3. Research-directed activities that provide insight in the supervisory process.

The major goal of training in supervision is mastery of "Competencies for Effective Clinical Supervision." Since competence in clinical services and work experience sufficient to provide a broad clinical perspective are considered essential to achieving competence in supervision, it is apparent that most preparation in supervision will occur following the preservice level. Even so, positive effects of preservice introduction to supervision have been described by both Anderson (1981) and Rassi (1983). Hence, the presentation of basic material about the supervisory process may enhance students' performance as supervisees, as well as provide them with a framework for later study.

The steadily increasing numbers of publications concerning supervision and the supervisory process indicate that basic information concerning supervision now is becoming more accessible in print to all speech-language pathologists and audiologists, regardless of geographical location and personal circumstances. In addition, conferences, workshops, and convention presentations concerning supervision in communication disorders are more widely available than ever before, and both coursework and supervisory practicum experiences are emerging in college and university educational programs. Further, although preparation in the supervisory process specific to communication disorders should be the major content, the commonality in principles of supervision across teaching, counseling, social work, business, and health care professions suggests additional resources for those who desire to increase their supervisory knowledge and skills.

To meet the needs of persons who wish to prepare themselves as clinical supervisors, additional coursework, continuing education opportunities, and other programs in the supervisory process should be developed both within and outside graduate education programs. As noted in an earlier report on the status of supervision (ASHA, 1978), supervisors themselves expressed a strong desire for training in supervision. Further, systematic study and investigation of the supervisory process is seen as necessary to expansion of the data base from which increased knowledge about supervision and the supervisory process will emerge.

The "Tasks of Supervision" and "Competencies for Effective Clinical Supervision" are intended to serve as the basis for content and outcome in preparation of supervisors. The tasks and competencies will be particularly useful to supervisors for self-study and self-evaluation, as well as to the consumers of supervisory activity, that is, supervisees and employees.

A repeated concern by ASHA membership is that implementation of any suggestions for qualifications of supervisors will lead to additional standards or credentialing. At this time, preparation in supervision is a viable area of specialized study. The competencies for effective supervision can be achieved and implemented by supervisors and employers.

Summary

Clinical supervision in speech-language pathology and audiology is a distinct area of expertise and practice. This paper defines the area of supervision, outlines the special tasks of which it is comprised, and describes the competencies for each task. The competencies are developed by special preparation, which may take at least three avenues of implementation. Additional coursework, continuing education opportunities and other programs in the supervisory process should be developed both within and outside of graduate education programs. At this time, preparation in supervision is a viable area for specialized study, with competence achieved and implemented for supervisors and employers.

BIBLIOGRAPHY

American Speech and Hearing Association. (1978). Committee on Supervision in Speech-Language-Pathology and Audiology. Current status of supervision of speech-language pathology and audiology [Special report]. *Asha, 20,* 478–486.

American Speech-Language Hearing Association (1980). *Standards for accreditation by the Education and Training Board.* Rockville, MD: ASHA.

American Speech-Language Hearing Association (1982). *Requirements for the certificates of clinical competence* (Rev.). Rockville, MD: ASHA.

American Speech-Language Hearing Association (1983). New standards for accreditation by the Professional Services Board. *Asha, 25, 6,* 51–58.

Anderson, J. (Ed.). (1980, July). *Proceedings: Conference on Training in the Supervisory Process in Speech-Language Pathology and Audiology.* Indiana University, Bloomington.

Anderson, J. (1981). A training program in clinical supervision. *Asha, 23,* 77–82.

Culatta, R., & Helmick, J. (1980). Clinical supervision: The state of the art—Part I. *Asha, 22,* 985–993.

Culatta, R., & Helmick, J. (1981). Clinical supervision: The state of the art—Part II. *Asha, 23,* 21–31.

Laney, M. (1982). Research and evaluation in the public schools. *Language, Speech, and Hearing Services in Schools, 13,* 53–60.

Rassi, J. (1983, September). *Supervision in Audiology.* Seminar presented at Hannemann University, Philadelphia.

CHAPTER FOUR

UNDERSTANDING THE SUPERVISORY PROCESS

*Both [teacher and supervisor] must learn a great deal about each other and
about their roles in clinical supervision before they can begin the process of
planning, teaching, observation, analysis, etc. in the cycle of supervision.*
—Cogan (1973, p. 78)

Regardless of their place on the continuum, supervisors and supervisees in all settings must engage in a special type of interpersonal interaction to accomplish their objectives. This interaction is so important in the supervisory process that it deserves all the effort and attention that can be brought to it to make it a satisfying and rewarding experience for all participants. The ability to facilitate an understanding of the clerical and supervisory process is the first competency in Task 1.0, establishing and maintaining an effective working relationship with the supervisee. Understanding may well be the most crucial component of the supervisory process.

There are many ways to teach people to swim. One is to toss them into the water and hope that they will suddenly acquire the necessary techniques to reach the edge of the pool. At one time, some clinicians were introduced to the clinical process in much the same way—sink or swim! This practice has been modified as a result of ASHA requirements for student observations prior to practicum and more specific requirements for

supervision. Higher education programs also include certain clinical courses and experiences in their curricula that orient the neophyte clinician to the intricacies of the clinical process. Introduction to the supervisory process, however, still appears to be "sink or swim" because few educational programs appear to teach about the supervisory process and there seems to be little discussion of the supervisory process in supervisory conferences at any experience level.

PURPOSE OF THE COMPONENT

This chapter will present ways to (1) prepare supervisees for meaningful participation in the supervisory process, and (2) communicate about the process throughout the entire period of interaction between supervisor and supervisee.

The premise for such preparation is that mutual understanding of the various components of the supervisory process will enrich the process, enable participants to better use the process to strengthen clinical performance, and promote professional growth. Further, the interaction will be most effective when all participants are able to observe, discuss, and analyze the process so that the experience can be designed to meet their needs. This mutual understanding will come from (1) a basic knowledge about the supervisory process, (2) the preliminary investigation of the expectations and needs of both participants, and (3) discussion of the dynamics of the ongoing interaction between participants. This continuous dialogue about what is happening in the supervisory interaction should *facilitate independent thinking and problem solving by the supervisee* (1.6) and help to maintain *a professional and supportive relationship that allows supervisor and supervisee growth* (1.7), which will ultimately result in better service to clients.

This first component of the continuum consists of several facets—an awareness of the possible roles of participants, the importance of supervisors and supervisees knowing and understanding each other's needs and expectations as they begin the process, the anxieties that supervisees and perhaps supervisors bring to the process, and the importance of self knowledge. What will be presented is a method and some strategies for preparing both supervisors and supervisees for an interaction the will best address the needs of all participants in the clinical and supervisory processes—client, clinician, supervisee, supervisor.

The Name of the Game

This Understanding component relates to learning about the basic principles of supervision, but should not be assumed to be relevant only to the beginning of the interaction. The understanding of such a complex set of behaviors is developmental. It is more than an induction phase or an orientation or introduction to the process. It is ongoing and applies across the continuum.

Interpreting is not a satisfactory descriptor of this phase because it is not inclusive enough and also seems to imply that the supervisor is the sole provider of information, a concept that is inconsistent with the theme of this book. *Rapport* is a term that is used frequently in describing the relationship between clinician and client. It is a desirable objective in the supervisory process; however, what is being discussed here requires a deeper understanding of each other than the usual concept of rapport. Understanding involves in-depth knowledge of and familiarity with the many facets of all the components of the supervisory process, including the thoughts and feelings of the partners in the relationship.

TREATMENT OF THE SUPERVISORY PROCESS IN CONFERENCES

Data from studies of supervisory conferences in speech-language pathology make it clear that conferences traditionally have not included much discussion of the supervisory process or of the needs and behaviors of the supervisees or supervisors who are participating in these conferences (Culatta et al., 1975; Culatta & Seltzer, 1977; Pickering, 1984; Roberts & Smith, 1982; Shapiro, 1985a, 1985b; Smith & Anderson, 1982b; Tufts, 1984). One can make certain assumptions about that fact. Such discussion may not be perceived as an important component and thus is intentionally excluded from discussion. It may be that the classic view of the supervisory process as evaluation or as a supervisor-dominated activity is so strong and so accepted that it is assumed that there is no need for discussion of the process. It may be that supervisors, who generally control the direction of the conference, do not have an understanding of the components of supervision, and feel inadequate to deal with the topic. Additionally, supervisees have probably not been prepared for supervision in such a way that they are able to either initiate or participate in meaningful discussion. Whatever the reason, the data consistently indicate that the focus of the conference is on the clinical process, mainly the client but not the clinician.

The appropriateness of this exclusive focus on the clinical process is highly questionable, given that the primary objective of supervision is to facilitate independent thinking and problem-solving skills of the supervisee. Expanding the focus to encourage interpretation of the supervisory process as a means of contributing to the growth and development of the supervisee and supervisor should enrich the clinical process as well.

Speech-language pathologists and audiologists have always been concerned about the ability of the client to generalize behaviors acquired in the clinical setting. Of equal concern should be the generalization of behaviors acquired by clinicians in supervisory interactions. However, it appears that supervisees are expected to extrapolate from discussion of the client's behavior to their own to determine the changes they should make in their own clinical performance. Such an approach limits the overall professional growth of clinicians.

Two strategies for altering this traditional approach to supervision seem plausible. The first and most obvious is to move beyond an individual focus on a particular client or clinician-client dyad to look for patterns of clinical behavior that can be generalized across the clinical process. Unable to resist the restatement of a well-worn piece of advice, Anderson (1988) cited the analogy, "Give me a fish and I eat for a day. Teach me to fish and I eat for a lifetime."

The second possibility is to attend to the behavior of clinicians as supervisees to try to determine if their participation is such that they obtain maximum benefits from the supervisory process, enabling them to learn problem-solving techniques they can use in other situations. Hopefully these two strategies will move supervisor and supervisee beyond an exclusive focus on the client.

UNDERSTANDING ROLES
IN THE SUPERVISORY PROCESS

Role is usually considered to be a set of expectations about the behavior of persons who occupy certain positions in social units or as actions that are perceived to be appropriate to certain positions. It is a set of prescriptions for behavior that are shaped by the rules and sanctions of others and by each person's conception of what his or her behavior should be in a certain situation (Biddle & Thomas, 1966).

Preconceived stereotypes about supervisors and supervision, together with the many roles that supervisors and supervisees have available to them and the fact that they may be performing several roles at one time, make it essential to examine the operative roles. If communication is to be open, objectives are to be met, and professional growth is to take place as a result of the supervisory process—that is, if supervision is to be productive—participants should be aware of the role perceptions they have for themselves and each other and the expectations they bring into the supervisory interaction.

Perceived Roles for Supervisors

Supervisors are viewed as assuming a variety of roles, among them that of teacher, overseer, controller, evaluator, counselor (Hatten, 1966), and decision maker (Schubert, 1978). Cogan (1973) listed six types of relationships between supervisor and supervisee, all of which would demand very different roles for each of the participants—the superior–subordinate relationship, the teacher–student relationship, the counselor–client relationship, the supervisor as evaluator or rater, the helping relationship, and the colleagueship relationship. Weller (1971), in discussing the three functions of "counselor, teacher, and trainer," made an important point when he said, "Supervisors can rarely expect to be equally competent in all three functions, yet neither can they afford to be ignorant of any one" (p. 8). Anderson (1988) noted that supervisor roles may include provider of information, questioner, problem-solver, evaluator, demonstrator, and facilitator. Roles should be assumed consciously and should be congruent with the goals of the supervisory process.

Techniques we have used to identify perceived roles for ourselves and our supervisees are to (1) write personal definitions of supervision and (2) list characteristics of a "good" supervisor and a "good" supervisee. Sharing and discussing these techniques enable us to understand each other's perspective about what we think supervision ought to be. If there is a mismatch between perceived roles and the goals for the supervisory process, this will become apparent in the discussion, and modifications can be made. Pannbacker, Middleton, and Lass (1993) surveyed 100 students to identify their perceptions of a "good supervisor." Results revealed that a good supervisor is available, consistent, fair, flexible, and provides feedback; a bad supervisor is late for appointments, has unrealistic expectations, doesn't respect students, and is not clinically competent. A number of researchers (Casey, 1985; Mournot, Siegle, & Solomon, 1985; Peaper & Mercaitis, 1989a) have developed instruments based on the 13 tasks and 81 associated competencies for effective clinical supervision to systematically assess supervisees' understanding of the supervisory process, needs, and expectations.

Importance of Shared Expectations

Expectations are the perceptions of appropriate behavior for one's own role or the role of others and, as such, are a potent influence on the individual's behavior as well as on how he or she believes others should behave. To speak of *shared expectations* implies that each individual perceives his or her own and others' roles similarly (Biddle & Thomas, 1966). This is considered an important prerequisite to communication and to meeting objectives, especially in the supervisory relationship. "Leaders must either change their style to coincide with followers' expectations or change followers' expectations" (Hersey & Blanchard, 1982, p. 132). If supervisors and supervisees operate from different sets of assumptions about what should take place between them, then communication barriers are raised even before the interaction begins (Blumberg et al., 1967).

Discrepancies between expectations and perceptions of what actually happened lead to confusion and conflict. Individuals expressing such role conflict have been found to be less effective than others, suggesting that the consequence of role conflict may be not only ineffectiveness for the institution within which they work, but also frustration for the individual (Cooper & Good, 1983: Getzel & Guba, 1954; Trow, 1960).

After an extensive review of the literature on education students' expectations, Tihen (1984) noted, "If there is a discrepancy between the supervisee's expectations and the supervisor's actual behavior, both the performance of the supervisee and the satisfaction which he or she derives from the supervisory process may be negatively affected" (p. 7). To avoid uncertainty, confusion, lack of direction, frustration, and stress, and to establish a positive supervisory relationship, it is imperative to clarify roles, expectations, and needs of both supervisees and supervisors. **In fact, sharing of goals and objectives, defining needs and expectations, and clarification of the differences and similarities in perceptions of roles may well be one of the most important components of the entire supervisory interaction, probably forming the pattern for the entire relationship.** It is also reasonable to assume that needs, expectations, and perceptions are not static and are altered by maturity, experience, and the influence of the many variables within each situation. Therefore, there is a need for *continuing exploration* of perceived role, as well as expectations and needs, in every supervisory relationship as it progresses through a semester, a year, or an ongoing situation such as an employment setting. The ability to establish joint communication regarding expectations and responsibilities in the clinical and supervisory processes (1.9) is an important competency for establishing and maintaining an effective relationship.

EXPECTATIONS FOR SUPERVISION

Speech-Language Pathology and Audiology Research

The literature contains many studies that identify the expectations and needs of supervisees and the extent to which they are met. Much of this literature is overlapping and some is contradictory and equivocal. A few important themes emerge and provide insights about the wide variety of expectations that may be present in any situation.

Supervisor Skills.　Russell (1976) asked student supervisees to indicate their perception of the importance of 65 different behaviors and also to indicate what behaviors were actually exhibited by their supervisors. Her subjects listed being treated fairly and impartially, being encouraged to question, disagree, and express their ideas, being guided to make clinical decisions, being provided with constructive feedback, having supervisors perceive and be responsive to clinician's feedback and evaluation, and having supervisors demonstrate flexibility and adaptability as the most valued supervisor behaviors. Interestingly enough, when Russell's supervisees were asked what supervisors *do* most frequently, "treating the clinician in a fair and impartial manner" was the only actual behavior that emerged from the most valued list. Discrepancies between expectations and reality were greatest in terms of supervisor's attention to clinician needs, feelings, and problems and to evaluation.

Some researchers have looked at needs or expectations of speech-language pathology students at different experience levels. Myers (1980) found beginning students ranked supervisor enthusiasm and interest, demonstration, and being provided the theoretical bases and rationales underlying therapy techniques as more important than did most advanced clinicians. As students gained experience, technical needs decreased in importance but affective needs remained constant throughout the educational program and across experience levels. Russell and Engle (1977) and Dowling and Wittkopp (1982) found differences between experienced and less experienced students, indicative of the changing needs of students. In their investigation across six universities, Dowling and Wittkopp (1982) found that assistance in writing lesson plans and the need for more frequent observations were given greater value by less-experienced clinicians, whereas the more-experienced clinicians wished to assume increased responsibility for the client.

Larson (1982) examined both need and expectations and found similar expectations in her inexperienced (no clinical hours) and experienced (over 150 hours) supervisees; inexperienced, however, had slightly higher expectations and stronger needs. Both groups expected to ask questions, participate in conferences, express opinions, have their ideas used, and have supervisors be supportive. Both needed to have their point of view considered and to have assistance with client goals and therapy strategies.

Tihen (1984) studied three levels of clinicians. He examined the importance attached to five categories of expectations and whether the clinicians perceived their supervisors attaching similar or dissimilar importance to the same categories. Tihen found, as did other investigators, that inexperienced clinicians expected more direction from supervisors than the more experienced groups. As clinicians gained experience, they placed greater value on the expectations related to their own responsibility in the supervisory process. Tihen concluded that clinicians enter the supervisory process without priorities for their expectations of supervisors and that their priorities develop as a function of supervised practica. Further, he proposed that knowledge of supervisees' expectations profiles would assist a supervisor in planning an experience that is more compatible with needs. Larson's and Tihen's scales (Appendix 4A, 4B, 4C) are useful tools for analyzing supervisee needs and expectations. Supervisees' responses can be compared to those of the supervisor and provide a focus for subsequent discussion and clarification.

These findings suggest that supervisees do change in terms of their perception of need and the expectations for supervision as they move along the continuum. Preferences for a direct or indirect style of supervision, which reflects the amount of supervisor involvement, has been studied extensively in education (Blumberg, 1974, 1980; Blumberg & Amidon, 1965; Copeland, 1980, 1982; Copeland & Atkinson, 1978) and somewhat in speech-language pathology (Nilsen, 1983; Smith, 1978; Wollman & Conover, 1979). Most novices seem to prefer a directive style, one in which their supervisors initiate, criticize, give suggestions and opinions, and help them reach immediate solutions to problems. With experience, however, supervisees appear to prefer a more indirect style, characterized by supervisor questioning, reflecting the supervisees' ideas and feelings, and listening. This is perhaps not surprising, but the question that supervisors must ask themselves is whether or not their supervisory approaches are compatible with these changes. The literature suggests that supervisory styles do not adjust to changing expectations of supervisees (Blumberg, 1980; Copeland, 1980, 1982; Culatta & Seltzer, 1977; Nilsen, 1983; Roberts & Smith, 1982; Smith, 1978). Supervisors continue to use a direct-active style, regardless of supervisee needs or preferences.

Mastriano, Gordon and Gottwald (1999) studied expectations from the beginning and end of a semester for 10 supervisors and 35 supervisees at two universities using an adaptation of Larson's (1982) scale. Factor analysis revealed four significant factors with regard to the roles assumed by a supervisor: instructor, mentor, personal facilitator, and the person who helps transfer responsibility for treatment to the supervisee. Interestingly, at the end of the semester the 52 dyads evidenced lower levels of agreement on items that described how actively involved the supervisor should be in the supervisory process but higher levels for how active the supervisee should be. The results substantiate "the need for supervisors and supervisees to engage in some formal assessment of each participant's expectations at the outset of any supervisory relationship" (p. 2) and to periodically review them throughout the supervisory experience.

Broyles, McNeice, et al. (1999) compared perceptions of effective supervision strategies for 49 supervisors and 197 graduate students from 11 universities. Neither years of supervisory experience nor accrued clock hours of experience influenced the perceptions of the groups. Of the 43 items examined, supervisors and student clinicians reported the following strategies as most effective: demonstrates/models clinical techniques during a therapy session, models professional behavior, and creates an atmosphere of mutual respect and sharing of attitudes, feelings, beliefs, and philosophies. Supervisors' and supervisees' perceptions of effective supervision strategies significantly differed on observation and self-evaluation strategies. At least 12 supervisors reported they did not use the following strategies: requires written agreement to ensure follow-through, gives a summary rating sheet within one week of a session, gives gestural guidance/cues during a session, holds regularly scheduled group supervision conferences, requires joint analysis of video/audiotaped sessions, holds supervision conferences upon clinician request, and observes through a closed-circuit television monitor. The scales developed for this study (Appendix 4D) could be helpful tools for checking perceptions at the onset and throughout a supervisory experience.

Learning Style Preferences. The ability to apply learning principles in the supervisory process is an acknowledged competency (1.4) for effective supervision and one aspect of this competency that has received attention in recent literature is that of learning style. A *learning style* is the habitual strategy used by an individual to process information for problem solving (Katz & Heimann, 1991, cited in Lincoln, McLeod, McAllister, et al., 1994). Early educational experiences, educational specialization, professional career choice, and current job role shape learning style (Kolb, 1984, cited in Lincoln et al., 1994). In a two-year longitudinal study involving more than 100 communication disorders students in Sydney, results revealed homogeneous learning styles (Lincoln, McLeod, McAllister, et al., 1994). The majority of students were *reflectors*—those who like to listen to different perspectives before drawing conclusions, or *activists*—those who learn by active experimentation and the challenge of novel experiences. Few were *theorists*—those who analyze and synthesize observations to formulate theories and attempt to form pieces of information into a whole, or *pragmatists*—those who experiment with new ideas, theories, and techniques and are interested in the practicality and application of information. Supervisors who are sensitive to the differences in styles can assist supervisees in using their dominant style and encourage them to explore learning opportunities using other styles. One way to facilitate learning is to discuss different styles and to instruct students about child and adult learning.

Farmer and Farmer (1995) recommended that learning styles be analyzed, profiled, and shared to enhance the interactions between supervisor and supervisee, as well as clients, families, and others involved in the clinical process. Identifying and discussing dominant intelligences for those involved in the process can effect mutual understanding and the likelihood of positive outcomes. Farmer and Farmer used Gardner's (1983, 1993) theory of multiple intelligences and classification of the different types of intelligence: body-kinesthetic, musical, logical, mathematical, linguistic, spatial, interpersonal, and intrapersonal.

Kayser (1993) and Battle (1995) discussed learning styles in terms of field dependent/holistic and field independent/analytic styles of learning. The salient characteristics of each are:

FIELD DEPENDENT	FIELD INDEPENDENT
Takes an integrative approach to information processing, organizes the world in terms of totalities, and is sensitive to the overall context of objects or events.	Responds to events and objects in the environment independently of the total field or context.
Prefers cooperative group work	Prefers competition and independent work
Prefers to operate in relative, holistic time units, often delaying task completion in lieu of personal and social obligations	Prefers to operate in discrete time units and completes tasks within a specific time frame.
Learns best when material is presented in a human, social framework—when concepts are humanized and illustrated with stories, anecdotes, and personal experiences.	Learns best in an analytical framework that requires conformity to rules, memorization, and recall of facts.
Desires models and demonstrations of tasks	Desires scientific reasoning to support practice
Values social, interpersonal relationships with peers and teachers. Seeks role models and mentors and thrives in a nurturing environment	Values personal achievement and tangible rewards. Relationships with teacher are formal.

Audiology and Speech-Language Pathology

Russell and Engle (1977) found some differences between expectations of audiology and speech-language pathology students. Audiology students perceived that it was important for supervisors to guide them in being nonthreatening to their clients, developing a clinical atmosphere, and helping them to be procedure-oriented and to provide oral feedback to the client. Audiology students placed great importance on receiving help when encountering difficulty. Speech-language pathology students valued flexibility and adaptability in their supervisors as well as guidance in developing clients' understanding of goals, providing feedback, and utilizing resources. These differences would appear to reflect the difference between the one-time diagnostic interaction and the technological requirements of audiology versus the ongoing and variable nature of the therapeutic interaction in speech-language pathology.

Rassi, Hoffman and Willie (1991) administered Larson's (1982) Expectations and Needs scales in two consecutive academic years to audiology and speech-language pathology master's students at their university who had different amounts and types of practicum experience. Needs and expectations were higher for first-year students than for second-year students. Hoffman and Willie (1992) compared *conference* needs and expectations for five audiology and eight speech-language pathology graduate students. They speculated that students' decreasing needs and expectations for a supervisor to be directive during conferences would indicate progression along the continuum in the direction of self supervision. Audiology students' needs and expectations to state the objectives of their conferences showed a mean increase over a one-year period, whereas those of SLP students decreased. The remaining needs and expectations [for having supervisors use their ideas in conferences, to provide information to their supervisors about the clinical sessions, to ask many questions during conferences, and to discuss ways to improve materials] decreased over time for both groups. These differences between audiology and speech-language pathology students would appear to reflect the difference between one-time diagnostic interaction and the technological requirements of audiology versus the ongoing and variable nature of the therapeutic interaction in speech-language pathology. Supervisors reported using information about supervisees' needs and expectations to set goals and plan for the clinical and supervisory processes.

Jones (1993) compared the needs of 12 audiology versus 12 speech-language pathology student clinicians, using Larson's (1982) needs and expectations scales. Both groups had similar expectations of the clinical supervisor and supervisory process, but audiology students had higher needs on 18 of the 23 items. Audiology students indicated a greater need to have supervisors discuss ways to improve their performance. Speech-language pathology students had a greater need to have the supervisor discuss *client's* performance (versus *their* performance).

Gender, Cultural, and Age-Related Variations

Differences in styles of thinking, problem-solving, and communicating have gained a great deal of popularity in recent years when books such as those by linguist Deborah Tannen, *You Just Don't Understand* (1990) and *Talking From 9 to 5* (1994), psychologist Mary Belenky and her colleagues, *Women's Ways of Knowing* (1986), and others hit the *New York Times* best-seller lists. Understanding cultural, cognitive, and communication style differences are important to consider in the preparation of our students as well as in the delivery of services to our clients (Battle, 1993; Sorensen, 1992).

Although sparse, there is some attention in the communicative sciences and disorders literature to the influence that gender, ethnicity, and age may have on expectations. These variables are important in light of the demographics apparent in ASHA membership. Data indicate that more than 90% of ASHA members are Caucasian women and about 30% are in the 35–44 year age range and about 35% are in the 45–54 year age range (ASHA, 2001b).

Understanding differences and similarities can lead to more effective outcomes.

Langellier and Natalle (1987) described the ways in which gender is a profound and pervasive influence on our work and on our self-expressions. Providing facts gleaned from research on gender and interpersonal communication, and integrating facts about the profession of speech-language pathology and the world of academe, Langellier and Natalle offered a number of strategies for analyzing and dealing with differences in conversational styles. Seymour (1992), Larkins (1992), and Pickering (1992) addressed "Women's Ways of Supervising," noting how gender may impact self-esteem, perceptions of roles, the ways we work and our preferences within our work settings. Pickering (1992) stated, "A woman's way of being in the world, whether the domestic, public, or professional world, is likely to be different from that of a man's" (p. 41).

DeVane (1992) offered multicultural strategies for quality improvement in the management/supervisory process, stressing the responsibility of supervisors to create a learning and work environment that uses the strengths and expertise of all participants. DeVane described underlying problems that interfere with successful management of diversity in academic and employment settings:

- Maintenance of the homogeneity theory/America as a "melting pot"
- Failure to differentiate between difference and deficit
- Cognitive and behavioral rigidity/ethnocentrism

Understanding is gained by examining what we have in common, how we are alike, and by sharing our values and developing common goals. Empathy and concern for others, evidenced by behaviors such as active listening, asking questions, and honest and open communication are imperative. It is also necessary to recognize the relationship between language and culture, and understand that experiences, concepts, values, beliefs, and attitudes are reflected in how language is used.

Kayser (1993) cited four training issues that are important when supervising Hispanic SLP students: (1) culture, (2) language proficiency, (3) mentoring, and (4) supervision and clinical management of minority clients. Culture is the knowledge that individuals must have to be functional members of a community and includes rules for interactions, appropriate behaviors, and regulations for interacting with people from different cultures (Saville-Troike, 1986, cited in Kayser, 1993). Acculturation involves adhering to certain rules for interaction and adopting some values of a second culture while preserving the rules and regulations of one's native culture. Assimilation involves accepting various ideas and values from a second culture but rejecting differing values and expectations of one's native culture. Kayser (1993) noted that "bilingual-bicultural graduate students come into graduate programs with differing levels of acculturation and assimilation" (p. 18). The variability within and between ethnic groups and the impact that cognitive, behavioral, and affective differences may have on interactions with peers, supervisors, clients, and their families, necessitates self-analysis. The self-awareness that is achieved through self-analysis provides the opportunity to recognize differences in styles and to identify those that enhance clinical effectiveness. Knowing that bilingual students are a heterogeneous group, Kayser recommends that the graduate program be designed to enable students to develop proficiency in assessment and clinical management in both languages. The issue of language proficiency is addressed in ASHA's (1989) position statement, which includes an operational definition for bilingual SLPs.

Murray and Owen (1991) defined *mentoring* as "a deliberate pairing of a more skilled or experienced person with a lesser skilled or experienced one, with the agreed-upon goal of having the lesser skilled person grow and develop specific competencies" (p. xiv). Mentoring is an unquestionable critical factor in the retention of culturally and linguistically different students. The paucity of persons of color in our professions makes cross-racial and cross-cultural matches inevitable. Further, it isn't fair to expect the one or few persons of color or ethnicity in an organization to assume the role of "minority in residence" or expert on all issues related to diversity (Brasseur, 1994).

Since the early '80s, numerous articles have stressed not only the importance of mentoring, but also have suggested strategies. For example, Murray and Owen (1991) suggested that a mutually developed action plan that includes professional, educational, and personal goals be constructed. For each goal the following should be detailed: (a) activities, (b) skills or knowledge to be achieved, and (c) timelines. The frequency of regular meetings should be addressed during the planning process. Confidentiality also needs to be addressed. The plan is a contract of sorts, and as such should specify the length of the formal relationship. Murray and Owen call this a "no-fault termination" clause and note that it is similar to a prenuptial agreement in that it provides for a civilized dissolution and a graceful ending. Supervisors who are unfamiliar with the body of literature on mentoring are advised to engage in some self study to assist in our professions' efforts to recruit and retain diverse professionals.

In describing supervisor and supervisee style differences and preferences, Kayser explains some of the behaviors associated with a "field dependent" learning style, which is fairly typical of Mexican Americans, as is a polychronic style of treatment. Battle (1995) expands the discussion of variation in learning styles and states that a field independent/analytic learning style is more typical of European American students while the field dependent/holistic learning style is often used by African American, Asian American/Pacific Islander, and Hispanic students. Naturally, no single style exists for all members of a particular ethnic group. Supervisors need to understand the distinctions and how to adjust their style to meet supervisee needs.

Inglebret (1996) described a model used at Washington State University for the recruitment and retention of Native American students. Recognizing learning style preferences and implementing those styles are essential to student success. Inglebret cited a body of literature that substantiates Native American students' preference for a cooperative versus competitive style. In applying this to supervision, supervisors will need to be familiar with group dynamics and the principles needed to form and facilitate effective functioning in learning groups.

ANXIETY IN THE SUPERVISORY PROCESS

The role of the emotions in the communication process and in the learning process is significant and should be considered in any study of the supervisory process. Gazda (1974), in discussing the emotional tone of the classroom, stated that although it is true that students who are emotionally involved learn best, it is the specific emotion and its intensity that may "either facilitate, distract from, or inhibit learning" (p. 10). Research and experience demonstrate that a little bit of anxiety is motivating and provides incentive for learning. However, too much anxiety can immobilize a learner. Further, "one's values, biases, preconceived notions of how things *'ought to be,'* basic philosophy, roles, etc., influence how a person perceives and interprets the behaviors of others" (Pickering & McCready, 1990, p. 25) Anxiety, fear, and confusion are emotions that are experienced by both supervisees and supervisors. A common anxiety for both is the feeling that we ought to know more than we do (Pickering & McCready, 1990).

Anxiety of Supervisees

Weller (1971) said that the initial years of teaching produce great stress, especially for persons who set high standards for themselves. One contributing factor is that the feedback about failures is often more obvious and persistent than feedback about successes. "This may be the first instance of failure for the novice who has had an academic history of success, and such perceptions of failure are frequently taken in an intensely personal way" (Weller, 1971, p. 8). This is probably equally true for speech-language pathology and audiology supervisees. In fact, the first practicum will probably

be the first time the supervisee has had his or her behavior subjected to the type of scrutiny received during observations and conferences.

Small wonder, then, that supervisees approach the experience with a broad range of emotions. Anyone who has overheard a conversation between students prior to their first practicum will be aware of the "jitters" that accompany this rite of passage. All professionals probably remember the great amount of anxiety, as well as time, that accompanied the preparation of lesson plans in the early days of their own practicum experiences. They also may remember the threat of the unseen, but nevertheless acknowledged, observer on the opposite side of the observation room window. Or they may remember the even worse, ever-present possibility of an unplanned interruption in the therapy session by a supervisor. For some, the anxiety produced by observations diminishes only slightly, even with experience.

Possible sources of anxiety for supervisees during their educational program, including off-campus experiences, no matter how good the interpersonal interaction may be, are such factors as evaluations, grades, and recommendations for graduate school or jobs. In the employment setting, anxiety over evaluations relates primarily to retention, promotions, or recommendations for other jobs. Additionally, in the work setting, anxieties are often apparent when supervisors are from another discipline. In every setting, supervisors have some power over supervisees and this can create anxiety.

Openness and the ability to communicate freely will certainly be affected by feelings of anxiety. Such feelings may result in hostility or an inability to think clearly or to be flexible, and will probably increase the amount of "selective listening." People hear what they want to hear or what their emotional state allows them to hear. Some may focus only on the negative; others may hear only the positive. Supervisors need to do what they can do to decrease the anxiety of supervisees.

The anxiety factor is discussed at length in relation to the colleagueship aspect of the clinical supervision model Cogan (1973) proposed. He said that teachers perceive supervisors as a threat for a variety of reasons. Some of these include the beliefs that: supervisors are searching for weaknesses, supervisors' criteria for good performance are unknown, and supervisees have a low estimation of supervisors' competencies. Energy dissipated through excessive anxiety is energy lost to the task at hand.

Kadushin (1968), in an article inspired by Berne's (1964) theory of gamesmanship, noted the anxieties of supervisees that may be generated by the need for change of behavior and, perhaps, personality, the threat to autonomy and sense of adequacy, the return to a relationship similar to the parent–child relationship, and the threat of evaluation and confrontation. Kadushin said that supervisees have developed some clearly identifiable games as a result of these anxieties and suggested, among others, the following games: "Be Nice to Me Because I Am Nice to You," "Protect the Sick and the Infirmed," "Treat Me, Don't Beat Me," "Evaluation Is Not for Friends," and the wonderful avoidance devices that may be familiar to supervisors—"I Have a Little List," which is, in turn, related to "Heading Them Off at the Pass." Sleight (1984) has suggested similar games for supervisees in speech-language pathology and audiology. The games concept tends to be a simplistic approach to the complexities of supervision, as indeed it is to life in general, but it does afford supervisors some amusing and insightful glimpses of themselves and their supervisees.

Studies of Supervisee Anxiety in Speech-Language Pathology and Audiology

The literature in our professions has addressed the anxieties of supervisees. Rassi (1978) included in her qualifications for audiology supervisors a practical knowledge of human behavior and the ability to deal with supervisees regarding their uncertainty about the future and other concerns. Oratio (1977), on the basis of informal interviews with students, related fear and anxiety experienced by students entering clinical practicum to three sources: anxiety about their inability to attain supervisory standards, the responsibility for the welfare of the client, and the fear that they will be unable to put academic knowledge into practice.

The *Sleight Clinician Anxiety Test* (SCAT) was developed to rate fears and anxieties of new practicum students (Sleight, 1985). The 40-item scale describes four areas of fears: (1) living up to supervisory standards and relationships between supervisors and supervisees, (2) responsibility for clients, (3) transferring theory into practice, and (4) general feelings about practicum. On the basis of a study in which the test was used with students, Sleight said that during the practicum, students decreased their anxieties and increased their confidence regarding supervisor/clinician interactions and general fears but not regarding client well-being or putting theory into practice. Decreases in anxiety about responsibility to clients was not apparent. This seems to be a continuing source of anxiety, as perhaps it should be. Feelings of confidence increased about their ability to put theory into practice and overall functioning in practicum only after students accrued experience in off-campus settings. Sleight (1985) stated, "It appears that additional experience in the same setting does not affect a student's confidence, but additional experience in a different setting increases confidence in some areas" (p. 41). The SCAT may prove to be useful in identifying the anxieties of individual supervisees.

Chan, Carter, and McAllister (1994) explored sources of anxiety in 127 students at different levels in their academic programs and concomitant differences in clinical practicum experience. Five factors contributed to anxiety across all student levels: (1) their ability to fulfill both clinical and academic demands, (2) the amount of preparation required for clinic, (3) the amount of relevant clinical experience they had to date, (4) their ability to apply theory to practice, and (5) high expectations of self. The authors stated that some student anxieties can be eliminated by modifying structural aspects of the training program—for example, rescheduling some courses, modifying the curriculum, and so on. The most significant solution is ongoing dialogue. Students must become skilled in professional and personal communication abilities to enable them to better negotiate their learning experiences with their supervisors (p. 131).

Although evaluation of clinical performance is only one of the thirteen tasks of supervision, it is a task that is evident in every setting in which supervision occurs and one that evokes anxiety for supervisees (Dowling & Wittkopp, 1982; Larson, Hoag & Schraeder-Neidenthal, 1987; Pickering, 1981a, 1981b; Russell & Halfond, 1985; Wollman & Conover, 1979). Russell and Halfond (1985) reported that graduate student clinicians perceived practicum grades as anxiety producing, subjective, non-negotiable, and based on inconsistent standards. Supervisors employ variable criteria and are often influenced by "student's potential," past experience, and level of client difficulty in assigning grades (Russell & Halfond, 1985). A variety of strategies has proven effective in explicitly defining supervisor expectations for performance and criteria for evaluation, for enhancing objectivity, and improving the consistency and specificity of feedback. These include: a contract-based system (Larson et al., 1987; Peaper & Mercaitis, 1989b), competency-based goal setting and evaluation (Rassi, 1987), and interactive and joint involvement in the analysis and assessment of clinical performance (Monnin & Peters, 1981; Strike-Roussos, Brasseur, Jimenez, O'Connor, & Boggs, 1991). Anxiety about evaluation can be diminished or eliminated with early discussion about how it will be handled and mutual involvement in the assessment process throughout the supervisory experience.

During the initial supervisory conference, supervisors should share their evaluation procedures and the evaluation instrument with supervisees to decrease anxiety and facilitate a positive relationship (Brasseur, 1987a). Additionally, Hutchinson, Uhl, and Weinrich (1987) demonstrated that "indepth explanation **prior to the initiation of practicum** of the clinical skills that supervisors expect clinicians to demonstrate, particularly those that will be evaluated, decreases the need for redundant supervisor feedback" (pp. 132–133, emphasis added). Supervisors who are clear and effective communicators increase supervisee satisfaction with the process (Peaper & Mercaitis, 1989a). Discussion about evaluation should continue into the planning phase as certain clinical skills and competencies are transformed into objectives for the supervisee's professional growth (Brasseur, 1987a).

Anxieties of Supervisors

One cannot assume that all the anxiety and apprehensions brought into the supervisory experience are brought there by supervisees. Most supervisors have not been prepared for the tasks they must perform as supervisors. Their perceptions of their roles have come from as many different sources as have those of their supervisees. Perhaps they bring even more stereotypes or preconceived notions because they have been supervised even if they have not supervised. In discussing supervisors' anxieties, Pickering and McCready (1990) noted that fear of failure, to varying degrees, and anxiety about being uninformed or being criticized "are simply part of the fabric of supervision" (p. 27).

Anderson noted that supervisors—in speech-language pathology and audiology at least—do not usually plan to be supervisors; their preparation, career objectives, and self-perception as professionals is that of a clinician. To be suddenly thrust into the new role of supervisor of professional adults, without preparation, may result in a difficult and stressful transition that requires the development of a new and different self-concept. Additionally, supervisors may begin work with little or no organizational assistance or support, such as job descriptions, models, or opportunity for in-service education to help them learn new skills or define their new role. Indeed, the importance of the role may be downgraded by the casual way in which supervisors are selected and the lack of guidance they receive. Off-campus supervisors, for example, may be provided with very little in the way of guidelines or support from the university for which they are supervising. Or the off-campus facility may need to establish policies and procedures for the organization to ensure compliance with accreditation standards and regulatory agencies (e.g., JCAHO, ASHA/CAA, HCFA, IDEA, etc.) while interns are earning clock hours at the facility. University supervisors or supervisors in a service delivery setting may receive no input about their responsibilities and thus may operate autonomously. These are only a few sources of anxieties for supervisors.

Most supervisors recognize the importance of their tasks along with their lack of preparation. Most are conscientious about fulfilling their roles. Some supervisors' perception of their role is of a professional who must have the answer to every possible clinical question, who must be able to solve every problem or issue that arises. That "heavy" self-perception, along with the inner knowledge that one does not really have that kind of information, skill, or power, will surely produce anxiety. This self-concept—that supervisors must have all the answers—has serious consequences in the development of the Collaborative Style. Sometimes the dispelling of this myth comes as a great surprise and a great relief. Every supervisor has the right—and the responsibility— to say, "I don't know."

This initial anxiety about role may continue. There are very few data in any of the areas where supervision is utilized that supports a particular methodology. Supervisors who want to find hard and fast answers about what they should be doing will search without much result. As with the clinical process, there is no "cookbook" for effective supervision, let alone a recipe for success. Cogan (1973) stated that professional uncertainties have existed for a long time and will probably persist for a long time.

Some supervisors experience difficulties in using the various types of authority inherent in their positions—administrative, evaluative, educational, and consultative. The attempt to deal with these difficulties may lead to two categories of games—games of abdication and games of power, neither of which resolves the problem. According to Hawthorne (1975), supervisors must examine their own feelings and needs concerning the authority of their professional role.

Supervisors, in their role as evaluators, often have to make or participate in life-altering decisions—retention or dismissal from an educational program or recommendations for a job, for promotion, or for tenure. If dealt with seriously and responsibly, these are awesome responsibilities that understandably create tension and anxiety.

What are the effects, then, of supervisor anxiety and what is its relationship to supervision at this stage of the continuum? Why insert it at this point in the discussion? If supervisors are, indeed, responsible for structuring the supervisory experience, they should have, in addition to information, some sense of comfort in the role. Excessive anxiety or uncertainty on the part of the supervisor will surely be communicated to the supervisee through various means—aggression, neglect of duties, uncertainty, erratic behavior. On the other hand, too much complacency about the role is not desirable.

Very little is known about the feelings of supervisors. Pickering (1984; Pickering & McCready, 1983) touched upon it in their studies, especially when they wrote about the use of journal writing by supervisors, as did McCready, Shapiro, and Kennedy (1987). Like most other aspects of the process, supervisor anxiety must be considered as thoughtfully as possible, without the benefit of a great many definitive answers. It is speculated that perhaps the judicial use of a modicum of self-disclosure might contribute to collegiality, encourage better communication, and possibly diminish anxieties of both supervisor and supervisee. The image of the supervisor who knows all is difficult to maintain; more reasonable is the image of the supervisor who knows how to problem-solve and is willing to enter into this type of activity with the supervisee.

IMPLICATIONS FOR PARTICIPANTS IN THE SUPERVISORY PROCESS

What does all this mean to the supervisor and supervisee facing each other for the first time or the fiftieth time? In implementing the Understanding component, supervisors are dealing with two distinct entities. The first is the interpersonal factor; the second a teaching factor—that is, teaching about supervision.

It has already been stated that the interpersonal component of the supervisory process will not be dealt with in great detail here other than to point out the wealth of information on this topic that is available from other sources and the importance of an in-depth knowledge of the interpersonal aspects of human relations. However, this component is one of the places where an understanding of the dynamics of interpersonal interaction is not only relevant but also essential. Competency 1.5 substantiates the importance of interpersonal communication in stipulating that supervisors should be able "to apply skills of interpersonal communication in the supervisory process."

The very essence of this component is mutual understanding, not only of the mechanics of the process, but also of the other person in the interaction. Therefore, supervisors will need to bring to bear all their knowledge, insight, and skills about interpersonal interactions to successfully accomplish the goals of this component. The interpersonal skills that supervisors have learned and taught clinicians to apply to clients are essentially the same ones that are applicable in the supervisory process. In one of their significant articles on preparing clinical personnel, Ward and Webster (1965a) stated that clinicians will tend to view others as they have been viewed, to treat others as they have been treated. "They can use knowledge with compassion and meaningfulness or they can apply techniques mechanically" (Ward & Webster, 1965a, p. 39). In describing the tasks of supervision, Ulrich (1990), who chaired the committee that drafted the ASHA Position Statement (1985b) that contained them, noted that it was no accident that Task 1, establishing and maintaining an effective working relationship with the supervisee, was first on the list and had the most competencies associated with it.

Pickering and McCready (1990) described certain skills as particularly relevant to the supervisory process. They advocated that supervisors study and develop, at minimum, basic listening, self-disclosure, and conflict management skills. Further, they noted that empathy should be a major component of supervisory interactions because it connotes/denotes accepting or confirming others as individuals. McCrea's dissertation study (1980), which revealed that empathy occurred at such miniscule levels in supervisory conferences that it could not be measured, suggests that empathy is a skill that supervisors need to be trained to use.

Immediacy

A substantive body of research in the speech communication literature indicates that the notion of immediacy has a positive influence on student–teacher interaction. Mehrabian (1969a, 1969b) characterized immediacy as the behaviors that reduce physical and psychological distance between interactants. Verbal and nonverbal immediacy are behaviorally demonstrated by eye contact, reduced physical distance, touch, smiling, humor, and the use of inclusive language and communication strategies (Mehrabian, 1981). Later, Gorham (1988) identified the use of personal examples, encouraging students to talk, discussing issues student bring up in class, and using humor as also being important to the demonstration of verbal immediacy of teachers. These behavioral correlates of verbal and nonverbal immediacy are conceptually related to empathy, facilitative genuineness, respect, and concreteness that have been identified in the counseling literature as being foundational to behavior change (Gazda, 1974).

Positive relationships have been found between student cognitive achievement and teacher clarity as well as between student affect and teacher immediacy (Powell & Harville, 1990). In a study involving 311 undergraduates at California State University Los Angeles, they asked the following questions: (1) to what extent are teacher nonverbal and verbal immediacy related to teacher clarity for white, Latino, and Asian American ethnic groups and (2) to what extent are teacher verbal immediacy, nonverbal immediacy, and teacher clarity related to (a) students' attitudes toward the class, (b) students' likelihood of engaging in behaviors taught in class, (c) students' willingness to enroll in a course of similar content, and (d) students' attitudes toward the instructor for white, Latino, and Asian American ethnic groups? Overall results indicated that verbal and nonverbal immediacy were related to teacher clarity. The strength of this association varied by ethnic group. In terms of magnitude, teacher clarity consistently maintained a positive and significant relationship with each of the outcome measures and the authors concluded that immediacy is related to teacher clarity, which itself is a significant contributor to student learning.

The term *immediacy* by itself is a high inference notion; however, now that research has indicated the behavioral correlates that signify it, the term has become concrete and does not require interpretation to infer what it implies. This, in turn, means that supervisors can become aware of and manipulate these behaviors in their interactions with students in an effort to enhance them.

Role Discrepancies

Literature on the importance of shared expectations has been reviewed and its application is critical to a positive supervisory experience. A lack of congruence about role expectations may be a major source breakdown in communication and there are many possible scenarios for this type of situation. Consider, for example, supervisees who have had little opportunity in previous family or educational experiences to participate in problem solving and decision making and who have learned to expect authority figures—parent, teacher, employer, and others—to tell them what to do and provide evaluative feedback. Such supervisees will probably expect supervisors to assume the same role. This will cause problems for supervisors who perceive their role as facilitators in joint problem solving and expect supervisees to gradually assume decision-making responsibilities. Supervisors likely expect super-

visees to be able to work effectively with increasing levels of independence, but it is essential that supervisors share that expectation with supervisees at the beginning of the relationship to alleviate the probability of frustration and negative experiences.

Learning about Discrepancies

If supervisors are to know about the discrepancies that exist between themselves and their supervisees or between expectations and reality, they must take the lead in talking about the supervisory process itself. To do this, they must first raise to a conscious level what it is that *they* believe about or expect from supervision. They also need to assist their supervisees in developing an ability to discuss their feelings, concerns, and expectations.

Further, supervisors must recognize the individuality of their supervisees. Each person is unique: novice clinicians who bring their anxiety, blatantly obvious in a variety of reactions or covered by false self-confidence, bravado, or hostility, into the conference; slightly more experienced, but nevertheless anxious, clinicians; supervisees who have been supervised often and frequently by supervisors with divergent styles and philosophies; the mature, competent supervisee—all have different needs and different expectations. Supervisors must learn all they can about each one while still dealing with their own anxieties.

Dealing with Discrepancies

Possible mismatches of expectations can be dealt with in several ways. One possibility is supervisory assignments made to avoid such situations. This alternative can be discarded almost immediately. Such variables as experience, ability, training needs, and organizational constraints make scheduling difficult enough in most settings as it is. Time, requirements for clinical hours, space, and availability of clients often dictate scheduling in educational programs. In most off-campus assignments, there are only limited numbers of supervisors in each setting and, in the service delivery setting, there is usually only one supervisor available, often for many supervisees. Furthermore, information is not available for making the "perfect" match for the most effective supervision even if it were logistically possible. More important, if supervisees are to grow professionally and move from the evaluation feedback position to the self-supervisory and consultation stage discussed previously, one cannot assume that the nature of the supervisory experience should not be determined by the supervisee's preferences or expectations alone. In other words, the supervisee who prefers or feels a need for guidance and direction from authority figures would not necessarily profit from being matched with a supervisor who will meet that need—very little growth is apt to take place. What supervisees perceive as their needs may not be what is best for their professional growth. Supervisees' preferences for supervisor behavior are not necessarily related to the effectiveness of supervision (Copeland & Atkinson, 1978). Children like and want candy, but it may, after all, produce dental cavities, hyperactivity, and weight gain. What is more consistent with the approach to supervision described in this text is that both participants in the process become aware of the other's role perceptions and expectations, and that there is communication about the incongruencies that exist and the changes that may be necessary for both the supervisee and supervisor if communication is to be enhanced and professional growth is to occur throughout the experience. Accommodations must be made where there are discrepancies if the interaction is to be successful (Hersey & Blanchard, 1982). This practice is congruent with competency 1.10 (ASHA, 1985b), which requires that the supervisor and supervisee evaluate the effectiveness of the ongoing supervisory relationship.

PREPARING FOR SUPERVISION

As stated previously, most supervisors have not studied the supervisory process. Basic to the approach presented here, however, is some understanding of the dynamics of the process. The first step is for supervisors to prepare themselves for the encounter, learning about themselves as well as the process. This will not only increase their understanding but should allay some of their anxieties as well.

Study of the Process by Supervisors

Although it is true that formal coursework has not been or may not now be available to many supervisors, there are ways for them to become more knowledgeable about the process. Speech-language pathologists and audiologists have an ethical responsibility to provide the best services possible to their clients. In shifting roles from clinician to supervisor, the same holds true. The list of tasks and competencies adopted by ASHA (1985b) is probably the best starting place for study. The position paper that contains the 13 tasks and 81 associated competencies also makes suggestions about ways for supervisors to become more knowledgeable about the process (see Chapter 3). Reading, coursework, conferences, and presentations at professional meetings are ways to begin. In many organizations or areas, supervisors have formed study groups and list servs. Additionally, self-study is a valuable tool for supervisors who wish to monitor their skills. Strategies for self-analysis and self-study will be detailed in Chapter 9.

Supervisor Self-Knowledge

The admonition to "know thyself" is as important in the approach to the supervisory process as it is in the many other situations in which it is wisely offered as a guideline. Self-knowledge in several categories is critical. Supervisors first must define, or raise to a conscious level, their basic philosophy of what supervision really is. They need to define the purpose of supervision and the principles on which they determine their supervisory techniques. They must be honest about the supervisory process and the values they bring to it.

Anderson (1988) recounted a discussion of supervisory techniques with a supervisor who described her use of indirect behaviors such as questioning and asking supervisees for ideas. These techniques were consistent with the supervisor's philosophy and her beliefs that indirect behaviors would facilitate supervisees' problem-solving and independent functioning. She shared, "The supervisee came up with a good idea, so I could go along with it. I don't know what I would have done if I hadn't been comfortable with it." Obviously, there were some discrepancies between what the supervisor *really* believed and what she perceived she was doing.

Supervisors need to understand their self-perceptions of their own roles. They need to analyze their own behavior to determine if it is consistent with their basic philosophy and must have a rationale for their behaviors. It is interesting that supervisors expect supervisees to be able to provide rationales for their clinical behaviors—the "whys" to support the strategies and techniques they plan to implement in clinical intervention. Yet a majority never think to ponder the rationales for their own supervisory behaviors. Supervisors must recognize the complexity of the supervisory process and determine if they see it as teaching, evaluation, modeling, collaboration, or any of the many other available models. They need to examine their belief in a scientific approach to observation, data collection, and analysis and their own dedication to maintaining a scientific approach. They must honestly analyze their own philosophical foundation for the practices in which they engage before they can expect to discuss the process with their supervisees.

A further area of self-knowledge is that of personal motivations in relation to supervision. Why do individuals become supervisors? Many would answer the question with noble statements about the professional growth and development of young professionals and the obligations of passing on that which they have learned to new generations, thereby contributing to their profession. Those are certainly valid reasons and, for the most part, sincere and honest motivations. The reality is, however, that most supervisors became such by accident. Rather than planning to be supervisors, they were in the right place at the right time and, voilà—they became a supervisor. As they continue in this role, however, there is always the specter of the seductiveness of power and authority lurking in the background. Brammer (1985) suggested that many people who are involved in the helping process do so "to meet their own unrecognized needs" (p. 3). This can also be true of supervisors. Supervisors need to be aware of their basic attitude toward people and their worth. If, in their role of supervisor/helper, they are going to step back and *permit* their supervisees to grow, then they must value them as autonomous individuals, believe fully in their ability to think and learn, and recognize these abilities when they are present. If they believe they are responsible for the supervisee's growth and development, if they do not believe that individuals can independently solve problems and formulate solutions to clinical dilemmas, they may become manipulative and self-serving in their supervisory role. They may perceive themselves as "rescuers" and the kinds of satisfactions they obtain from this so-called helping relationship are not likely to be healthy. Supervisors can determine their values and attitudes only after considerable soul-searching, but it is an essential prerequisite to assuming the role of supervisor.

TEACHING SUPERVISEES ABOUT THE SUPERVISORY PROCESS

Introducing the student to the supervisory process may take several forms, organizationally or individually based, between supervisor and supervisee. The approach is analogous to the first experiences students have in observing therapy and in observing therapy in a new, distinct setting. Without guidance, many students look at clinical intervention globally, unable to identify individual behaviors or patterns of behavior, much less understand their significance. The same holds true for the supervisory process.

In teaching about the clinical process, various methods are used by different programs. In addition to a great amount of coursework related to normal and abnormal speech and language development, the student is introduced to the clinical process through discussion of clinical issues and case studies in academic courses and clinical process courses (i.e., Introduction to Clinic, Methods of Clinical Practice, etc.). Students are gradually introduced to therapy through observation and participation prior to their first hands-on supervised experience. This important component of the educational process is substantiated by ASHA/CAA requirements.

Certain techniques are used to teach about the clinical behaviors in the early observations before the student enters the clinical world—joint observations, guided observations, check lists, interaction analysis systems, followed by reports and analysis of observed behaviors. Once the practicum is begun, the focus is on the clinical process in a wide variety of ways.

If students or employed professionals are to be successful as supervisees, it is just as important that they be introduced to the supervisory process in a similar manner. It is imperative that they understand their dual roles and responsibilities as clinician/clinician assistant and supervisee. Ideally, this preparation should begin at the undergraduate level, prior to the first practicum. Subsequently, the supervisory process needs to be examined and analyzed throughout all supervisory experiences, whether in university training programs or professional settings. Because many universities and employment settings do not provide formal training such as courses or in-service workshops, the responsibility for preparing supervisees to participate in the supervisory process usually falls on individual supervisors. The supervisor has the responsibility for setting the stage and directing the supervisory interaction. The supervisor is accountable for preparing the supervisee to participate. In discussing the colleagueship relationship of the clinical supervision model, Cogan (1973) maintained that the supervisor is responsible for structuring the framework of discussion but not the total content of interaction. Supervisors must get the study of the process started while still making it clear that the supervisee has equal responsibility in the relationship.

Preparing supervisees for the supervisory process is expected to contribute to their professional growth and, thus, to facilitate more effective clinical practice and better services for our clients. It should also contribute to more effective clinical supervision. All 13 tasks and most of the associated competencies (ASHA, 1985b) are related to the initial preparation of supervisees—and certainly provide a structure for the ongoing analysis and discussion of the supervisory process, regardless of the setting in which supervision is occurring or the previous experience of supervisees.

Introducing the Supervisory Process

An introduction to the process that addresses the objectives of supervision, the roles of the participants, and the components of the process is essential regardless of the setting in which supervision is to take place. Whether the process is treated in coursework or workshops or not at all, *each supervisor should take time at the beginning and throughout each interaction* to talk about supervision as the situation dictates. Topics for discussion at the beginning of the experience might include any of the following, in any order:

1. *Components of the Supervisory Process.* This discussion will reflect a content approach to supervision based on the components defined by Anderson (1988) and detailed in this text. It should include both the supervisor's philosophy about supervision and the supervisee's impressions about the process.

2. *Perceptions of Supervisees about Supervision.* Information about the perceptions of roles (i.e., preconceived stereotypes derived from various sources) should be shared. Personal biases, previous experience, theoretical perspectives, information from friends, information derived from the literature, and the complexities of the supervisory process itself make many roles available to both supervisors and supervisees. Supervisors will want to know what supervisees' role expectations are for them. Are they perceived as helpers, teachers, counselors, evaluators, trainers, overseers, and so on? And, what do these titles means to supervisees? For example, do supervisees perceive the supervisor as the expert—someone who has all the answers and can provide any and all of the information they might need? Or is the supervisor's role that of evaluator—someone to tell them what they did right or wrong, point out their weaknesses, and then tell them the correct way to do it?

Supervisees' perceptions of their own roles must be discussed. Do they perceive themselves as passive participants in the process—following directives provided by the supervisor? Do they have insight about their responsibilities in problem solving—for their own professional development? Do they have confidence in their ability to establish objectives for their clients and to devise methods for achieving those objectives?

Techniques we have used to clarify perceived roles for ourselves and our supervisees include the following, done independently and without collaboration:

- Write your personal definition of supervision
- List the characteristics of a "good supervisor"
- List the characteristics of a "good supervisee"

Share and discuss what you've written.

3. *Goals and Objectives for Supervision.* Setting goals and objectives for the supervisory process will be addressed in Chapter 5. During the introductory phase, supervisees need to know that goals will be established not only for clients, but also for them as supervisees and clinicians, *and* for supervisors. Goals may be long-term ones, which include overall, broad objectives related to general patterns, or short-term ones that are specific to a particular interaction.

4. *Prior Experiences in Supervision.* Supervisors and supervisees need to discuss supervisees' past experiences in supervision, the types of interactions they have had with supervisors, their feelings about supervision, and what they learned about the process. Important questions to pose include: How much previous experience have supervisees had? What was the nature of previous

experiences? What positive and negative feelings, likes and dislikes, about supervision does the supervisee have?

5. *Supervisee Style Preference.* It is important to decide whether supervisees prefer a direct-active supervisor style, which is characterized by a higher proportion of supervisor talk during interactions and involves telling, giving opinions, giving suggestions, critiquing, and so on, or an indirect style, which is characterized by supportive supervisor statements, active listening, asking for opinions and suggestions, and reflecting supervisee feelings and ideas (Blumberg, 1974). Whether supervisees can accurately differentiate behaviors characteristic of these styles is also important to establish (Brasseur & Anderson, 1983). Further, the consequences of preferred style in relation to supervisee growth and independence need to be explored. Specifically, how style influences placement and movement on the continuum needs to be discussed. If the preferences of the supervisor and supervisee are not congruent, differences should be examined at the beginning of the relationship.

6. *Supervisee Anxieties.* Cogan (1973) maintained that, during the initial conferences, supervisors need to deal with supervisees' anxieties and uncertainties. This is especially critical for novice supervisees or those working with a new type of client. While a little anxiety is motivating, too much is incapacitating. For some, identifying anxieties and their sources will be a sufficient technique for diffusing them. For others, the process will be more involved. Possible sources of anxiety may include preparing lesson plans, the threat of being continuously observed, the possibility of unplanned interruption/intervention, evaluations, recommendations, grades, inability or lack of confidence regarding one's ability to manage clinical problems, and a host of other concerns. Based on our experience, "fear of the unknown" is often a source of anxiety. Oratio (1977) and Sleight (1985) state that beginning clinicians' anxieties primarily concern their ability to attain supervisory standards, the supervisory relationship itself, responsibility for client welfare, and the ability to apply academic information to the clinical process.

7. *Supervisee Baseline Needs and Competencies.* The fact that data will be collected should be conveyed in one of the first conferences. Actual data collection procedures and timelines will be thoroughly addressed in the planning stage as supervisors introduce the continuum perspective and the appropriate style of supervision relative to placement on the continuum.

Notice that discussion of the client has not yet been suggested. This is appropriate because this is the time for the supervisee to become aware of his or her own feelings and to share expectations with the supervisor. Once preliminary rapport is established, the supervisor and supervisee can move on to the more traditional planning for the client and then for the clinician, supervisee, and supervisor.

Learning How to Talk about Supervision

The discussion described previously may be elicited and enhanced in a variety of ways. First and foremost, the supervisor must be a skilled listener. Scattered throughout the literature on supervisees' expectations are references to the supervisee wanting the supervisor to listen and to take seriously what they say (Kayser, 1993; Larson, 1982; Peaper & Mercaitis, 1989a, 1989b; Russell, 1976; Tihen, 1984). As Anderson noted, the fact that this is stated at all is significant. Have supervisors communicated to supervisees that they are not taking supervisees seriously? That they do not respect their ideas and abilities? The supervisor who takes time to *hear* what the supervisee expresses about needs, expectations, and anxieties will learn valuable information and enhance the relationship immeasurably.

Good communication and interpersonal skills, including active listening, are vital supervisor competencies. Specific supervisor behaviors that need to be demonstrated include accepting and using the supervisees' ideas in discussions, reflecting the content and feelings of supervisee utterances, and skilled questioning. Modeling a supportive, collegial communication style may be more important than what is actually said (Anderson, 1988). Both verbal and nonverbal behaviors must be monitored to ensure that what a supervisors espouse as their philosophy of supervision is consistent with actual practice.

Supervisors may wish to give students some reading material about the supervisory process. The NSSLHA monograph (Casey, Smith, and Ulrich, 1988), *Self Supervision: A Career Tool for Audiologists and Speech-Language Pathologists,* is a particular favorite of ours.

Getting accurate statements of how supervisees feel at this point may be difficult. They may not know how to express their ideas. The supervisor or the total situation may be so threatening that supervisees' reactions will be inhibited. The supervisor may not be able to resist loaded questions in which the expected answer is obvious. It is sometimes gratifying or easier to hear what one wishes to hear, but it is not productive in the effort to learn supervisees' real feelings. Also, some supervisees may have learned through the grapevine what a particular supervisor likes or expects and may play the game, "Tell the supervisor what she wants to hear." The skill and sensitivity of supervisors in asking questions determines much of the outcome here.

Some supervisors find questionnaires and scales such as Larson's (1982) and Tihen's (1984) scales (Appendix 4A, 4B, 4C) helpful for facilitating honest discussions about supervision. A scale developed and validated by Powell (1987) to measure attitudes toward Cogan's clinical supervision model could also be used at this stage to learn more about the supervisee's ideas and provide a basis for discussion (Appendix 4E). Indeed, supervisors who have not yet worked out their own personal beliefs about the process might also find it useful. A supervisory conference rating scale developed by Smith (1978; Smith & Anderson, 1982a) and modified by Brasseur (1980a) may also be helpful to obtain specific information about supervisees' perceptions of individual conferences (Appendix 4F). Both supervisor and supervisees might complete part of Casey's scale (1985, 1988) to delineate the relative importance of the 13 tasks and 81 associated competencies and discuss their responses (Appendix 4G).

Some supervisors ask students to write an informal statement about their feelings at the beginning of the interaction. Others ask students to keep a journal (Laccinole & Shulman, 1985; Lubinsky & Hildebrand, 1996; Maloney, 1994; Pickering & McCready, 1990; Schill & Swanson, 1993) to reflect on or to evaluate their clinical performance throughout a term. This may be difficult for some students so, if the supervisor perceives that a student is somewhat intimidated or is reluctant to share their feelings early on, these writings can be maintained by the supervisee until a climate of trust and openness is firmly established in the relationship.

From the outset, supervisees need to see supervision as a larger issue than "What do I do with my client?" The concept of setting objectives for themselves as a supervisee and as a clinician may never have entered their mind. Even students with prior clinical and supervisory experience may have had supervisors who focused exclusively on the clinical process and ignored the supervisory process. So, the concept that supervision is *not* just about and for the client's welfare may be new.

Information from supervisors about what to expect from the situation is helpful in allaying anxieties of supervisees. More of this will be discussed in the planning section, but supervisees deserve to know the organizational requirement, as well as those of the individual supervisor, the format under which they will be operating, and the criteria for success in each experience. Supervisors should not only be cognizant of their biases, quirks, idiosyncrasies, and personal operating procedures but they should also share these with supervisees in the first conference.

Because supervisors do evaluate supervisees in every type of supervisory interaction, from university training programs to employment setting, obtaining *honest* feedback from supervisees during the course of the experience, or after the fact, can be difficult. If supervisors genuinely want it though, they will be able to devise ways to obtain it. To illustrate, common supervisee complaints include: "My supervisor is always late," "My supervisor talks on the phone during our conferences," "My supervisor talks too much during conferences," or "I feel like I'm getting mixed messages." Obviously these things are difficult for supervisees to share with their supervisor unless the supervisor has set the stage for receiving feedback, exhibits high-level interpersonal skills that enable supervisees to take risks, and reacts in a nondefensive manner when supervisees provide honest feedback. It will take *time* to develop the trust and rapport needed to be honest and candid. It is also helpful to teach supervisees some types of communicative behaviors that can decrease the risk of supervisor defensiveness or the possibility of conflict. For example, the use of "I" statements and indirect requests are particularly useful techniques (e.g., "I wonder if it might be possible to take the phone off the hook during our conferences? I have trouble concentrating when interruptions happen," or, "I'm not sure I understand…I think I'm hearing two different things—X and Y—I'm a little confused").

Although discussion about the general process of supervision is initiated in the first conference, **it continues throughout the entire experience.** Once objectives have been established for the clinician/supervisee and the supervisor, they must be assessed to see if they are being met, and revised if necessary. A prerequisite to talking about the ongoing interaction is gathering data, which will serve as the nucleus of a discussion. Data should include attitudes, perceptions, needs, and actual behaviors. Once collected, data can be analyzed. A data-based, analytical focus also facilitates open and honest communication.

The use of some exercises, scales, and other tools discussed previously are good ways to set the tone and get the process of talking about supervision established as a norm for the relationship. Formulating goals and strategies for collecting and analyzing data relative to the supervisory process will be discussed in subsequent chapters. We have not provided comprehensive coverage of the topic nor an exhaustive list of techniques for preparing supervisees for the process. However, we hope readers have a better understanding of the importance of preparation, as well as a basic framework for this task. Further, we hope you see how this Understanding, as a component of the supervisory process, will help supervisors achieve the competencies for effective clinical supervision (ASHA, 1985b).

SUMMARY

The foundation of a productive supervisory relationship is a basic understanding of the supervisory process and effective communication between supervisor and supervisee about philosophies, expectations, perceptions, and objectives. This is more than merely an introduction to the process; it requires ongoing discussion about the continuing interaction.

RESEARCH ISSUES AND QUESTIONS

The 10 competencies associated with Task 1, "Establishing and maintaining an effective working relationship with the supervisee," offer an excellent starting point for validating the effectiveness of supervisory behaviors and practices related to Understanding. Casey, Smith, and Ulrich (1988) suggested that Casey's Supervisory Skills Self-Assessment (Appendix 4G) offers a method of profile comparison. This instrument is applicable across settings and experience levels of supervisors and supervisees. Respondents rate each task and competency by answering two questions: "How important is this competency for effectiveness in my program?" and "How satisfied am I with my (my supervisor's) ability to perform this skill?" After completing the ratings, a "gap score" is calculated. For example, an item rated as "9" in importance but "3" in satisfaction with ability to perform yields a gap score of 6. Items with gap scores of 3 or more are listed in priority order on an "action item list." The top few items on the list become targets for change. Knowing that supervisors have a difficult time changing behaviors and their style of interacting with super-

visees, it would be interesting to investigate the length of time needed to effect self-selected areas for change (i.e., their prioritized action list) versus ones based on supervisees' needs and expectations (i.e., supervisees' prioritized gap score list)—or to examine the process for negotiating and mutually agreeing on targets for change and measuring the impact that the supervisor change has on clinicians' professional growth.

Follow-up studies and partial replications are essential for establishing the validity of certain practices. For example, Strike-Roussos (1988) demonstrated that supervisors could be trained to use open-ended questions and the literature reveals that supervisees also expect to ask questions in conferences (Larson, 1982; Russell, 1976). Thus, it would be logical to explore the extent to which supervisees can be trained to ask high-level questions or how they can be trained to use certain interpersonal skills when asking "risky" questions and looking at the impact that supervisee questioning has on clinical competence. For that matter, any number of supervisee expectations could be actualized and manipulated to assess their impact on the professional growth of the supervisees. It may be that some contribute to professional growth while others impede it or positive clinical outcomes. That is, what an individual wants isn't always what is best for him or her.

Multiple variables and behaviors need to be simultaneously manipulated in single studies (Naremore, 1984). Schiavetti and Metz (1997) noted that parametric designs are usually more appropriate for the kinds of questions that need to be answered in our professions. For example, if we want to research the "ability to apply skills of interpersonal communication in the supervisory process," a study that involves training supervisors using a variety of skills (e.g., empathy, active listening, genuineness, etc.), then measuring how skills enhance supervisee growth, could be completed.

Supervisors have reported that they are not sure how to develop effective working relationships, have limited time available to put into developing and maintaining relationships, and encounter supervisees who are passive and do not share in relationship variables (Pickering, 1990). Thus, it appears that identifying a core set of interpersonal skills/behaviors that can be acquired with relative ease should be a research priority. The question is, "What are the basic behaviors/skills that every supervisor should be able to employ in their interactions with supervisees that are essential to an effective working relationship?" Pickering and McCready (1990) have suggested that basic listening skills, basic self-disclosure skills, basic conflict management skills, and empathy are "particularly relevant to the supervisory process" (p. 29). Unconditional positive regard, contact, empathy, congruence, authenticity, genuineness, and concreteness have been cited as integral interpersonal dimensions supervisory relationships (Caracciolo, Rigrodsky, & Morrison, 1978a, 1978b; Farmer & Farmer, 1989; McCrea, 1980; Pickering, 1977, 1987a). These skills, frequently cited in the literature, give us a starting point.

Larson's Supervisory Expectations Rating Scale

Please give your assessment of what you expect will happen during your future individual supervisory conferences. Circle the number that best represents the expected *level of occurrence* of the behaviors suggested by each item. The numbers correspond to the following categories:

Rating Description	
1 — To a very little extent	4 — To a great extent
2 — To a little extent	6 — To a very great extent
3 — To some extent	

1. Do you expect your supervisors will help you set goals for your client?   1   2   3   4   5

2. Do you expect your supervisors will use conference time to discuss ways to improve materials?   1   2   3   4   5

3. Do you expect your supervisors will motivate you to perform at your highest potential?   1   2   3   4   5

4. Do you expect you will state the objectives of your conferences?   1   2   3   4   5

5. Do you expect your supervisors will pay attention to what you are saying whenever you talk with them?   1   2   3   4   5

6. Do you expect you will ask many questions during your conferences?   1   2   3   4   5

7. Do you expect your supervisors will use your ideas in discussion during conferences?   1   2   3   4   5

8. Do you expect your supervisors will function as teachers who are instructing you?   1   2   3   4   5

9. Do you expect you will inform your supervisors of your needs?   1   2   3   4   5

10. Do you expect your supervisors will tell you the weaknesses in your clinical behavior?   1   2   3   4   5

11. Do you expect you will use conference time to provide information about the clinical session to your supervisors?   1   2   3   4   5

12. Do you expect your supervisors will be willing to listen to your professional problems?   1   2   3   4   5

13. Do you expect your supervisors will be available to talk to you immediately following clinical sessions?   1   2   3   4   5

14. Do you expect your supervisors will be the superiors and you the subordinate in the relationship?   1   2   3   4   5

15. Do you expect you will give value judgments about your clinical behavior?   1   2   3   4   5

16. Do you expect your supervisors will give suggestions on therapy techniques to be used in subsequent clinical sessions?   1   2   3   4   5

17. Do you expect your supervisors will be supportive of you?   1   2   3   4   5

(continued)

18. Do you expect discussions with your supervisors will be focused on clients' behaviors rather than on your behavior?

1   2   3   4   5

19. Do you expect your supervisors will give a rationale for their statements or suggestions?

1   2   3   4   5

20. Do you expect your supervisors will demonstrate how to improve your performance?

1   2   3   4   5

21. Do you expect your supervisors will give you the opportunity to express your opinions?

1   2   3   4   5

22. Do you expect your supervisors will ask you to think about strategies that might have been done differently or that may be done in the future?

1   2   3   4   5

23. Do you expect your supervisors will be willing to listen to your personal problems?

1   2   3   4   5

24. How often do you expect your supervisors will meet with you for an individual conference?

1 — most expected
5 — least expected

_____ weekly throughout practicum   1   2   3   4   5

_____ weekly at beginning and end of practicum   1   2   3   4   5

_____ at your request   1   2   3   4   5

_____ at supervisor's request   1   2   3   4   5

25. What information sources have influenced your responses to the previous questions?

Please check all applicable sources and then rate only those sources checked according to level of *influence.*

1 — most influential
5 — least influential

_____ peer group (students at same training level)   1   2   3   4   5

_____ graduate student clinicians (at more advanced level than you) 1   2   3   4   5

_____ clinical supervisors   1   2   3   4   5

_____ academic courses   1   2   3   4   5

_____ training program policies (i.e., practicum manual)   1   2   3   4   5

_____ other (please specify) _____ 1   2   3   4   5

26. Do you have any expectations about supervision that have not been covered in the previous questions? If so, please specify in the space below.

Reprinted with permission from Larson, L. (1982). Perceived supervisory needs and expectations of experienced vs. inexperienced student clinicians. (Doctoral dissertation, Indiana University, 1981). *Dissertation Abstracts International, 42,* 4758B. (University Microfilms No. 82-11, 183)

Larson's Supervisory Needs Rating Scale

Regardless of what you indicated about your expectations, now indicate to what extent you need the same behaviors to occur during your future individual supervisory conferences. Circle the number that best represents the *level of occurrence* at which the behaviors suggested by each item are needed. The numbers correspond to the following categories:

Rating Description	
1 — To a very little extent	4 — To a great extent
2 — To a little extent	6 — To a very great extent
3 — To some extent	

1. To what extent do you need your supervisors to give suggestions on therapy techniques to be used in subsequent clinical sessions?   1   2   3   4   5

2. To what extent do you need your supervisors to pay attention to what you are saying whenever you talk with them?   1   2   3   4   5

3. To what extent do you need to inform your supervisors of your needs?   1   2   3   4   5

4. To what extent do you need your supervisors to use your ideas in discussion during conferences?   1   2   3   4   5

5. To what extent do you need your supervisors to be available to talk to you immediately following clinical sessions?   1   2   3   4   5

6. To what extent do you need your supervisors to ask you to think about strategies that might have been done differently or that may be done in the future?   1   2   3   4   5

7. To what extent do you need your supervisors to function as teachers who are instructing you?   1   2   3   4   5

8. To what extent do you need to give value judgments about your clinical behavior?   1   2   3   4   5

9. To what extent do you need your supervisors to demonstrate how to improve your performance?   1   2   3   4   5

10. To what extent do you need discussions with your supervisors to be focused on clients' behaviors rather than on your behavior?   1   2   3   4   5

11. To what extent do you need your supervisors to be willing to listen to your professional problems?   1   2   3   4   5

12. To what extent do you need to use conference time to provide information about the clinical session to your supervisors?   1   2   3   4   5

13. To what extent do you need your supervisors to tell you the weaknesses in your clinical behavior?   1   2   3   4   5

14. To what extent do you need to ask many questions during your conferences?   1   2   3   4   5

15. To what extent do you need your supervisors to give a rationale for their statements or suggestions?   1   2   3   4   5

(continued)

16. To what extent do you need your supervisors to be the superiors and you the subordinate in the relationship?	1	2	3	4	5
17. To what extent do you need your supervisors to give you the opportunity to express your opinions?	1	2	3	4	5
18. To what extent do you need your supervisors to use conference time to discuss ways to improve materials?	1	2	3	4	5
19. To what extent do you need your supervisors to be willing to listen to your personal problems?	1	2	3	4	5
20. To what extent do you need to state the objectives of your conferences?	1	2	3	4	5
21. To what extent do you need your supervisors to help you set goals for your client?	1	2	3	4	5
22. To what extent do you need your supervisors to be supportive of you?	1	2	3	4	5
23. To what extent do you need your supervisors to motivate you to perform at your highest potential?	1	2	3	4	5

24. How often do you need your supervisors to meet with you for an individual conference?

1 — most needed
5 — least needed

_____ weekly throughout practicum	1	2	3	4	5
_____ weekly at beginning and end of practicum	1	2	3	4	5
_____ at your request	1	2	3	4	5
_____ at supervisor's request	1	2	3	4	5

25. What information sources have influenced your responses to the previous questions?

Please check all applicable sources and then rate only those sources checked according to level of *influence*.

1 — most influential
5 — least influential

_____ peer group (students at same training level)	1	2	3	4	5
_____ graduate student clinicians (at more advanced level than you)	1	2	3	4	5
_____ clinical supervisors	1	2	3	4	5
_____ academic courses	1	2	3	4	5
_____ training program policies (i.e., practicum manual)	1	2	3	4	5
_____ other (please specify) _____	1	2	3	4	5

26. Do you have any supervisory needs that have not been covered in the previous questions? If so, please specify in the space below.

Reprinted with permission from Larson, L. (1982). Perceived supervisory needs and expectations of experienced vs. inexperienced student clinicians. (Doctoral dissertation, Indiana University, 1981). *Dissertation Abstracts International, 42,* 4758B. (University Microfilms No. 82-11, 183)

Tihen's Expectations Scale

Student:

Please complete both sections of this scale.

Section I contains a number of possible expectations that a student may have of his/her clinical practicum supervisor(s). Each expectation is to receive both a "Student" and "Supervisor" rating. The "Student" rating represents the importance that you, as a student, *presently* attach to the expectation. The "supervisor" rating represents the importance that you perceive your clinical supervisor(s), by their actions, as having attached to the expectation. On both the "student" and "supervisor" scales, the relative importance of each expectation is to be rated from one (1) to seven (7), with (1) representing a *Very Unimportant* expectation, and seven (7) representing a *Very Important* expectation. A rating of four (4) would represent a neutral rating of the expectation. The following example is provided for clarification purposes.

The supervisor should grade my lesson plans.

(Student)	Very UNimportant	1	②	3	4	5	6	7	Very Important
(Supervisor)	Very UNimportant	1	2	3	4	5	⑥	7	Very Important

In the above example, the student's circled rating of two (2) on the "student" scale indicates that the student places relatively little importance on having the supervisor grade his/her lesson plans. The student's circled rating of six (6) on the "supervisor" scale indicates that the student perceives his/her supervisor as attaching greater importance to the grading of lesson plans.

Since you will be attaching relative importance to the expectations, with some being more important to you than others, READ ALL OF THE POSSIBLE EXPECTATIONS IN SECTION I CAREFULLY BEFORE RATING ANY ITEMS. AFTER READING ALL THE POSSIBLE EXPECTATIONS, RETURN TO ITEM ONE, AND RATE EACH EXPECTATION.*

Students completing Section I who have not yet begun their clinical practicum should provide ratings on the "student" scale ONLY. They would not enter any information on the "supervisor" scale.

Supervisor:

This scale contains a number of possible expectations that a student may have of his/her practicum supervisor(s). Each expectation is to receive both a "student" and "supervisor" rating.

The "supervisor" rating represents the importance that you presently attach to the expectation.

The "student" rating represents the importance that you perceive your student(s), by their actions, as having attached to that expectation.

Since you will be attaching relative importance to the expectations, with some being more important than others, PLEASE READ ALL ITEMS CAREFULLY FIRST, RETURN TO ITEM ONE, AND CIRCLE YOUR CHOICES.

STUDENT EXPECTATIONS OF THEIR CLINICAL SUPERVISOR(S)

	Rating Description	
1 — Very UNimportant		5 — Low Importance
2 — Medium UNimportance		6 — Medium Importance
3 — Low UNimportance		7 — Very Important
4 — Neutral		

I expect that:

1. The supervisor should provide me with suggestions during the supervisory conference.

| (Student) | Very UNimportant | 1 | 2 | 3 | 4 | 5 | 6 | 7 | Very Important |
| (SOR) | Very UNimportant | 1 | 2 | 3 | 4 | 5 | 6 | 7 | Very Important |

2. The supervisor should demonstrate behavior modification techniques to control inappropriate behavior by my clients.

| (Student) | Very UNimportant | 1 | 2 | 3 | 4 | 5 | 6 | 7 | Very Important |
| (SOR) | Very UNimportant | 1 | 2 | 3 | 4 | 5 | 6 | 7 | Very Important |

3. The supervisor should function as a teacher during my clinical practicum.

| (Student) | Very UNimportant | 1 | 2 | 3 | 4 | 5 | 6 | 7 | Very Important |
| (SOR) | Very UNimportant | 1 | 2 | 3 | 4 | 5 | 6 | 7 | Very Important |

4. The supervisor should relate academic information to therapy situations.

| (Student) | Very UNimportant | 1 | 2 | 3 | 4 | 5 | 6 | 7 | Very Important |
| (SOR) | Very UNimportant | 1 | 2 | 3 | 4 | 5 | 6 | 7 | Very Important |

5. The supervisor should evaluate my performance during the clinical practicum.

| (Student) | Very UNimportant | 1 | 2 | 3 | 4 | 5 | 6 | 7 | Very Important |
| (SOR) | Very UNimportant | 1 | 2 | 3 | 4 | 5 | 6 | 7 | Very Important |

6. The supervisor should provide the opportunity for me to express my opinions during supervisory conferences.

| (Student) | Very UNimportant | 1 | 2 | 3 | 4 | 5 | 6 | 7 | Very Important |
| (SOR) | Very UNimportant | 1 | 2 | 3 | 4 | 5 | 6 | 7 | Very Important |

7. The supervisor should provide the opportunity for me to evaluate my performance during the clinical practicum.

| (Student) | Very UNimportant | 1 | 2 | 3 | 4 | 5 | 6 | 7 | Very Important |
| (SOR) | Very UNimportant | 1 | 2 | 3 | 4 | 5 | 6 | 7 | Very Important |

8. The supervisor and I should work together in determining the therapy goals and objectives for my client.

    (Student)   Very UNimportant   1   2   3   4   5   6   7   Very Important
    (SOR)   Very UNimportant   1   2   3   4   5   6   7   Very Important

9. The supervisor should be patient with me.

    (Student)   Very UNimportant   1   2   3   4   5   6   7   Very Important
    (SOR)   Very UNimportant   1   2   3   4   5   6   7   Very Important

10. The supervisor should provide the opportunity for me to identify my clinical weaknesses.

    (Student)   Very UNimportant   1   2   3   4   5   6   7   Very Important
    (SOR)   Very UNimportant   1   2   3   4   5   6   7   Very Important

11. The supervisor should provide the opportunity for me to identify my clinical strengths.

    (Student)   Very UNimportant   1   2   3   4   5   6   7   Very Important
    (SOR)   Very UNimportant   1   2   3   4   5   6   7   Very Important

12. The supervisor should function as an evaluator during my clinical practicum.

    (Student)   Very UNimportant   1   2   3   4   5   6   7   Very Important
    (SOR)   Very UNimportant   1   2   3   4   5   6   7   Very Important

13. The supervisor should provide the opportunity for me to regulate my own professional conduct.

    (Student)   Very UNimportant   1   2   3   4   5   6   7   Very Important
    (SOR)   Very UNimportant   1   2   3   4   5   6   7   Very Important

14. The supervisor should encourage me to discuss my personal feelings about the clinical practicum.

    (Student)   Very UNimportant   1   2   3   4   5   6   7   Very Important
    (SOR)   Very UNimportant   1   2   3   4   5   6   7   Very Important

15. The supervisor and I should work together in identifying my clinical strengths.

    (Student)   Very UNimportant   1   2   3   4   5   6   7   Very Important
    (SOR)   Very UNimportant   1   2   3   4   5   6   7   Very Important

16. The supervisor and I should work together in identifying my clinical weaknesses.

    (Student)   Very UNimportant   1   2   3   4   5   6   7   Very Important
    (SOR)   Very UNimportant   1   2   3   4   5   6   7   Very Important

17. The supervisor should provide the opportunity for me to develop therapy lesson plans.

    (Student)   Very UNimportant   1   2   3   4   5   6   7   Very Important
    (SOR)   Very UNimportant   1   2   3   4   5   6   7   Very Important

18. The supervisor should evaluate my lesson plans.

| (Student) | Very UNimportant | 1 | 2 | 3 | 4 | 5 | 6 | 7 | Very Important |
| (SOR) | Very UNimportant | 1 | 2 | 3 | 4 | 5 | 6 | 7 | Very Important |

19. The supervisor should evaluate me primarily for the purpose of making appropriate modifications in my clinical performance.

| (Student) | Very UNimportant | 1 | 2 | 3 | 4 | 5 | 6 | 7 | Very Important |
| (SOR) | Very UNimportant | 1 | 2 | 3 | 4 | 5 | 6 | 7 | Very Important |

20. The supervisor should keep me informed of my progress throughout the clinical practicum.

| (Student) | Very UNimportant | 1 | 2 | 3 | 4 | 5 | 6 | 7 | Very Important |
| (SOR) | Very UNimportant | 1 | 2 | 3 | 4 | 5 | 6 | 7 | Very Important |

21. The supervisor and I should work together in the writing of my clients' clinical reports.

| (Student) | Very UNimportant | 1 | 2 | 3 | 4 | 5 | 6 | 7 | Very Important |
| (SOR) | Very UNimportant | 1 | 2 | 3 | 4 | 5 | 6 | 7 | Very Important |

22. The supervisor should provide me with the clinical techniques/strategies to be used with my client.

| (Student) | Very UNimportant | 1 | 2 | 3 | 4 | 5 | 6 | 7 | Very Important |
| (SOR) | Very UNimportant | 1 | 2 | 3 | 4 | 5 | 6 | 7 | Very Important |

23. The supervisor should be a warm, accepting person.

| (Student) | Very UNimportant | 1 | 2 | 3 | 4 | 5 | 6 | 7 | Very Important |
| (SOR) | Very UNimportant | 1 | 2 | 3 | 4 | 5 | 6 | 7 | Very Important |

24. The supervisor should provide me with well-defined, objective criteria that will be used to determine my success in the clinical practicum.

| (Student) | Very UNimportant | 1 | 2 | 3 | 4 | 5 | 6 | 7 | Very Important |
| (SOR) | Very UNimportant | 1 | 2 | 3 | 4 | 5 | 6 | 7 | Very Important |

25. The supervisor should provide me the opportunity to determine the therapy goals and objectives for my client.

| (Student) | Very UNimportant | 1 | 2 | 3 | 4 | 5 | 6 | 7 | Very Important |
| (SOR) | Very UNimportant | 1 | 2 | 3 | 4 | 5 | 6 | 7 | Very Important |

26. The supervisor and I should work together in developing therapy lesson plans.

| (Student) | Very UNimportant | 1 | 2 | 3 | 4 | 5 | 6 | 7 | Very Important |
| (SOR) | Very UNimportant | 1 | 2 | 3 | 4 | 5 | 6 | 7 | Very Important |

27. The supervisor's comments and suggestions should be directed to my clinical behavior.

| (Student) | Very UNimportant | 1 | 2 | 3 | 4 | 5 | 6 | 7 | Very Important |
| (SOR) | Very UNimportant | 1 | 2 | 3 | 4 | 5 | 6 | 7 | Very Important |

28. The supervisor should diagnose the client's problems/needs.

(Student)	Very UNimportant	1	2	3	4	5	6	7	Very Important
(SOR)	Very UNimportant	1	2	3	4	5	6	7	Very Important

29. The supervisor should regulate my professional conduct.

(Student)	Very UNimportant	1	2	3	4	5	6	7	Very Important
(SOR)	Very UNimportant	1	2	3	4	5	6	7	Very Important

30. The supervisor should provide the opportunity for us to contribute information during supervisory conferences.

(Student)	Very UNimportant	1	2	3	4	5	6	7	Very Important
(SOR)	Very UNimportant	1	2	3	4	5	6	7	Very Important

31. The supervisor should tell me which diagnostic instruments are to be used with my client.

(Student)	Very UNimportant	1	2	3	4	5	6	7	Very Important
(SOR)	Very UNimportant	1	2	3	4	5	6	7	Very Important

32. The supervisor should make positive value judgments about my clinical competence (praise).

(Student)	Very UNimportant	1	2	3	4	5	6	7	Very Important
(SOR)	Very UNimportant	1	2	3	4	5	6	7	Very Important

33. The supervisor should provide me behavior modification techniques to control inappropriate behavior by the client.

(Student)	Very UNimportant	1	2	3	4	5	6	7	Very Important
(SOR)	Very UNimportant	1	2	3	4	5	6	7	Very Important

34. The supervisor should evaluate my clinical reports.

(Student)	Very UNimportant	1	2	3	4	5	6	7	Very Important
(SOR)	Very UNimportant	1	2	3	4	5	6	7	Very Important

35. The supervisor should have a sense of humor.

(Student)	Very UNimportant	1	2	3	4	5	6	7	Very Important
(SOR)	Very UNimportant	1	2	3	4	5	6	7	Very Important

36. The supervisor should provide the opportunity for me to write my clients' clinical reports.

(Student)	Very UNimportant	1	2	3	4	5	6	7	Very Important
(SOR)	Very UNimportant	1	2	3	4	5	6	7	Very Important

37. The supervisor should provide the opportunity for me to make suggestions during the supervisory conference.

| (Student) | Very UNimportant | 1 | 2 | 3 | 4 | 5 | 6 | 7 | Very Important |
| (SOR) | Very UNimportant | 1 | 2 | 3 | 4 | 5 | 6 | 7 | Very Important |

38. The supervisor and I should work together in regulating my own professional conduct.

| (Student) | Very UNimportant | 1 | 2 | 3 | 4 | 5 | 6 | 7 | Very Important |
| (SOR) | Very UNimportant | 1 | 2 | 3 | 4 | 5 | 6 | 7 | Very Important |

39. The supervisor should talk more than me during supervisory conferences.

| (Student) | Very UNimportant | 1 | 2 | 3 | 4 | 5 | 6 | 7 | Very Important |
| (SOR) | Very UNimportant | 1 | 2 | 3 | 4 | 5 | 6 | 7 | Very Important |

40. The supervisor should demonstrate diagnostic techniques/procedures with my client.

| (Student) | Very UNimportant | 1 | 2 | 3 | 4 | 5 | 6 | 7 | Very Important |
| (SOR) | Very UNimportant | 1 | 2 | 3 | 4 | 5 | 6 | 7 | Very Important |

41. The supervisor and I should work together in determining the clinical techniques/strategies to be used with my client.

| (Student) | Very UNimportant | 1 | 2 | 3 | 4 | 5 | 6 | 7 | Very Important |
| (SOR) | Very UNimportant | 1 | 2 | 3 | 4 | 5 | 6 | 7 | Very Important |

42. The supervisor should provide the opportunity for me to develop behavior modification procedures to control inappropriate behavior by my clients.

| (Student) | Very UNimportant | 1 | 2 | 3 | 4 | 5 | 6 | 7 | Very Important |
| (SOR) | Very UNimportant | 1 | 2 | 3 | 4 | 5 | 6 | 7 | Very Important |

43. The supervisor should provide me with therapy goals and objectives for my client.

| (Student) | Very UNimportant | 1 | 2 | 3 | 4 | 5 | 6 | 7 | Very Important |
| (SOR) | Very UNimportant | 1 | 2 | 3 | 4 | 5 | 6 | 7 | Very Important |

44. The supervisor should provide the opportunity for me to ask questions during the supervisory conference.

| (Student) | Very UNimportant | 1 | 2 | 3 | 4 | 5 | 6 | 7 | Very Important |
| (SOR) | Very UNimportant | 1 | 2 | 3 | 4 | 5 | 6 | 7 | Very Important |

45. The supervisor and I should work together in determining which diagnostic instruments are appropriate for use with my clients.

| (Student) | Very UNimportant | 1 | 2 | 3 | 4 | 5 | 6 | 7 | Very Important |
| (SOR) | Very UNimportant | 1 | 2 | 3 | 4 | 5 | 6 | 7 | Very Important |

46. The supervisor should identify my clinical strengths.

(Student)	Very UNimportant	1	2	3	4	5	6	7	Very Important
(SOR)	Very UNimportant	1	2	3	4	5	6	7	Very Important

47. The supervisor should provide the opportunity for me to determine the clinical techniques/strategies to be used with my client.

(Student)	Very UNimportant	1	2	3	4	5	6	7	Very Important
(SOR)	Very UNimportant	1	2	3	4	5	6	7	Very Important

48. The supervisor should be an understanding person.

(Student)	Very UNimportant	1	2	3	4	5	6	7	Very Important
(SOR)	Very UNimportant	1	2	3	4	5	6	7	Very Important

49. The supervisor should be considerate of me.

(Student)	Very UNimportant	1	2	3	4	5	6	7	Very Important
(SOR)	Very UNimportant	1	2	3	4	5	6	7	Very Important

50. The supervisor should identify my clinical weaknesses.

(Student)	Very UNimportant	1	2	3	4	5	6	7	Very Important
(SOR)	Very UNimportant	1	2	3	4	5	6	7	Very Important

51. The supervisor should respect my individuality.

(Student)	Very UNimportant	1	2	3	4	5	6	7	Very Important
(SOR)	Very UNimportant	1	2	3	4	5	6	7	Very Important

52. The supervisor should provide supervision that is free of anxiety.

(Student)	Very UNimportant	1	2	3	4	5	6	7	Very Important
(SOR)	Very UNimportant	1	2	3	4	5	6	7	Very Important

53. The supervisor should provide the opportunity for me to diagnose the clients' problems/needs.

(Student)	Very UNimportant	1	2	3	4	5	6	7	Very Important
(SOR)	Very UNimportant	1	2	3	4	5	6	7	Very Important

54. The supervisor should maintain confidentiality about my performance during the clinical practicum.

(Student)	Very UNimportant	1	2	3	4	5	6	7	Very Important
(SOR)	Very UNimportant	1	2	3	4	5	6	7	Very Important

55. The supervisor and I should work together in the application of my academic work to therapy situations.

| (Student) | Very UNimportant | 1 | 2 | 3 | 4 | 5 | 6 | 7 | Very Important |
| (SOR) | Very UNimportant | 1 | 2 | 3 | 4 | 5 | 6 | 7 | Very Important |

56. The supervisor and I should work together in evaluating my performance during the clinical practicum.

| (Student) | Very UNimportant | 1 | 2 | 3 | 4 | 5 | 6 | 7 | Very Important |
| (SOR) | Very UNimportant | 1 | 2 | 3 | 4 | 5 | 6 | 7 | Very Important |

57. The supervisor should provide demonstration therapy with my client.

| (Student) | Very UNimportant | 1 | 2 | 3 | 4 | 5 | 6 | 7 | Very Important |
| (SOR) | Very UNimportant | 1 | 2 | 3 | 4 | 5 | 6 | 7 | Very Important |

58. The supervisor and I should work together in developing behavior modification procedures to control inappropriate behavior by my clients.

| (Student) | Very UNimportant | 1 | 2 | 3 | 4 | 5 | 6 | 7 | Very Important |
| (SOR) | Very UNimportant | 1 | 2 | 3 | 4 | 5 | 6 | 7 | Very Important |

59. The supervisor should provide me with therapy lesson plans.

| (Student) | Very UNimportant | 1 | 2 | 3 | 4 | 5 | 6 | 7 | Very Important |
| (SOR) | Very UNimportant | 1 | 2 | 3 | 4 | 5 | 6 | 7 | Very Important |

60. The supervisor should provide the opportunity for me to select the appropriate diagnostic instruments to use with my clients.

| (Student) | Very UNimportant | 1 | 2 | 3 | 4 | 5 | 6 | 7 | Very Important |
| (SOR) | Very UNimportant | 1 | 2 | 3 | 4 | 5 | 6 | 7 | Very Important |

61. The supervisor should provide the opportunity for me to relate my academic work to therapy situations.

| (Student) | Very UNimportant | 1 | 2 | 3 | 4 | 5 | 6 | 7 | Very Important |
| (SOR) | Very UNimportant | 1 | 2 | 3 | 4 | 5 | 6 | 7 | Very Important |

62. The supervisor should provide me with information during supervisory conferences.

| (Student) | Very UNimportant | 1 | 2 | 3 | 4 | 5 | 6 | 7 | Very Important |
| (SOR) | Very UNimportant | 1 | 2 | 3 | 4 | 5 | 6 | 7 | Very Important |

Reprinted with permission from Tihen, L. (1984). Expectations of student speech/language clinicians during their clinical practicum. (Doctoral dissertation, Indiana University, 1983). *Dissertation Abstracts International, 44,* 3048 B. (University Microfilms No 84-01, 620)

Broyles et al. Supervision Surveys

CLINICAL SUPERVISOR SURVEY I

Perceived Effectiveness of Various Supervision Strategies

The following is a list of supervision strategies obtained through reviewing the literature and interviewing supervisors and student clinicians. Please rate each strategy according to its perceived effectiveness in facilitating student clinicians' clinical and professional growth. If a strategy is not familiar to you, please rate it according to how effective you perceive it would be. For supervision strategies you have used, rate to the left; for supervision strategies you have not used, rate to the right.

Rating Scale

5 Highly Effective	4 Effective	3 Moderately Effective	2 Minimally Effective	1 Not Effective

Perceived effectiveness of strategies I HAVE USED in supervision					Strategy	Perceived effectiveness of strategies I HAVE NOT USED in supervision				
5	4	3	2	1	Provide reading material (i.e., articles, journals, student manual, previously completed paperwork) as examples	5	4	3	2	1
5	4	3	2	1	Provide information regarding legal and ethical issues	5	4	3	2	1
5	4	3	2	1	Model professional behavior	5	4	3	2	1
5	4	3	2	1	Assist in the development of goals and objectives	5	4	3	2	1
5	4	3	2	1	Request information from clinician to test retention of given information	5	4	3	2	1
5	4	3	2	1	Provide specific guidelines to adhere to (i.e., time constraints, dress code, paperwork format)	5	4	3	2	1
5	4	3	2	1	Adhere to specific guidelines/timelines as a supervisor	5	4	3	2	1
5	4	3	2	1	Create an atmosphere of mutual respect and sharing of attitudes, feelings, beliefs, and philosophies	5	4	3	2	1
5	4	3	2	1	Demonstrate/model clinical techniques during conference (role play)	5	4	3	2	1
5	4	3	2	1	Demonstrate/model clinical techniques during a session with client	5	4	3	2	1
5	4	3	2	1	Focus on student clinician's overall clinical performance (e.g., clinical strengths/weaknesses)	5	4	3	2	1
5	4	3	2	1	Focus on client behaviors as opposed to clinician behaviors	5	4	3	2	1
5	4	3	2	1	Give gestural guidance, cues using gestures (i.e., head nod, hand motion) during a session	5	4	3	2	1

(continued)

CLINICAL SUPERVISOR SURVEY I   *(continued)*

5 4 3 2 1		Strategy	5 4 3 2 1	
5 4 3 2 1		Give verbal guidance during a session	5 4 3 2 1	
5 4 3 2 1		Review session plans before each session	5 4 3 2 1	
5 4 3 2 1		Make general suggestions for revisions in paperwork	5 4 3 2 1	
5 4 3 2 1		Make specific written corrections on paperwork for revisions	5 4 3 2 1	
5 4 3 2 1		Encourage student clinician to express opinions and ideas	5 4 3 2 1	
5 4 3 2 1		Turn most of the responsibility for the client over to the student clinician	5 4 3 2 1	
5 4 3 2 1		Observe in therapy room (actually inside the room or sitting outside with door slightly open)	5 4 3 2 1	

CLINICAL SUPERVISOR SURVEY II

Perceived Effectiveness of Various Supervision Strategies

Rating Scale

5 Highly Effective	4 Effective	3 Moderately Effective	2 Minimally Effective	1 Not Effective

Perceived effectiveness of strategies I HAVE USED in supervision	Strategy	Perceived effectiveness of strategies I HAVE NOT USED in supervision
5 4 3 2 1	Observe through a two-way mirror	5 4 3 2 1
5 4 3 2 1	Observe through a closed-circuit television monitor	5 4 3 2 1
5 4 3 2 1	Observe by viewing a video/audio taped session	5 4 3 2 1
5 4 3 2 1	Require joint-analysis of video/audio taped sessions	5 4 3 2 1
5 4 3 2 1	Require a written agreement to ensure follow through after suggestions have been given	5 4 3 2 1
5 4 3 2 1	Hold regularly scheduled individual conferences (e.g., weekly)	5 4 3 2 1
5 4 3 2 1	Hold regularly scheduled group supervision conferences	5 4 3 2 1
5 4 3 2 1	Hold supervision conferences upon clinician request	5 4 3 2 1
5 4 3 2 1	Interact with the supervisee in planning, executing, and analyzing assessment and treatment sessions.	5 4 3 2 1
5 4 3 2 1	Give written rating in numerical form immediately after a session	5 4 3 2 1
5 4 3 2 1	Give written feedback in narrative form immediately after a session	5 4 3 2 1
5 4 3 2 1	Give written feedback during conference	5 4 3 2 1
5 4 3 2 1	Give oral feedback immediately after a session	5 4 3 2 1
5 4 3 2 1	Give a summary rating sheet within one week of a session	5 4 3 2 1
5 4 3 2 1	Give oral feedback during conference	5 4 3 2 1

CLINICAL SUPERVISOR SURVEY II *(continued)*

5 4 3 2 1	Ensure confidentiality when clinical feedback is provided	5 4 3 2 1
5 4 3 2 1	Use subjective evaluations	5 4 3 2 1
5 4 3 2 1	Use a comprehensive evaluation system that takes into account clinicians' level of experience.	5 4 3 2 1
5 4 3 2 1	Give rationale for statements and suggestions	5 4 3 2 1
5 4 3 2 1	Require student to rate their own performance during a clinical session	5 4 3 2 1
5 4 3 2 1	Require student to self-evaluate with video/audio tape	5 4 3 2 1
5 4 3 2 1	Require student to evaluate supervisor performance	5 4 3 2 1

Please indicate your total years experience as a clinical supervisor: _____

GRADUATE STUDENT SUPERVISION SURVEY I

Perceived Effectiveness of Various Supervision Strategies

The following is a list of supervision strategies obtained through reviewing the literature and inter-viewing supervisors and student clinicians. Please rate each strategy according to its perceived ef-fectiveness in facilitating student clinicians' clinical and professional growth. If a strategy is not familiar to you, please rate it according to how effective you perceive it would be. For supervision strategies your supervisors have used, rate to the left; for supervision strategies your supervisors have not used, rate to the right.

Rating Scale

5 Highly Effective	4 Effective	3 Moderately Effective	2 Minimally Effective	1 Not Effective

Perceived effectiveness of strategies my supervisors HAVE USED in supervision	Strategy	Perceived effectiveness of strategies my supervisors HAVE NOT USED in supervision
5 4 3 2 1	Provides reading material (i.e., articles, journals, student manual, previously completed paperwork) as examples	5 4 3 2 1
5 4 3 2 1	Provides information regarding legal and ethical issues	5 4 3 2 1
5 4 3 2 1	Models professional behavior	5 4 3 2 1
5 4 3 2 1	Assists in the development of goals and objectives	5 4 3 2 1
5 4 3 2 1	Requests information from clinician to test retention of given information	5 4 3 2 1
5 4 3 2 1	Provides specific guidelines to adhere to (i.e., time constraints, dress code, paperwork format)	5 4 3 2 1

GRADUATE STUDENT SUPERVISION SURVEY I   *(continued)*

5	4	3	2	1	Adheres to specific guidelines/timelines as a supervisor	5	4	3	2	1
5	4	3	2	1	Creates an atmosphere of mutual respect and sharing of attitudes, feelings, beliefs, and philosophies	5	4	3	2	1
5	4	3	2	1	Demonstrates/models clinical techniques during conference (role play)	5	4	3	2	1
5	4	3	2	1	Demonstrates/models clinical techniques during a session with client	5	4	3	2	1
5	4	3	2	1	Focuses on student clinician's overall clinical performance (e.g., clinical strengths/weaknesses)	5	4	3	2	1
5	4	3	2	1	Focuses on client behaviors as opposed to clinician behaviors	5	4	3	2	1
5	4	3	2	1	Gives gestural guidance, cues using gestures (i.e., head nod, hand motion) during a session	5	4	3	2	1
5	4	3	2	1	Gives verbal guidance during a session	5	4	3	2	1
5	4	3	2	1	Reviews session plans before each session	5	4	3	2	1
5	4	3	2	1	Makes general suggestions for revisions in paperwork	5	4	3	2	1
5	4	3	2	1	Makes specific written corrections on paperwork for revisions	5	4	3	2	1
5	4	3	2	1	Encourages student clinician to express opinions and ideas	5	4	3	2	1
5	4	3	2	1	Turns most of the responsibility for the client over to the student clinician	5	4	3	2	1
5	4	3	2	1	Observes in therapy room (actually inside the room or sitting outside with door slightly open)	5	4	3	2	1

GRADUATE STUDENT SUPERVISION SURVEY II

Perceived Effectiveness of Various Supervision Strategies

Rating Scale

5 Highly Effective	4 Effective	3 Moderately Effective	2 Minimally Effective	1 Not Effective

Perceived effectiveness of strategies my supervisors HAVE USED in supervision	Strategy	Perceived effectiveness of strategies my supervisors HAVE NOT USED in supervision
5 4 3 2 1	Observes through a two-way mirror	5 4 3 2 1
5 4 3 2 1	Observes through a closed-circuit television monitor	5 4 3 2 1
5 4 3 2 1	Observes by viewing a video/audio taped session	5 4 3 2 1
5 4 3 2 1	Requires joint-analysis of video/audio taped sessions	5 4 3 2 1
5 4 3 2 1	Requires a written agreement to ensure follow through after suggestions have been given	5 4 3 2 1

GRADUATE STUDENT SUPERVISION SURVEY II *(continued)*

5	4	3	2	1		5	4	3	2	1
5	4	3	2	1	Holds regularly scheduled individual conferences (e.g., weekly)	5	4	3	2	1
5	4	3	2	1	Holds regularly scheduled group supervision conferences	5	4	3	2	1
5	4	3	2	1	Holds supervision conferences upon clinician request	5	4	3	2	1
5	4	3	2	1	Interacts with the supervisee in planning, executing, and analyzing assessment and treatment sessions.	5	4	3	2	1
5	4	3	2	1	Gives written rating in numerical form immediately after a session	5	4	3	2	1
5	4	3	2	1	Gives written feedback in narrative form immediately after a session	5	4	3	2	1
5	4	3	2	1	Gives oral feedback immediately after a session	5	4	3	2	1
5	4	3	2	1	Gives a summary rating sheet within one week of a session	5	4	3	2	1
5	4	3	2	1	Gives written feedback during conference	5	4	3	2	1
5	4	3	2	1	Gives oral feedback during conference	5	4	3	2	1
5	4	3	2	1	Ensures confidentiality when clinical feedback is provided	5	4	3	2	1
5	4	3	2	1	Uses subjective evaluations	5	4	3	2	1
5	4	3	2	1	Uses a comprehensive evaluation system that takes into account clinicians' level of experience.	5	4	3	2	1
5	4	3	2	1	Gives rationale for statements and suggestions	5	4	3	2	1
5	4	3	2	1	Requires student to rate their own performance during a clinical session	5	4	3	2	1
5	4	3	2	1	Requires student to self-evaluate with video/audio tape	5	4	3	2	1
5	4	3	2	1	Requires student to evaluate supervisor performance	5	4	3	2	1

Please indicate your total number of clinical clock hours completed to date: _____

Powell's Attitudes toward Clinical Supervision Scale

This scale is designed to measure attitudes toward clinical supervision. Please read each item carefully and circle the response that best describes your attitude for that item.

SA	=	Strongly Agree
A	=	Agree
U	=	Undecided
D	=	Disagree
SD	=	Strongly Disagree

1. Supervisees should analyze their own behavior.   SA A U D SD
2. The supervisor and the supervisee should strive for a collegial relationship rather than   SA A U D SD
   a superior–subordinate relationship.
3. The supervisor should be more responsible for the client than the supervisee.   SA A U D SD
4. Supervisees should play an active role in the supervisory process.   SA A U D SD
5. The supervisee should be subordinate to the supervisor.   SA A U D SD
6. The supervisee should be more responsible for the client than the supervisor.   SA A U D SD
7. Written feedback should consist of the supervisor's opinions.   SA A U D SD
8. The supervisor and the supervisee should plan jointly for the supervisory conference.   SA A U D SD
9. Self-analysis by the supervisee is more important than the supervisor's analysis of the   SA A U D SD
   supervisee.
10. The supervisor should dominate the supervisory conference.   SA A U D SD
11. The supervisory conference should focus on the supervisee rather than on the client.   SA A U D SD
12. The supervisory conference should focus on the client's behavior.   SA A U D SD
13. The supervisor should select goals for the supervisee.   SA A U D SD
14. Problems in therapy should be solved by the supervisor.   SA A U D SD
15. Supervisee's ideas are less important than the supervisor's ideas.   SA A U D SD

Directions for Administration and Scoring of the Clinical Supervision Attitude Scale

1. Respondents should be asked to read each item and mark whether they strongly agree, agree, are undecided, disagree, or strongly disagree with the statement.
2. For positively worded items (i.e., items 1, 2, 4, 6, 8, 9, 11), assign values as follows:

   5 points: Strongly Agree
   4 points: Agree
   3 points: Undecided
   2 points: Disagree
   1 point: Strongly Disagree

3. For negatively worded items (i.e., items 3, 5, 7, 10, 12, 13, 14, 15), assign values as follows:

   1 point: Strongly Agree
   2 points: Agree
   3 points: Undecided
   4 points: Disagree
   5 points: Strongly Disagree

4. Once point values have been assigned to each item, sum the points across all 15 items. The total should be between 15 (lowest possible score corresponding to one point per item) and 75 (highest possible score corresponding to five points per item.)

Reprinted with permission from Powell, T. (1987). A rating scale for measurement of attitudes toward clinical supervision. *SUPERvision, 11,* 31–34.

Supervisory Conference Rating Scale

Your Name: _____ Date: _____

Name of Supervisor or Supervisee: _____

Circle one: Individual   Client   Group

Circle one: Individual   Individual conference   Group (N =   )

Directions: Please give your assessment of what happened in the conference just completed by rating the following items. Circle the number that best represents the *level of occurrence* of the activity suggested by each item. You can rate each item anywhere from 1 to 7.

Please do not confer with the other participants while you are completing this task.

	DEFINITELY NO		NEUTRAL			DEFINITELY YES	
1. The supervisee asks many questions.	1	2	3	4	5	6	7
2. The supervisor provides justification for statements or suggestions.	1	2	3	4	5	6	7
3. The supervisor uses conference time to discuss ways to improve materials.	1	2	3	4	5	6	7
4. The supervisor offers suggestions on therapy techniques during the conference.	1	2	3	4	5	6	7
5. The supervisor uses the supervisee's ideas in discussion during the conference.	1	2	3	4	5	6	7
6. The supervisor responds to statements, questions, or problems presented by the supervisee.	1	2	3	4	5	6	7
7. The supervisee uses the conference time to provide feedback to the supervisor about the clinical session.	1	2	3	4	5	6	7
8. The supervisor and supervisee participate in a teacher–student relationship.	1	2	3	4	5	6	7
9. The supervisor uses a supportive style.	1	2	3	4	5	6	7
10. The supervisor helps the supervisee set realistic goals for the clients.	1	2	3	4	5	6	7
11. The supervisee verbalizes needs.	1	2	3	4	5	6	7
12. The supervisor uses conference time to discuss weaknesses in the supervisee's clinical behavior.	1	2	3	4	5	6	7
13. The supervisor presents value judgments about the supervisee's clinical behavior.	1	2	3	4	5	6	7
14. During the conference, the supervisee requests a written copy of the supervisor's behavioral observations.	1	2	3	4	5	6	7
15. The supervisor and supervisee participate in a superior–subordinate relationship.	1	2	3	4	5	6	7
16. The supervisor states the objectives of the conference.	1	2	3	4	5	6	7
17. The supervisor asks the supervisee to analyze or evaluate something that has occurred or may occur in the clinical sessions.	1	2	3	4	5	6	7
18. The supervisor asks the supervisee to think about strategies that might have been done differently, or that may be done in the future.	1	2	3	4	5	6	7

Reprinted with permission from Brasseur, J., & Anderson, J. (1983). Observed differences between direct, indirect, and direct/indirect videotaped supervisory conferences. *Journal of Speech and Hearing Research, 26,* 349–355. Adapted from Smith, K., & Anderson, J. (1982). Development and validation of an individual supervisory conference rating scale for use in speech-language pathology. *Journal of Speech and Hearing Research, 25,* 252–261.

Casey's Supervisory Skills Self-Assessment

Instruction

The supervisory skills self-assessment guide contains a number of supervisory Tasks and Competencies that may or may not be appropriate to your specific working setting. Select the Task(s) that you want to explore in your supervision development program and complete the self-assessment as follows:

Step 1.
For each supervision Competency within the selected Task(s) ask, "How important is this competency for effectiveness in my program?"

0	1	2	3	4	5	6	7	8	9	10
Not Important or Not Applicable			Minimally Important		Somewhat Important		Rather Important			Extremely Important

Insert your rating (0–10) under Column 1 to the left of each item. Rate each item before going on to Step 2.

Step 2.
For each supervision Competency ask, "How satisfied am I with my ability to perform this skill?"

0	1	2	3	4	5	6	7	8	9	10
No Experience or Training in this Area			Not Quite Satisfied		Moderately Satisfied		Well Satisfied			Highly Satisfied

Insert your rating (0–10) under Column 2 to the left of each item. Rate each item before going on to Step 3.

Step 3.
Calculate your GAP score for each item by subtracting the number in Column 2 from the number in Column 1. Insert the GAP score in the column labeled G. Note that some GAP scores will turn up as negative numbers and they should be recorded as such.

Step 4.
Record your scores on the scoring sheets. Go on to Step 5 to obtain your Ideal (I) and Present Scores (P) for each Task. Record these scores on the bottom of each Task sheet.

Step 5.
For each of the targeted tasks, add up the scores in Column 1 and place the total on the line marked "Ideal Score" (I) at the bottom of the page.

Add up the scores in Column 2 and place the total on the line marked "Present Score" (P) at the bottom of the page.

Divide the Present Score (P) by the Ideal Score (I).

Enter the percentage figure in the space provided at the bottom of page. Ex: P/I = _____ %

90–100%	= You are satisfied and on top of the demands of Task area.
80–89%	= You are getting by. Develop skill to higher degree.
70–79%	= You are struggling—Task area should become a target for change.
0%–60%	= You are struggling more than you should. Target change immediately.

Scoring:

Step 1.
Examine the numbers in the GAP columns for the Task(s) you selected and circle any score +3 or greater. This suggests a discrepancy exists between the importance of that competency and your present performance.

Step 2.
Prioritize discrepant competencies by listing them (highest point value to lowest point value) on the lines below labeled "ACTION ITEMS."

ACTION ITEMS

Score

_____   _____

_____   _____

_____   _____

_____   _____

_____   _____

_____   _____

_____   _____

_____   _____

_____   _____

_____   _____

_____   _____

Score Interpretation

+6, +7, +8, +9	Needs immediate action NOW
+4, +5	Needs action sometime soon
+3	Needs action

Step 3.
Examine the numbers in the GAP columns for each of the Task(s) you selected and place an "X" over any score –3 or greater. This means you are "overqualified" in light of your present needs.

Step 4.

Prioritize the skills that you are most qualified in by listing them on the lines below labeled "AREA OF STRENGTH." Examine the numbers in Column 2 for each of the selected Tasks. List all competencies for which you scored an 8, 9, or 10.

AREA OF STRENGTH

Score

_____   _____

_____   _____

_____   _____

_____   _____

_____   _____

_____   _____

_____   _____

_____   _____

_____   _____

_____   _____

_____   _____

Interpretation

Congratulations! These are your areas of greatest strength as a supervisor. You should feel qualified to help other supervisors develop skills in these competency areas.

1.0 Establishing and Maintaining an Effective Working Relationship

<u>1 / 2 / G</u>

__/__/__ **1.** Ability to facilitate an understanding of the clinical and supervisory processes.

__/__/__ **2.** Ability to organize and provide information regarding the logical sequences of supervisory interaction (i.e., joint setting of goals and objectives, data collection and analysis, evaluation).

__/__/__ **3.** Ability to interact from a contemporary perspective with the supervisee in both the clinical and supervisory process.

__/__/__ **4.** Ability to apply learning principles in the supervisory process.

__/__/__ **5.** Ability to apply skills of interpersonal communication in the supervisory process.

__/__/__ **6.** Ability to facilitate independent thinking and problem solving by the supervisee.

__/__/__ **7.** Ability to maintain a professional and supportive relationship that allows supervisor and supervisee growth.

__/__/__ **8.** Ability to interact with the supervisee objectively.

__/__/__ **9.** Ability to establish joint communication regarding expectations and responsibilities in the clinical and supervisory processes.

__/__/__ **10.** Ability to evaluate, with the supervisee, the effectiveness of the ongoing supervisory relationship.

Ideal Score (I)   _____   P/I = _____ %

Present Score (P)   _____

2.0 Assisting in Developing Clinical Goals and Objectives

1 / 2 / G

__/__/__ **1.** Ability to assist the supervisee in planning effective client goals and objectives.

__/__/__ **2.** Ability to plan, with the supervisee, effective goals and objectives for clinical and professional growth.

__/__/__ **3.** Ability to assist the supervisee in using observation and assessment in preparation of client goals and objectives.

__/__/__ **4.** Ability to assist the supervisee in using self-analysis and previous evaluation in preparation of goals and objectives for professional growth.

__/__/__ **5.** Ability to assist the supervisee in assigning priorities to clinical goals and objectives

__/__/__ **6.** Ability to assist the supervisee in assigning priorities to goals and objectives for professional growth.

Ideal Score (I)   _____   P/I = _____ %

Present Score (P)   _____

3.0 Assisting in Developing and Refining Assessment Skills

1 / 2 / G

__/__/__ **1.** Ability to share current research findings and evaluation procedures in communication disorders.

__/__/__ **2.** Ability to facilitate an integration of research findings in client assessment.

__/__/__ **3.** Ability to assist the supervisee in providing rationale for assessment procedures.

__/__/__ **4.** Ability to assist supervisee in communicating assessment procedures and rationales.

__/__/__ **5.** Ability to assist the supervisee in integrating findings and observations to make appropriate recommendations.

__/__/__ **6.** Ability to facilitate the supervisee's independent planning of assessment.

Ideal Score (I)   _____   P/I = _____ %

Present Score (P)   _____

4.0 Assisting in Developing and Refining Management Skills

1 / 2 / G

__/__/__ **1.** Ability to share current research findings and management procedures in communication disorders.

__/__/__ **2.** Ability to facilitate an integration of research findings in client management.

__/__/__ **3.** Ability to assist the supervisee in providing rationale for treatment procedures.

__/__/__ **4.** Ability to assist the supervisee in identifying appropriate sequences for client change.

__/__/__ **5.** Ability to assist the supervisee in adjusting steps in the progression toward a goal

__/__/__ **6.** Ability to assist the supervisee in the description and measurement of client and clinician change.

__/__/__ **7.** Ability to assist the supervisee in documenting client and clinician change.

__/__/__ **8.** Ability to assist the supervisee in integrating documented client and clinician change to evaluate progress and specify future recommendations.

Ideal Score (I) _____   P/I = _____ %

Present Score (P) _____

5.0 Demonstrating and Participating in Clinical Process

1 / 2 / G

__/__/__ **1.** Ability to determine jointly when demonstration is appropriate.

__/__/__ **2.** Ability to demonstrate or participate in an effective client–clinician relationship.

__/__/__ **3.** Ability to demonstrate a variety of clinical techniques and participate with the supervisee in clinical management.

__/__/__ **4.** Ability to demonstrate and use jointly the specific materials and equipment of the profession.

__/__/__ **5.** Ability to demonstrate or participate jointly in counseling of clients or family/ guardian of clients.

Ideal Score (I) _____   P/I = _____ %

Present Score (P) _____

6.0 Assisting in Observing and Analyzing Assessment and Treatment

1 / 2 / G

__/__/__ **1.** Ability to assist the supervisee in learning a variety of data collection procedures.

__/__/__ **2.** Ability to assist the supervisee in selecting and executing data collection procedures.

__/__/__ **3.** Ability to assist the supervisee in accurately recording data.

__/__/__ **4.** Ability to assist the supervisee in analyzing and interpreting data objectively.

__/__/__ **5.** Ability to assist the supervisee in revising plans for client management based on data obtained.

Ideal Score (I) _____   P/I = _____ %

Present Score (P) _____

7.0 Development and Maintenance of Clinical and Supervisory Records

1 / 2 / G

__/__/__ **1.** Ability to assist the supervisee in applying record-keeping systems to supervisory and clinical records.

__/__/__ **2.** Ability to assist the supervisee in effectively documenting supervisory and clinically related interactions.

__/__/__ **3.** Ability to assist the supervisee in organizing records to facilitate easy retrieval of information concerning clinical and supervisory interactions.

__/__/__ **4.** Ability to assist the supervisee in establishing and following policies and procedures to protect the confidentiality of clinical and supervisory records.

__/__/__ **5.** Ability to share information regarding documentation requirements of various accrediting and regulatory agencies and third-party funding sources

Ideal Score (I)   _____   P/I = _____ %

Present Score (P)   _____

8.0 Planning, Executing, and Analyzing Supervisory Conferences

1 / 2 / G

__/__/__ **1.** Ability to determine with the supervisee when a conference should be scheduled.

__/__/__ **2.** Ability to assist the supervisee in planning a supervisory conference agenda.

__/__/__ **3.** Ability to involve the supervisee in jointly establishing a conference agenda.

__/__/__ **4.** Ability to involve the supervisee in joint discussion of previously identified clinical or supervisory data or issues.

__/__/__ **5.** Ability to interact with the supervisee in a manner that facilitates the supervisee's self-exploration and problem solving.

__/__/__ **6.** Ability to adjust conference content based on the supervisee's level of training and experience.

__/__/__ **7.** Ability to encourage and maintain supervisee in making commitments or changes in clinical behavior.

__/__/__ **8.** Ability to assist the supervisee in making commitments for changes in clinical behavior.

__/__/__ **9.** Ability to involve the supervisee in ongoing analysis of supervisory interactions.

Ideal Score (I)   _____   P/I = _____ %

Present Score (P)   _____

9.0 Assisting in Evaluation of Clinical Performance

1 / 2 / G

__/__/__ **1.** Ability to assist the supervisee in the use of clinician evaluation tools.

__/__/__ **2.** Ability to assist the supervisee in the description and measurement of his/her progress and achievement.

__/__/__ **3.** Ability to assist the supervisee in developing skills of self-evaluation.

__/__/__ **4.** Ability to evaluate clinical skills with the supervisee for purposes of grade assignment, completion of Clinical Fellowship Year, professional advancement, and so on.

Ideal Score (I)   _____   P/I = _____ %

Present Score (P)   _____

10.0 Developing Skills of Verbal Reporting, Writing, and Editing

<u>1 / 2 / G</u>

__/__/__ **1.** Ability to assist the supervisee in identifying appropriate information to be included in a verbal or written report.

__/__/__ **2.** Ability to assist the supervisee in presenting information in a logical, concise, and sequential manner.

__/__/__ **3.** Ability to assist the supervisee in using appropriate professional terminology and style in verbal and written reporting.

__/__/__ **4.** Ability to assist the supervisee in adapting verbal and written reports to the work environment and communication situation.

__/__/__ **5.** Ability to alter and edit a report as appropriate while preserving the supervisee's writing style.

Ideal Score (I) _____   P/I = _____ %

Present Score (P) _____

11.0 Sharing Ethical, Legal, Regulatory, and Reimbursement Information

<u>1 / 2 / G</u>

__/__/__ **1.** Ability to communicate to the supervisee a knowledge of professional codes of ethics (e.g., ASHA).

__/__/__ **2.** Ability to communicate to the supervisee an understanding of legal and regulatory documents and their impact on the practice of the profession (licensure, PL 94-142, Medicare, medical, etc.).

__/__/__ **3.** Ability to communicate to the supervisee an understanding of reimbursement policies and procedures of the work setting

__/__/__ **4.** Ability to communicate a knowledge of supervisee rights and appeal procedures specific to the work setting.

Ideal Score (I) _____   P/I = _____ %

Present Score (P) _____

12.0 Modeling and Facilitating Professional Conduct

<u>1 / 2 / G</u>

__/__/__ **1.** Ability to assume responsibility.

__/__/__ **2.** Ability to analyze, evaluate, and modify own behavior.

__/__/__ **3.** Ability to demonstrate ethical and legal conduct.

__/__/__ **4.** Ability to meet and respect deadlines.

__/__/__ **5.** Ability to maintain professional protocols (respect for confidentiality, etc.).

__/__/__ **6.** Ability to provide current information regarding professional standards (PSB, ESB, licensure, teacher certification, etc.).

__/__/__ **7.** Ability to communicate information regarding fees, billing procedures, and third-party reimbursement.

__/__/__ **8.** Ability to demonstrate familiarity with professional issues.

__/__/__ **9.** Ability to demonstrate continued professional growth.

Ideal Score (I) _____ P/I = _____ %

Present Score (P) _____

13.0 Research Skills in Clinical or Supervisory Process

<u>1 / 2 / G</u>

__/__/__ **1.** Ability to read, interpret, and apply clinical and supervisory research.

__/__/__ **2.** Ability to formulate clinical or supervisory research questions.

__/__/__ **3.** Ability to investigate clinical or supervisory research questions.

__/__/__ **4.** Ability to support or refute clinical or supervisory research findings.

__/__/__ **5.** Ability to report results of clinical or supervisory research and disseminate as appropriate (e.g., inservice, conference, publications).

Ideal Score (I) _____ P/I = _____ %

Present Score (P) _____

CASEY'S CLINICIAN/SUPERVISEE SKILLS SELF-ASSESSMENT INSTRUMENT

Instruction

The clinician/supervisee self-assessment guide contains a number of supervisory Tasks and Competencies that may or may not be appropriate to your specific working setting. Select the Task(s) that you want to explore in your supervision development program and complete the self-assessment as follows:

Step 1.
For each clinician/supervisee Competency within the selected Task(s) ask, "How important is this competency for effectiveness in my program?"

0	1	2	3	4	5	6	7	8	9	10
Not Important or Not Applicable			Minimally Important		Somewhat Important		Rather Important			Extremely Important

Insert your rating (0–10) under Column 1 to the left of each item. Rate each item before going on to Step 2.

Step 2.
For each clinician/supervisee competency ask, "How satisfied am I with my ability to perform this skill?"

0	1	2	3	4	5	6	7	8	9	10
No Experience or Training in this Area			Not Quite Satisfied		Moderately Satisfied		Well Satisfied			Highly Satisfied

Insert your rating (0–10) under Column 2 to the left of each item. Rate each item before going on to Step 3.

Step 3.
Calculate your GAP score for each item by subtracting the number in Column 2 from the number in Column 1. Insert the GAP score in the column labeled G. Note that some GAP scores will turn up as negative numbers and they should be recorded as such.

Step 4.
Record your scores on the scoring sheets. Go on to step 5 to obtain your Ideal (I) and Present Scores (P) for each Task. Record these scores on the bottom of each Task sheet.

Step 5.
For each of the targeted Task(s) add up the scores in Column 1 and place the total on the line marked "Ideal Score" (I) at the bottom of the page.

Add up the scores in Column 2 and place the total on the line marked "Present Score" (P) at the bottom of the page.

Divide the Present Score (P) by the Ideal Score (I).

Enter the percentage figure in the space provided at the bottom of page. Ex: P/I = _____ %

90–100% = You are satisfied and on top of the demands of Task area.
80–89%   = You are getting by. Develop skill to higher degree.
70–79%   = You are struggling. Task area should become a target for change.
0%–60%   = You are struggling more than you should. Target change immediately.

Scoring:

Step 1.
Examine the numbers in the GAP columns for the Task(s) you selected and circle any score +3 or greater. This suggests a discrepancy exists between the importance of that competency and your present performance.

Step 2.
Prioritize discrepant competencies by listing them (highest point value to lowest point value) on the lines below labeled "ACTION ITEMS."

ACTION ITEMS

Score

_____   _____

_____   _____

_____   _____

_____   _____

_____   _____

_____   _____

_____   _____

_____   _____

_____   _____

_____   _____

Score Interpretation

+6, +7, +8, +9   Needs immediate action NOW
+4, +5   Needs action sometime soon
+3   Needs action

Step 3.
Examine the numbers in the GAP columns for each of the Task(s) you selected and place an "X" over any score –3 or greater. This means you are "overqualified" in light of your present needs.

Step 4.
Prioritize the skills you are most qualified in by listing them on the lines below labeled "AREA OF STRENGTH." Examine the numbers in Column 2 for each of the selected Tasks. List all competencies for which you scored an 8, 9, or 10.

AREA OF STRENGTH

Score

_____   _____

_____   _____

_____   _____

_____   _____

_____   _____

_____   _____

_____   _____

_____   _____

_____   _____

_____   _____

Interpretation

Congratulations! These are your areas of greatest strength as a clinician/supervisee. You should feel qualified to help other supervisees develop skills in these competency areas.

1.0 Establishing and Maintaining an Effective Working Relationship

__/__/__ **1.** Ability to demonstrate an understanding of the clinical and supervisory processes.

__/__/__ **2.** Ability to demonstrate knowledge of the logical sequences of clinical interaction and supervisory interaction (i.e., joint setting of goals and objectives, data collection and analysis, evaluation).

__/__/__ **3.** Ability to interact from a contemporary perspective with the supervisor in both the clinical and supervisory process.

__/__/__ **4.** Ability to apply learning principles in the clinical process.

__/__/__ **5.** Ability to apply skills of interpersonal communication in the clinical and the supervisory process.

__/__/__ **6.** Ability to demonstrate independent thinking and problem solving.

___/___/___ **7.** Ability to maintain a professional and supportive relationship that allows supervisor and supervisee growth.

___/___/___ **8.** Ability to interact with the supervisor objectively.

___/___/___ **9.** Ability to demonstrate joint communication regarding expectations and responsibilities in the clinical and supervisory processes.

___/___/___ **10.** Ability to evaluate, with the supervisor, the effectiveness of the ongoing supervisory relationship.

Ideal Score (I) _____   P/I = _____ %

Present Score (P) _____

2.0 Developing Clinical Goals and Objectives

1 / 2 / G

___/___/___ **1.** Ability to plan effective client goals and objectives.

___/___/___ **2.** Ability to plan effective goals and objectives for clinical and professional growth.

___/___/___ **3.** Ability to use observation and assessment in preparation of client goals and objectives.

___/___/___ **4.** Ability to use self-analysis and previous evaluation in preparation of goals and objectives for professional growth.

___/___/___ **5.** Ability to assign priorities to clinical goals and objectives.

___/___/___ **6.** Ability to assign priorities to goals and objectives for professional growth.

Ideal Score (I) _____   P/I = _____ %

Present Score (P) _____

3.0 Developing and Refining Assessment Skills

1 / 2 / G

___/___/___ **1.** Ability to share knowledge of current research findings and evaluation procedures in communication disorders.

___/___/___ **2.** Ability to integrate and demonstrate knowledge of research findings in client assessment.

___/___/___ **3.** Ability to provide a rationale for assessment procedures.

___/___/___ **4.** Ability to communicate assessment procedures and rationales.

___/___/___ **5.** Ability to integrate findings and observations to make appropriate recommendations.

___/___/___ **6.** Ability to demonstrate independent planning of assessment.

Ideal Score (I) _____   P/I = _____ %

Present Score (P) _____

4.0 Developing and Refining Management Skills

1 / 2 / G

___/___/___ **1.** Ability to share current research findings and management procedures in communication disorders.

___/___/___ **2.** Ability to demonstrate an integration of research findings in client management.

__/__/__ **3.** Ability to provide a rationale for treatment procedures.

__/__/__ **4.** Ability to identify appropriate sequences for client change.

__/__/__ **5.** Ability to adjust steps in the progression toward a goal.

__/__/__ **6.** Ability to describe and measure client and clinician change.

__/__/__ **7.** Ability to document client and clinician change.

__/__/__ **8.** Ability to integrate documented client and clinician change to evaluate progress and specify future recommendations.

Ideal Score (I)   _____   P/I = _____ %

Present Score (P)   _____

5.0 Interacting in the Clinical Process

 1 / 2 / G

__/__/__ **1.** Ability to determine jointly when demonstration is appropriate.

__/__/__ **2.** Ability to demonstrate an effective client–clinician relationship.

__/__/__ **3.** Ability to demonstrate the use of a variety of clinical techniques and participate with the supervisor in clinical management.

__/__/__ **4.** Ability to demonstrate and use the specific materials and equipment of the profession.

__/__/__ **5.** Ability to demonstrate or participate jointly in counseling of clients or family/ guardian of clients.

Ideal Score (I)   _____   P/I = _____ %

Present Score (P)   _____

6.0 Observing and Analyzing Assessment and Treatment

 1 / 2 / G

__/__/__ **1.** Ability to demonstrate knowledge of a variety of data collection procedures

__/__/__ **2.** Ability to select and execute data collection procedures.

__/__/__ **3.** Ability to accurately record data.

__/__/__ **4.** Ability to analyze and interpret data objectively.

__/__/__ **5.** Ability to revise plans for client management based on data obtained.

Ideal Score (I)   _____   P/I = _____ %

Present Score (P)   _____

7.0 Developing and Maintaining Clinical and Supervisory Records

 1 / 2 / G

__/__/__ **1.** Ability to apply record-keeping systems to supervisory and clinical records.

__/__/__ **2.** Ability to effectively document supervisory and clinically related interactions.

__/__/__ **3.** Ability to organize records to facilitate easy retrieval of information concerning clinical and supervisory interactions.

__/__/__ **4.** Ability to establish and follow policies and procedures to protect the confidentiality of clinical and supervisory records.

__/__/__ **5.** Ability to demonstrate knowledge regarding documentation requirements of various accrediting and regulatory agencies and third-party funding sources.

Ideal Score (I) _____ P/I = _____ %

Present Score (P) _____

8.0 Planning, Executing, and Analyzing Supervisory Conferences

1 / 2 / G

__/__/__ **1.** Ability to determine with the supervisor when a conference should be scheduled.

__/__/__ **2.** Ability to plan a supervisory conference agenda.

__/__/__ **3.** Ability to demonstrate involvement in jointly establishing a conference agenda.

__/__/__ **4.** Ability to jointly discuss with the supervisor previously identified clinical or supervisory data or issues.

__/__/__ **5.** Ability to demonstrate self-exploration and problem solving.

__/__/__ **6.** Ability to communicate level of training and experience.

__/__/__ **7.** Ability to maintain motivation for continued self-growth.

__/__/__ **8.** Ability to make commitments for changes in clinical behavior.

__/__/__ **9.** Ability to demonstrate ongoing analysis of supervisory interactions.

Ideal Score (I) _____ P/I = _____ %

Present Score (P) _____

9.0 Evaluating Clinical Performance

1 / 2 / G

__/__/__ **1.** Ability to use clinician evaluation tools.

__/__/__ **2.** Ability to describe and measure progress and achievement.

__/__/__ **3.** Ability to develop and demonstrate skills of self-evaluation.

__/__/__ **4.** Ability to evaluate clinical skills with the supervisor for purposes of grade assignment, completion of Clinical Fellowship Year, professional advancement, and so on.

Ideal Score (I) _____ P/I = _____ %

Present Score (P) _____

10.0 Demonstrating Skills of Verbal Reporting, Writing, and Editing

1 / 2 / G

__/__/__ **1.** Ability to identify appropriate information to be included in a verbal or written report.

__/__/__ **2.** Ability to present information in a logical, concise, and sequential manner.

__/__/__ **3.** Ability to use appropriate professional terminology and style in verbal and written reporting.

__/__/__ **4.** Ability to adapt verbal and written reports to the work environment and communication situation.

__/__/__ **5.** Ability to alter and edit a report as appropriate.

Ideal Score (I) _____ P/I = _____ %

Present Score (P) _____

11.0 Demonstrating Knowledge of Ethical, Legal, Regulatory, and Reimbursement Information

1 / 2 / G

__/__/__ **1.** Ability to communicate a knowledge of professional codes of ethics (e.g., ASHA, State Licensure boards, etc.).

__/__/__ **2.** Ability to communicate an understanding of legal and regulatory documents and their impact on the practice of the profession (licensure, PL 94-142, Medicare, medical, etc.).

__/__/__ **3.** Ability to communicate an understanding of reimbursement policies and procedures of the work setting

__/__/__ **4.** Ability to communicate a knowledge of rights and appeal procedures specific to the work setting.

Ideal Score (I) _____   P/I = _____ %

Present Score (P) _____

12.0 Demonstrating Professional Conduct

1 / 2 / G

__/__/__ **1.** Ability to assume responsibility.

__/__/__ **2.** Ability to analyze, evaluate, and modify own behavior.

__/__/__ **3.** Ability to demonstrate ethical and legal conduct.

__/__/__ **4.** Ability to meet and respect deadlines.

__/__/__ **5.** Ability to maintain professional protocols (respect for confidentiality, etc.).

__/__/__ **6.** Ability to demonstrate knowledge of current information regarding professional standards (PSB, ESB, licensure, teacher certification, etc.).

__/__/__ **7.** Ability to communicate information regarding fees, billing procedures, and third-party reimbursement.

__/__/__ **8.** Ability to demonstrate familiarity with professional issues.

__/__/__ **9.** Ability to demonstrate continued professional growth.

Ideal Score (I) _____   P/I = _____ %

Present Score (P) _____

13.0 Demonstrating Research Skills in Clinical Process

1 / 2 / G

__/__/__ **1.** Ability to read, interpret, and apply clinical research.

__/__/__ **2.** Ability to formulate clinical research questions.

__/__/__ **3.** Ability to investigate clinical research questions.

__/__/__ **4.** Ability to support or refute clinical research findings.

__/__/__ **5.** Ability to report results of clinical research and disseminate as appropriate (e.g., inservice, conference, publications).

Ideal Score (I) _____   P/I = _____ %

Present Score (P) _____

Reprinted with permission from Casey, P. (1985). Casey's Supervisory Skills Self-Assessment Instrument. Whitewater, WI; University of Wisconsin–Whitewater. Also published in Casey, P., Smith, K., & Ulrich, S. (1988). Self supervision: A career tool for audiologists and speech-language pathologists (Clinical Series No. 10). Rockville, MD: National Student Speech Language Hearing Association.

CHAPTER FIVE

PLANNING THE SUPERVISORY PROCESS

The planning conference sets the stage for effective communication.
—Acheson and Gall (1980, p. 42)

Planning in one form or another has long been a major task of professionals in speech-language pathology and audiology. Historically, the main thrust appears to have been planning for the client, for example, IEPs and SOAP notes. However, reflection on the complexity of the needs and expectations of the clinician/supervisee leads to the conclusion that, if all participants in the supervisory process are to grow and develop professionally, clinical teaching cannot take place haphazardly or spontaneously. Every facet of it must be thoughtfully considered and planned.

FOURFOLD PLANNING

Professional growth for all participants comes as a result of careful, systematic, fourfold planning: for the client, the clinician, the supervisee, and the supervisor. In other words, it is not enough to plan the clinical process, the process through which the client learns; the supervisory process, through which the supervisee and supervisor learn, must also be planned if maximum growth is to be achieved. This concept is supported in two ASHA

tasks for supervisors (ASHA, 1985b): Task 2—Assisting the supervisee in developing clinical goals and objectives; and Task 8—Interacting with the supervisee in planning, executing, and analyzing supervisory conferences. The concept is also supported by associated competencies that describe the ability to assist the supervisee in: planning effective client goals and objectives (2.1); planning effective goals and objectives for clinical and professional growth (2.2); using observation and assessment in preparing client goals and objectives (2.3); assigning priorities to clinical goals and objectives (2.5); assigning priorities to goals and objectives for professional growth (2.6.); providing rationales for assessment and treatment procedures (3.3, 4.3); adjusting steps in the progression toward a goal (4.5); jointly determining when demonstration is appropriate (5.1); determining when a conference should be scheduled (8.1); and planning a conference agenda (8.2) (pp. 58–59).

Fourfold planning must be seen as the very foundation of the ongoing supervisory process. All future action in the process and its evaluation are based on what is done during the planning component. All activities for all participants are planned—not only clinical activities but also observation, data collection, methods of analysis, participation in conferences, self-analysis, and evaluation. Planning, then, is a continuous process from the first interaction between supervisor and supervisee to the last. It is always integrated with data collection and analysis. Predictions are made on the basis of the data about what will and will not work; the accuracy of these predictions will form the basis for further planning in each set of plans coming out of the data from the previously planned activities. Furthermore, this component is considered necessary in all settings where supervision takes place—clinics in educational settings, off-campus practicum sites, and service delivery settings—although the procedures may differ in each.

Importance of Planning

Planning is a basic and important activity of supervisors; however, the focus of the planning has most often been on the client. This type of planning has been frequently discussed in the literature (Flower, 1984; Goldberg, 1997; Hegde and Davis, 1995; Irwin et al., 1961; Kleffner, 1964; Knight, Hahn, Ervin, & McIsaac, 1961; Miner, 1967; Prather, 1967; Van Riper, 1965; Villareal, 1964). Although all of these authors recognize the importance of planning for appropriate service delivery to clients, their discussion does not mention the importance of also planning for the clinician, supervisee, or supervisor.

Cogan (1973) talked about joint lesson planning for the teacher and took a long-range view of planning in which the daily lesson plan is only one element of a continuum of planning. He believed that the daily lesson plan produces episodic, discontinuous supervision and preferred to take a long view while at the same time checking to see that the daily lesson plan is "in tune" with the larger objectives. Planning for supervision of teachers was presented by Goldhammer and colleagues (1980) as the preobservation conference. They stressed the importance of mutual understanding of the plans and how each participant is to function. This col-

laborative phase of the process includes goal setting, developing rationales for instruction, and deciding on instructional methods with an emphasis on teacher behavior.

Planning was so important to Acheson and Gall (1980) that they differentiated between planning conferences and feedback conferences. The planning conference, the first phase of supervision in Acheson and Gall's framework, includes (1) identifying the teacher's concerns about instruction, (2) translating these concerns into observable behaviors, (3) identifying procedures for improving instruction, (4) assisting the teacher in setting self-improvement goals, and (5) arranging the details of the observation (time, observational instruments, behaviors to be recorded, context in which behaviors will be recorded). Although Cogan (1973), Goldhammer and colleagues (1980), and Acheson and Gall (1980) referred to the supervision of teachers who are working in the schools, the ideas are also applicable in speech-language pathology and audiology.

Perceptions about Planning

The literature in the professions documents differing perceptions about the extent of planning that occurs and its value. Anderson and Milisen (1965) and, ten years later, Cullatta and his colleagues (1975) both documented discrepancies between supervisors' perception of the value of planning via lesson plans and the value placed on this activity by their supervisees. Eighty-eight percent of supervisors ranked the preparation of lesson plans as important, but only 60% of their students reported that their plans were returned to them.

Peaper and Wener (1984) collected extensive early data in speech-language pathology about the frequency and perceived value of various types of planning required in educational programs and professional settings. They administered a 55-item questionnaire to 219 clinical supervisors, students, and working professionals. Not surprisingly, differences in perception were found between educational and professional settings and between supervisors and supervisees. In summarizing their results, Peaper and Wener speculated that their analysis indicated that all types of written planning need to be included in the preparation process, especially written long-term goals, and they suggested an alternative to daily lesson planning: first-year students might be required to write fairly detailed weekly lesson plans to develop skills in identifying short-term goals and accompanying procedures. Second-year students might eliminate the weekly lesson plan after the projected treatment plan has been submitted, with a brief lesson plan being required if goals and procedures are revised. Based on the continuum proposed in this book, it seems more appropriate to base planning requirements on individual competencies of supervisees and their place on the continuum. Emphasis should also be placed on projected treatment plans and therapy logs with special attention to writing long-term goals because many professional settings require them, such as schools/IEPs. Despite what has seemed to be a recent trend toward the writing of long-term programs in service delivery settings, this study reflected an opinion held by many supervisors in educational programs that the detailed writing of lesson plans is a necessary phase of the preparation of students for the future planning they will need to do—an initial step in the ability to formulate comprehensive long-term service plans.

Planning as a Joint Process

The principle that all direction and input in the supervisory process should not come from the supervisor is tested most rigorously in the planning stage. Planning begins as soon as the supervisor, presumably the more knowledgeable of the dyad, has introduced the supervisee to the supervisory process or has provided the opportunity for discussion of the process, as discussed in the previous chapter. The supervisor is responsible for operationalizing the planning process and for involving the supervisee at whatever level of the continuum she or he is to participate. In addition, it is the major responsibility of the supervisor to help the supervisee increase the amount of participation in planning over time in a manner that reflects the supervisee's capabilities. The planning component is particularly important in encouraging and assisting supervisees to develop a sense of ownership of and responsibility for their own clinical and professional behavior as well as for the outcomes achieved with a client/patient. Many supervisory programs are ineffective in this regard because their design does not involve supervisees directly; therefore, supervisees are not committed to them because they are the supervisors' programs, not theirs (Champagne & Morgan, 1978). Planning should be approached as a joint effort by supervisor and supervisee to determine what is best for the client and for themselves to ensure professional growth.

The early part of the planning component is the place to begin avoiding situations that encourage supervisee's dependence on the supervisor. It is a time for encouraging and accepting supervisee's ideas, being sensitive to their feelings of insecurity and threat, and fostering a sense of responsibility. Here, as in the previous component, is another place where the supervisor models the communication style that will probably become the standard for subsequent interactions.

Perhaps the **process** is equally, if not more, important than the product at this point. The way in which the planning is carried out lets supervisees know that supervisors really mean it when they talk about supervisee's participation, that supervisors are really planning *with* them, not *for* them (Cogan, 1973). It is a time when supervisors can demonstrate to their supervisees that it is possible for them to hold back in the conference and *allow* supervisees to problem solve and participate.

ASSESSMENT OF SUPERVISEES

References have been made elsewhere to analogies between the clinical and supervisory processes, but nowhere is that analogy clearer than it is in this early stage, which might be thought of as the assessment phase of supervision. Speech-language pathologists and audiologists respect the essential role of thorough assessment in planning treatment procedures that will meet the individual needs of every client. Why, then, when they become supervisors do they neglect to apply the same principle of assessment to supervisees and assume that one style of supervision can meet the needs of all supervisees?

Part of the planning process, basic to the successful implementation of the supervisory methodology presented here, is the accurate determination of the point on the continuum at which the supervisees are capable of functioning and the appropriate supervisory style to be used for each point. This aspect of the planning process takes on even greater importance in light of the revision of the ASHA standards for accreditation of academic programs (ASHA, 2000a) and ultimately for certification in either in speech-language pathology or audiology. These new standards specifically state that the amount of supervision of clinical practicum "must be appropriate to the student's level of knowledge, experience, and competence" (p. 7). Several issues need to be resolved in making this determination:

- The supervisee's ability to problem solve
- The degree of dependency/independency of the supervisee as clinician *and* supervisee
- The ability of the supervisee to self-observe and analyze
- The supervisor's flexibility in adapting his or her style to supervisee levels of development

Fourfold planning cannot be accomplished until these issues are resolved. Only then can the supervisor and supervisee break away from the traditional patterns revealed in the data and place themselves properly on the continuum.

This expanded need for planning adds a new dimension to what is probably the traditional procedure in which the supervisor spends some time at the beginning of the interaction obtaining information about the *clinical* experience of the supervisee. This new dimension makes it necessary for the supervisor to learn what kinds of supervisory experiences the supervisee has had. Rockman (1977) supported an assessment approach to the supervisory process when she pointed out that the parallels between the clinical and the supervisory process and emphasized the importance of the as-

sessment of the clinical skills of the supervisee prior to the beginning of the treatment program and supervision.

> The most fundamental area in which to begin the comparison between clinician and supervisor is that of initial assessment or diagnostic evaluation. Just as the clinician does not begin a treatment program without an overview of the client's behavior, the supervisory process should be preceded by the supervisor's "evaluation" or "assessment" of the students assigned for supervision. The supervisor engages in a diagnostic-like process for each assigned clinician examining the background, experience, and skills that the student brings to the situation. (Rockman, 1977, pp. 2–3)

Rockman continued to say that the supervisor must rely on questionnaires, personal interview, and direct observation for this entry-level evaluation. She suggested "exploration of academic background, prior clinical experiences, personal experiences, and work history" (p. 3) and stressed the importance of early observation in obtaining information about basic clinical skills. Although directed mainly toward clinical skills, this procedure can be extended to obtain information about the individual as a supervisee.

Obtaining Information about Supervisees

Assuming that the supervisor and supervisee have engaged in some preliminary discussion of the supervisory process, each supervisory interaction will begin with an assessment procedure, as does every clinical interaction.

The following outline is a brief overview, certainly not exhaustive, of information needed *before* the point on the continuum can be determined. Some supervisors will want to explore further in certain situations. As soon as this information is collected, planning can begin.

1. Clinician information
   a. General clinical experience
   b. Experience with clients with the disorder
   c. Academic background in disorder area

d. Other experiences relevant to the client or the disorder

e. Clinician's perception of strengths and needs in terms of the client

f. Anxieties about this client or disorder

g. Understanding the needs of the client

2. Supervisee information

a. Type(s) of supervisory interaction experienced previously

b. Perception of self in terms of dependence/independence in general and with client

c. Prior responsibility in data collection and analysis of client behavior

d. Experience in data collection and analysis of own clinical behavior prior to conferences

e. Perceptions of responsibility for bringing data and questions to the conference, assisting in problem solving, and decision making

f. Expectations for learning or modification of clinical skills from the current situation.

g. Perception of need for feedback (amount and type)

3. Supervisor information

a. General clinical and supervisory experience

b. Experience with type of client and disorder

c. Theoretical and practical approach to the disorder as compared to that of supervisee

d. Preferred or customary supervisory style

e. Expectations for the supervisee as a clinician and as a supervisee

f. Expectations for the supervisory interaction

g. Self-perception of role

Determining Dependence/Independence. Shriberg and colleagues (1974, 1975) have provided a valuable instrument for use at this point. Over several years, Shriberg and several members of the clinical staff at the University of Wisconsin–Madison developed and validated the Wisconsin Procedure for Appraisal of Clinical Competence (W-PACC) (Appendix 5A). This appraisal form will be discussed later under the topic of evaluation, but it is relevant here because of its basic approach. Rather than using client or clinician change as the criterion for effectiveness, this instrument "appraises the extent to which effectiveness is dependent upon continued supervisory input" (Shriberg et al., 1975, p. 160). The instrument is concerned not just with the fact that a supervisee is able to competently demonstrate a range of clinical skills but also with the amount and degree of supervisory support that was required to achieve this competence. The instrument provides for clinicians to be identified as operating at one of four levels at the beginning of the supervisory interaction and that might be different across settings. The criteria for assigning levels, as suggested by Shriberg and colleagues, are hours of experience, number of clients, experience with the disorder area or management approach, and the supervisor's judgment of the supervisee's academic preparation. Although these criteria are more relevant to the clinical process than to the items suggested for the supervisory assessment, the part of the W-PACC relevant to diagnosing the needs or skills of supervisees is the scale used to identify the level of dependence or independence of the supervisee. The scale consists of the following levels of scoring: Score 1—Specific direction from supervisor does not alter unsatisfactory performance and inability to make changes; Scores 2–3–4—Needs specific direction and/or demonstration from supervisor to perform effectively; Scores 5–6–7—Needs general direction from supervisor to perform effectively; and Scores 8–9–10—Demonstrates independence by taking initiative, making changes when appropriate, and is effective. Each of the 10 Interpersonal Skills and 28 Professional-Technical Skills that make up the instrument is scored using this scale.

The listed scales are mainly directed toward the clinician/client interaction but a few are related to the action of the clinician-as-supervisee. For example, Item 6—Listens, asks questions, participates with supervisor in therapy and/or client related discussions—is not defensive, and Item 7—Requests assistance from supervisor and/or other professionals when appropriate—are both focused on behavior important to the supervisory process.

Indiana University has developed a tool (Appendix 5B) (IUESP) for evaluating students' progress in practicum that is similar to the W-PACC in that the basis for evaluation is the dependence/ independence demonstrated by the supervisee in accomplishing the 64 items encompassed by it. It is procedurally less complex than the W-PACC and only considers student experience as a diagnostic variable.

In addition to the maturity and demonstrated independence of a student's technical skill, Whalen (2001) suggests that there are other aspects of behavior that are equally as important to their education and training. She describes the results of a study conducted at the University of Wisconsin physical therapy training program (May et al., 1995), which identified 10 "generic abilities" and 4 levels of behavioral criteria (beginning level, developing level, entry level, post-entry level) that define them. Although demonstrated independence is not specifically identified as part of the levels of these behavioral criteria, it is implied by them. Generic abilities are behaviors, attributes, or characteristics that are not explicitly part of a profession's core of knowledge and technical skill but nevertheless are required for success in the profession. These abilities include:

■ *Commitment to learning.* The ability to self-assess, self-correct, and self-direct; to identify needs and sources of learning and to continually seek new knowledge and understanding

■ *Interpersonal skills.* The ability to interact effectively with patients, families, colleagues, other health care professionals, and the community and to deal effectively with cultural and clinic diversity issues

■ *Communication skills.* The ability to communicate effectively (i.e., speaking, body language, reading, writing, listening) for varied audiences and purposes

■ *Effective use of time and resources.* The ability to obtain the maximum benefit from a minimum investment of time and resources

■ *Use of constructive feedback.* The ability to identify sources of and seek out feedback and to effectively use and provide feedback for improving personal interaction

■ *Problem-solving.* The ability to recognize and define problems, analyze data, develop and implement solutions, and evaluate outcomes

■ *Professionalism.* The ability to exhibit appropriate professional conduct and to represent the profession effectively

■ *Responsibility.* The ability to fulfill commitments and to be accountable for actions and outcomes

■ *Critical thinking.* The ability to question logically; to identify, generate, and evaluate elements of logical argument; to recognize and differentiate facts, illusions, assumptions, and hidden assumptions; and to distinguish relevant from irrelevant

■ *Stress management.* The ability to identify sources of stress and to develop effective coping behaviors (May et al., 1995)

According to Whalen, mastery of this repertoire of generic abilities facilitates the entry-level (beginning graduate practicum) professional's ability to:

■ Generalize from one context to another
■ Integrate information from different sources
■ Successfully apply knowledge and skills in practice settings
■ Synthesize cognitive, affective, and psycho-motor behaviors
■ Interact effectively with clients, families, the community, and other professionals

Whalen (2001) describes a process in the University of Cincinnati Physical Therapy (PT) Training Program in which each PT student assesses her- or himself according to the 10 generic abilities along with a simultaneous assessment by a member of the faculty. If the student demonstrates skills that are not the Developing Level, an action plan that contains goals, timelines, benchmarks, and consequences is implemented by the student in collaboration and consultation with their supervisor(s) to address the deficiencies, often before the student can begin practicum.

These abilities continue to be monitored for sustained growth by both the student and his or her supervisor(s) throughout the student's training. If at any time, they are found to be deficient, an action plan is again implemented that requires active involvement of both student and supervisor(s) in engaging these behaviors in the context of their professional training experiences.

It is important not only during student training but in professional settings as well to document continued development, through self-assessment or peer review, of these generic abilities in and among staff members. Accordingly, Henri (2001) incorporates aspects of Goldman's (1995) Emotional Intelligence Competence Framework in performance review of professional staff for whom he has responsibility. This framework, although organized differently than the 10 generic abilities, contains many of the same aspects of an individual's behavior. This framework includes:

- Self-awareness (knowing one's internal states, preferences, resources, intuitions)
- Self-regulation (managing one's internal states, impulses, resources)
- Motivation (emotional tendencies that guide/ facilitate reaching goals)
- Empathy (awareness of others' feelings and concerns)
- Social skills (adeptness at inducing desirable responses in others)

All of these instruments are of value in several ways. They can be used as diagnostic tools to determine level of student dependence. They can be used by supervisees at any level of training or professional practice as a self-appraisal of their perception of their own independence and professional maturity as well as a means to define their own goals. They can be used by the supervisor and supervisee together, in total or in part, for the same purpose. Furthermore, if all supervisors in an organization used them, and could maintain agreement, appraisals from previous semesters or work periods could provide a ready basis for determining the stage of dependence/independence, and therefore the need for an action plan to ad-

dress areas of need. These notions—longitudinal tracking along with independent and competent skill documented through formative assessment strategies—are at the heart of the new ASHA supervision standards (ASHA, 2000a) for program accreditation and certification. Tools such as the W-PACC, the IUESP, and the 10 generic abilities can contribute to this process with perhaps some minor modification. Finally, the continued use of instruments such as these could help both supervisors and supervisees focus on the general goal of clinician/supervisee independence and professional maturity rather than on individual client behavior. This focus is fundamental to progress along the continuum of supervision at any level of practice.

IMPLEMENTING THE PLANNING COMPONENT

Supervisors must orchestrate all the various aspects of the fourfold planning in collaboration with the supervisee. The fourfold planning expands that basic responsibility to a shared responsibility between supervisor and supervisees to plan for all participants. Methodologies for planning for each will be discussed in this section. Because planning for the client is discussed first, each method will be treated in somewhat greater detail in that section than in following discussions. It should be remembered, however, that any method described for clients can also be applied to planning for other participants as an extension of planning for the client. For example, behavioral objectives should be set for all participants. Written plans, programs, or contracts should include planning for more than the client.

Influence of Behavioral Objectives

Whatever the format, it seems that nearly all planning has been strongly influenced by a movement that has come from business management, education, and psychology—the setting of behavioral objectives. "A behavioral objective is any educational objective which is stated in terms of behaviors which can be observed and measured" (Mowrer, 1977, p. 146). This approach has been treated generously in the literature in several fields, particularly education, where the value of setting behavioral objectives has been stressed repeatedly (Baker & Popham, 1973; Mager, 1962, 1972; Mager & Pipe, 1970; Popham & Baker, 1970).

Such objectives have become standard in planning for clients in speech-language pathology and audiology. Although the principles are often included in clinical coursework, supervisors are usually responsible for implementing their use during practicum. Andrews (1971) described their importance to the student in clinical practicum, not only in measuring progress, but also in learning to rely on something other than intuition and subjective impression. "Among the advantages," he said, "are that both the student and the supervisor know exactly the purpose of each therapy session and whether or not the purpose has been accomplished" (p. 387).

It has been assumed that there are advantages in using behavioral objectives—that it makes the session more conducive to learning, that the therapy session is more focused, that it is necessary to state objectives for therapy sessions so that change can be documented and measured and results evaluated, and that it makes it easier to establish appropriate procedures and devise materials for use in therapy sessions.

On a practical level, behavioral objectives keep clinicians directed toward what is to be taught rather than first planning an activity and making what is to be learned fit the activity. It puts the cart and the horse in the correct sequence. If clinicians are unsure of what is to be learned and how to achieve it, writing it in a behavioral objective often helps clarify it in their minds.

Written Plans

Traditionally, supervisors in speech-language pathology and audiology have worked on the assumption that written plans are important and indeed necessary for the adequate preparation of students and for appropriately meeting the needs of clients (Peaper & Wener, 1984). However, these written plans can become ordeals for students, sometimes requiring much more time in their preparation than in their execution. Supervisors need to balance the intensity of their feedback on such plans and the semantics with which it is provided with the need to allow students their own initiative and perhaps even the dubious pleasure of learning through their mistakes. Intense and directive feedback from supervisors do not facilitate the assumption of responsibility for appropriate planning by the student because "my supervisor will change it anyway." The nature of feedback to students about their written plans should be determined by their place on the continuum.

The practice of students writing plans that are revised and altered by supervisors also does not encourage the joint participation advocated for all phases of the supervisory process. A more desirable approach would be to allow time for joint planning during the conference when there is input from both supervisor and supervisee based on data collected in previous therapy sessions and analyzed by either or both of the participants. This approach was supported by Peaper and Wener (1984). Verbal planning can be formalized into a written plan if it is needed for the clinician's guidance during the next session. Verbal planning also provides the foundation for the observation and analysis phases. At some point on the continuum it may also lead to setting long- and short-term objectives or to the use of other methods instead of a detailed written plan.

Contracts

Joint discussion and joint planning lend themselves to another form of written plan—contracts, which are mentioned frequently in the literature on supervision in other professions. Goldhammer and colleagues (1980) stressed the importance of agreement between supervisor and supervisee on the plans that have been discussed in the preobservation conference and suggested that a supervisory contract is a good way to reach such agreement, assuming that both are willing to modify the contract at a later time if it should become necessary. The contract, as they perceive it, is an agreement between the teacher and the supervisor that includes objectives of the lesson and their relationship to the overall learning program, activities to be observed, possible changes to which supervisor and supervisee may agree, feedback desired by the teacher, and methods of evaluation. The contract may be short-term for a specific lesson or long-term, covering a specified period of time. This type of contract can easily be modified to include planning the other three aspects of the fourfold planning.

Contracts based on goals are seen as a powerful tool for supervision in social work by Fox (1983). The contract is an agreement between supervisor and supervisee that includes

> purpose, targets issues, clarifies goals and objectives, states procedures and constraints, identifies participants roles, describes techniques and sets limitations on time. Incorporated directly into the supervisory process, goal oriented contract supervision promotes genuine collaboration in exploring needs and identifying goals between the supervisor and worker. (pp. 37–38)

It is performance oriented, goes beyond "tell me what to do" to mobilize the resources of the worker in self-directed activity, and enlists the worker's cooperation in identifying and determining to a significant degree the shape of supervision. "Furthermore, the goal oriented contract for supervision provides a concrete and objective means for measuring and documenting progress and performance" (p. 37).

Three studies in speech-language pathology have studied the use of contracts to structure the practicum experiences of students. Shapiro (1985b) addressed the effectiveness of written commitments, essentially a form of contract between the supervisor and supervisee. He classified commitments into five types: clinical procedures, clinical process administration, supervisory procedures, supervisory process administration, and academic information. The greatest number of commitments involved planning, analysis, and evaluation of the clinical process with a particular focus on the behavior of the client (47%) with the second most fre-

quent being commitments related to specific therapy or diagnostic techniques, again focusing on behavior of the client (39%). Shapiro contrasted two types of commitments made by supervisees: verbal (reached through discussion in the conference) and written (again reached through discussion but agreed on in writing by supervisor and supervisee), in essence a contract. The documentation also included the specification of the observable behaviors that the supervisee needed to demonstrate to indicate follow through of each commitment. Data analysis indicated that inexperienced clinicians completed more commitments when written documentation was required and experienced clinicians completed more when no written documentation was required. This study indicated the value of structured written documentation as a productive supervisory methodology, especially for beginning clinicians and for the supervisory dyad as well.

Larson, Hoag, and Schraeder-Neidenthal (1987) investigated both supervisor and supervisee satisfaction with a contract-based system for grading practicum. The data indicated that there were positive impressions about objectivity, explicitness, and clarity of expectations as well as feedback consistency for most of the student participants, which led to supervisees understanding the relationship between contract objectives and expectations for performance. This enabled supervisees to understand the relationship between contract objectives and expectations for performance.

Peaper and Mercaitis (1989b) used a variation of Fox's (1983) work. They developed a process for participation by both the supervisor and supervisee in determining baseline levels of behavior, for identification of goals, priorities, roles of both supervisor and supervisee, and establishment of measurement criteria. In a rank ordering of 16 factors contributing to a satisfactory supervisory experience, the item ranked as most important by the participating students was "their input is encouraged and valued." Peaper notes that "the contract is an excellent vehicle to encourage student input and participation" (p. 27).

A contract or written agreement between supervisor and supervisee will vary in its content depending on the situation, but if approached as a plan that will be followed to help both participants have a clear understanding of their goals and the procedures that will be followed to meet those goals, it is a natural way to approach collaborative supervision. The process of agreeing on the specifics of the contract forces discussion. If goals are mutually written and agreed on, there should be much less opportunity for incongruency between the expectations of both supervisor and supervisee. There will also be direction for the supervisory process that may not otherwise exist.

Planning for the Client

Planning for clients is one of the activities that most beginning clinicians spend considerable amounts of time and energy on completing. The early literature on this aspect of the clinical process was heavily influenced by the work of Skinner (1954), and programmed instruction, as it was then called, went through a period of evolution before being adapted to speech-language pathology and audiology. Costello (1977) defined it as "a systematically designed remediation plan which specifies *a priori* the teaching and learning behaviors required of both the teacher and the learner" (p. 3). She presented principles and procedures that would enable clinicians and experimenters to develop their own programmed instruction and in doing so, contributed a resource to enable clinicians to design and evaluate the success of their treatment services for their clients.

The passage of the Education for All Handicapped Children Act of 1975 (Public Law 94-142) and its subsequent revisions, Individuals with Disabilities Education Act (IDEA 1990 and 1997) mandated Individual Educational Plans (IEPs) for all children receiving a free and appropriate education under this legislation. This requirement formalized what most speech-language pathologists and audiologists had been taught to do in one form or another: set individual long-term behavioral objectives, including criteria for evaluation of completion. Public Law 99-457, which was passed in 1986, made comprehensive services available to identified infants and toddlers and their families at no cost and required the development of an Individual Family Service Plan (IFSP). The IFSP is modeled after the IEP and requires the development and monitoring of intervention goals for both the child and their family, if needed.

Hospital and medical settings require different kinds of planning than that for schools (Flower, 1984). Kent (1977) and Kent and Chabon (1980) modified a system for medical record keeping and planning (the Problem-Oriented Medical Record [POMR]), which they implemented in a small, university-based speech and hearing clinic. The system includes four components: (1) the collection of a database for each client, (2) identification of specific problems from the database, (3) design of written plans to favorably affect or resolve each problem, and (4) record of progress in therapy. This system of planning is very much like the SOAP (Subjective-Objective-Analysis-Plan) note that is currently so often used to document services provided to clients in medical settings.

Whatever form the planning and documentation takes, it results in improved accountability, better communication between supervisor and supervisee, and continuity of service to clients, as well as increased ability of students to draft effective treatment objectives and develop a professional writing style (Lemmer & Drake, 1983). Students develop a clearer understanding of the therapeutic process and clinical expectations. Here as in traditional lesson planning, the dependence or independence of the supervisee may determine the supervisor's style of participation.

Planning for the Clinician

The previous discussion of planning objectives and activities for the client is only one component of the planning needed for the fourfold approach to supervision. Similar documentation and planning of objectives and procedures for the clinician are equally important.

Plans for the clinician must include the planning of specific clinician behaviors that are needed to modify client behavior. This may seem as if the obvious is being stated. However, student clinicians often say, "My supervisor never talks about *my* behavior—just the client's." Although this may be the result of errors in student clinician perception, the analyses of conference content have repeatedly established that the *client, not the clinician,* is the focus of most discussion (Culatta & Seltzer, 1976; McCrea, 1980; Pickering, 1979, 1984; Roberts & Smith, 1982; Shapiro, 1985a, 1985b; Tufts, 1984). Some studies (Blumberg, 1980; Culatta & Seltzer, 1977; Roberts & Smith, 1982; Tufts, 1984) have also indicated that evaluation is not frequently included in the content of conference interaction.

Lack of specific discussion of clinician behavior probably had its beginning in the traditional concept of planning as it is reflected in the literature: plans are for the client, not the clinician, and goals are set for clients. This is particularly incongruous when several points are considered: (1) supervisees' expectations for supervision, (2) the types of evaluation forms used by supervisors that focus on clinician behavior and skill, and (3) the notion that clinical education is more than just evaluation of clinicians in their work with clients.

Planning as Related to Expectations. Expectations of supervisees are initially related to their own needs. Supervisees in Russell's (1976) study, for example, indicated that they wanted fair treatment in terms of *their* evaluation. Similar studies have consistently indicated a desire by supervisees not only to learn what to do with clients, but also for feedback about their own behavior, that is, to know if they are doing what they should be doing (Larson, 1982; Tihen, 1984). Although these expectations will have been addressed during the first component (interpreting and helping the supervisee to understand the supervisory process), such expectations are important in planning activities. If specific behavioral objectives have been set for clinician activities, if data have been collected and analyzed, clinicians will be able to determine more clearly the progress they have made and whether their expectations have been met. If the approach to supervision presented here is to become reality, specific attention must be given to the behavior, growth, and needs of *clinicians* in the clinical process, as well as to clients.

Indeed, it is this attention that begins to develop the self-awareness on the part of clinicians that lays the foundation for their growth and increasing independence.

Planning as Related to Evaluation. Although not the topic of this chapter, evaluation must be considered here in terms of setting objectives. Evaluation forms, for the most part, consist of lists of clinician, not client, behaviors (Dopheide et al., 1984; Klevans & Volz, 1974; Shriberg et al., 1975). If discussion in the conference is about client behavior but evaluation is based on clinician behavior, where is the bridge between the two? Certainly, clinicians should be aware of the criteria for themselves on evaluation forms and, if they are to be used in the total evaluation process, they should be considered in whatever planning is done.

Rockman (1977) cited the need for identifying both short- and long-range goals for the student clinicians' behavior.

Objectives may be as specific as improving the accuracy of phoneme judgments or learning to administer a specific test battery, or as general as "ability to plan therapy" or "ability to analyze therapy interaction." Obviously, the more specific the objective, the easier it is to document the achievement of that objective.

If the supervisor is as stringent in evaluating her or his objectives for the student as in evaluation of the student's objectives for the client, she or he will have difficulty in recognizing appropriate behavioral objectives. Basically, we have to ask ourselves the same questions we ask the clinicians. Are the objectives we have selected clear, unambiguous, reasonable, appropriate, and capable of being achieved? (Rockman, 1977, p. 4).

The importance of planning the role of the clinician was stressed also by Hunt and Kauzlarich in an ASHA presentation (1979) in which they reaffirmed that the base of the supervisory interaction triad is between the supervisor and clinician rather than the client and the clinician. They also discussed the importance of objectively defining the competencies of clinicians, which will form the basis for their evaluation. Further support for the need to attend to more than client behavior is also found in the task and competency list for clinical supervision (ASHA, 1985b), which places a major focus on assisting the supervisee to develop certain skills and abilities.

This setting of objectives for the clinician is related to subsequent steps in the supervisory process—observation, analysis, further planning, and certainly, evaluation. These components will be more fully developed if they are based on stated objectives and procedures. Evaluation is more objective and fair if based on specified behaviors and quantified progress toward goals. If attention continues to be on client behavior, evaluation of clinicians will continue to be imprecise. Clinician progress can only be measured adequately if clear objectives have been set and behaviors relating to those objectives quantified.

Long-Term Planning. Generalization of clinician behavior to a variety of situations should receive fully as much attention as does the generalization of client behavior. Generalization is considered by Elbert and Gierut (1986) to be the "hallmark of a 'successful' remediation program" and is defined as the "accurate production and use of trained target sounds in other untrained contexts or environments" (p. 121). Generalizations of clinician behavior should be of equal importance in the supervisory process and might be defined as "the appropriate use of trained clinical behaviors in other untrained clinical contexts or environments" (Elbert & Geirut, 1986, p. 121). This generalization is dependent on a comprehensive planning process and is necessary for the total professional development of independent, analytical, problem-solving, self-evaluating clinicians, which is the goal of the revised ASHA standards (ASHA, 2000a) requiring ongoing formative assessment in terms of both knowledge and skill.

Clinicians' ability to objectively observe, to analyze their own behavior, to problem-solve, and to set objectives for themselves is what will enable them to generalize across situations and to be increasingly effective in each. The ability to problem-solve, to devise solutions/techniques for each situation, and to determine what may or may not have produced change seems equally as important and probably more far-reaching, in terms of professional development, than assembling a series of techniques that work in individual instances. Specific solutions may never be used again, or more unfortunately, used at the wrong time, but self-knowledge is transferable from one situation to another.

Supervisors need to be aware of their broader responsibility beyond simply session-to-session planning. They should assist clinicians/supervisees in setting objectives for ongoing professional growth. Moreover, when general professional development is considered as the overriding purpose of the total supervisory process, short-term objectives must be seen as fitting into this larger perspective of total professional growth. In the educational program, where interaction with any one supervisee may be fragmented because of short-term assignments, it is easy to lose sight of general long-term professional development. Students, too, may not see the relationship between today's events and tomorrow's professional responsibilities unless they see the day-to-day activities against a framework of long-range goals.

The site where supervision takes place may have a major impact on this issue. In all service delivery settings, the first and foremost responsibility is the client. Immediate concerns about delivery of service to clients may make the urgency of the moment seem more important than the growth of the clinician. In the educational program, however, and in off-campus or CF settings, supervisors have a dual responsibility: preparation of clinicians and service to clients. They must learn to balance the needs of supervisees with the needs of clients. Awareness by both supervisor and supervisee of the status of the supervisee's overall professional competencies and goals will make it easier to coordinate them with client needs. This is best dealt with in all settings during the planning component. Setting long- and short-term goals and objectives for client, clinician/supervisee, and supervisor makes it clear throughout the interaction what each person's responsibility will be.

Clinicians who have been involved in the planning of their own goals and objectives and who have learned self-analysis and self-evaluation skills should be able to carry their long-term objectives from one client to the next, from one semester to another, from one practicum site to another, and then into employment settings where professional development continues. Such planning with clinicians is not a separate and additional activity that necessarily requires more time. It is not a different process, but rather a change of focus from customary planning with its client-centered focus and it is included naturally as a counterbalance to planning for the client.

Short-Term Planning.   Short-term planning for clinicians focuses on current, session-to-session interaction between the clinician and the client. It includes: (1) identification of clinician competencies or needs related to specific clinical sessions, the current client, or specific clinical problems; (2) determining how a baseline of clinician behaviors related to these competencies will be obtained; (3) identifying clinician strategies to be used to modify the client's behavior; and (4) planning observation, including (a) identification of data to be collected on the clinician's behavior by both supervisor and clinician, (b) planning the logistics of the observation, and (c) the identification of data collection methods.

Identification of Clinician Skill and Need.   In educational programs and professional settings, supervisors may be familiar with clinicians' skills from previous supervisory situations, from evaluations of previous experiences, or from the proverbial "grapevine." The ever-present danger here is in the possible bias from other opinions in the absence of one's own experiential "data" (Andersen, 1981). The emphasis on the Collaborative or the Consultative Style embodied in the continuum model of supervision mandates that clinicians themselves assume some responsibility for identifying their own strengths and weaknesses. Further, equal emphasis should be placed on competencies as well as needs. This is a more positive approach than the philosophy that directs the supervisor to attend only to the weaknesses of the clinicians and is underscored by clinicians who almost beg for "balanced feedback and evaluation."

The challenge of the new ASHA standards (ASHA, 2000a) to provide supervision that is "appropriate to the student's level of knowledge, experience, and competence" will require supervisors to develop a methodology for determining exactly what is "appropriate" supervision. What factors should be considered in making this determination—number of client contact hours, previous grades in practicum, supervisor's standard practice? Is it the supervisor alone or in collaboration with the student who will make this determination? Can the intensity of supervision, along with supervisory strategies, change over the course of a practicum experience? All of these questions, and probably others, need to be asked and answered during this planning phase.

Areas of competency and need may be identified in three primary ways. Some may be identified during the first conference as the supervisor and clinician progress through the understanding component. The discussion of items from evaluation forms has already been discussed and may help clinicians who are unsure of their competencies and needs. Not all competencies and needs can be identified prior to beginning the clinical experience. Others will be identified after clinical work has begun through a process of observation, data collection, and analysis of clinical sessions. As a part of the planning process, supervisor and clinician will need to decide what data will be collected on the clinician. These data will be studied in the analysis phase, and areas of competency and need confirmed.

Determining Baselines of Clinician Behavior. The same procedures used for determining baselines for clients are relevant for determining baselines for clinicians. The evaluation systems for practicum described previously, clinician-stated needs or preferences, and information obtained from interaction analysis systems (see Chapter 6 on Observation) are all sources of baseline data on clinician behavior that may need modification. Methods of obtaining baselines on clinical behaviors described by Brookshire (1967) would also be helpful to clinicians and supervisors at this stage.

Identification of Clinician Strategies for Modifying Client Behavior. Clinicians need different amounts of assistance in planning strategies for clinical sessions. It is tempting to supervisors, however, to provide too much from their own experience, at this point, and thus discourage creative participation by the clinician in the planning of clinical activities.

This is a crucial point in the process of supervision and the point at which the role of the clinical educator can be fully realized. It is where supervisors must use all of their skills in assisting the clinician to develop clinical strategies, in allowing the clinician to try and succeed or fail, to assume responsibility for the results of their plans and subsequent behavior, and, most importantly, to be a participant in the discussion of why the strategy succeeded or failed. This is the point at which clinicians can begin to become participants in the supervisory process and not just receivers of information. Certainly, supervisor input is necessary during this period, but it should not dominate the process unless the supervisee exhibits major inadequacies and clients are disadvantaged.

Setting Clinical Development Objectives. An example of clinician planning has been contributed by the second author:

> After my clinicians have completed baseline testing on the client (usually two or three sessions) and three therapy sessions, I require them to complete the W- PACC (Shriberg et al., 1974). This independent self-evaluation enables me to see how they perceive their own strengths and weaknesses. They are also required to write three personal goals on the back of the W-PACC at the same time. During our next conference we discuss and refine these goals to ensure that they are measurable and attainable (i.e., reasonable expectations for the semester).
>
> Some typical first-time goals may be (1) to feel more comfortable with my client and not feel nervous in my sessions, (2) to make sure I have enough things to do to keep my client interested and involved for the entire session, (3) to help my client improve, and (4) to be an effective clinician. When I get this type of general

> goal, we talk so I can identify sources of anxiety and get more specificity. For example, related to the first goal, the comfort factor may involve (a) identifying appropriate long-term/short-term goals, (b) developing and searching for activities that are motivating and productive and that lead to goal attainment, (c) overplanning—trying to ensure that they don't run out of activities, (d) developing branching steps for each step of the program in case the client is unable to perform the planned tasks, and (e) the fear of making mistakes; for example, incorrectly evaluating client responses.

Just as client objectives are planned together, based on baseline data, so are clinician objectives. Based on the general goals previously stated, specific goals may be:

- The clinician will formulate a hierarchy of short-term goals (number is specified) for each semester objective. The appropriateness will be measured by intra- and intersession percentages of correct/incorrect responses.
- The clinician will incorporate at least X number (usually one or two) of new activities or materials into the therapy session weekly.
- The clinician will use at least X number of activities for each session goal. Appropriateness will be determined by his or her subjective evaluation of client interest and objectively by the number of elicited responses (number to be determined as a part of the planning).
- The clinician will plan at least X number of activities for each session.
- The clinician will develop X branch steps for each major/primary step. A branch step will be implemented when the client's level of success is below 60% in X number of consecutive responses.
- The clinician will evaluate client responses during a 10-minute audio- or videotaped segment(s) of each therapy session until he or she achieves 90% or more intrarater agreement in three consecutive sessions. This will be completed for each new target behavior/response.

■ The clinician and supervisor (this then becomes a supervisor objective) will independently evaluate and record client responses for selected 10-minute portions of each therapy session until a 90% or more point-by-point interrater agreement is achieved for three consecutive sessions. (We mutually decide whether to do this live, via audio- or videotaped, or a combination of both.)

This example is predicated on a highly structured therapy sequence, presumably at the beginning of both the clinician's clinical experience and the client's participation in therapy. However, it illustrates the process of targeting specific aspects of behavior and skill, which can then be observed and measured. This same procedure can be adapted across disorders, levels of clinician experience, and settings to help clinicians actively and objectively engage their own behavior, understand it, and gain control over it. It is this process of learning to understand how behavior can be objectified and measured that is foundational to becoming independent, competent, and able to solve one's own problems. Khami (1995) advocates specific planning for the professional growth of clinicians and setting goals and developing plans to achieve them. Supervisors' mediation of planning and developing clinical development goals with supervisees is pivotal in the clinical education process and in implementing the continuum model of supervision.

Planning the Observation.   The essential factor in the ongoing identification of competencies and needs is in the collection of appropriate data and their interpretation. The next chapter will detail the principles and operationalizing strategies for observation, but what needs to be emphatically stated here is the **need to plan the observation.** Traditionally, supervisors have decided what data will be collected, but often this decision is made after the observation has begun-and it is often based on the supervisor's "square boxes." Clinicians, then, have no opportunity to participate in the decision or have their concerns considered. Bernthal and Beukelman (1975) stressed the importance of providing specific information to clinicians about their

own behaviors. The list of behaviors on which data may be collected is endless—statements of instruction or direction, use of client cues, on-task behaviors, talk behaviors of all types, types of questions. In order for this information to be most beneficial to clinicians and to ensure that it addresses their clinical development needs, it must come directly out of the goal-planning process.

Basically, the purpose of planning the observation is to allow input from clinicians and to ensure that the observation time is spent profitably and that appropriate data are collected that will make it possible for clinicians to begin to understand their behavior and skill. Whatever form the planning takes—written plans, contracts, programs, verbal agreements—it should include clearly understood objectives for the clinician, and perhaps, the supervisor. In addition to "The client will _____," a portion of the plan should always include "The clinician will _____" and, as necessary, "The supervisor will _____." Such statements give clinicians more direction for self-observation, data collection, and self-analysis and for modification of their own behavior. They also clearly state the supervisors' contribution to the clinician's clinical education. They are measurable, if appropriately written, and are much more meaningful than a subjective statement from either clinician or supervisor that "it went better today."

PLANNING THE SUPERVISORY PROCESS

The Supervisee

This is the point in the process at which clinicians begin to change roles. In terms of a superior/subordinate paradigm, they shift from a superior role with the client in which they are "in charge" to the subordinate role of the supervisee. This is the point in the process that is defined, and redefined, as they develop and demonstrate skill and competency. In the Direct-Active Style of the Evaluation-Feedback Stage, supervisees will play mainly passive roles and will need assistance in planning and assuming expanded roles in conferences and the supervisory process. In the Collaborative and

Consultative Styles, supervisees will be much more directly involved. If the Understanding component has been developed thoroughly, supervisees will understand their role in supervision and the purpose of planning their participation in it.

The literature from education provides a range of suggestions concerning the importance of involving supervisees in planning for the supervisory process. Cogan (1973) said, "The lesson planning session is not complete until the teacher has been prepared for the role he will take in the supervisory conference to follow" (p. 130). Maintaining the collegial role, as implied in the clinical supervision model, requires that supervisees understand their role as active participants in the conference, that they are not just passive respondents to supervisors' input, that they do not abdicate responsibility in joint problem solving that is important in any type of cooperative supervision. The historical literature indicates that supervisees are not active in conferences: they do not ask questions and only provide raw data while supervisors provide strategies and suggestions. One may conjecture about the reason. Perhaps they are burdened with stereotypes of their role as supervisees. Perhaps supervisees do not know how to be active even though it has been indicated in the expectancy studies that they want to be. Perhaps supervisors are too overpowering or do not set the stage properly for them to be active. At any rate, there is often a discrepancy between what supervisors say they want to do in the conference and what actually happens (Tihen, 1984). The solution to this may be in the planning stage.

Planning for the role of supervisee will include (1) setting objectives for the supervisory process, (2) planning the data to be collected from the conference by the supervisee, (3) planning the self-analysis of the conference data by the supervisee, (4) planning what the supervisee will bring into the conference on the basis of those data, and (5) planning the role of each participant in the conference, that is, planning an agenda for the conference.

Planning for the supervisee will become clearer in subsequent chapters of the book. For now, examples of overall long-term goals for supervisees might include: more active participation in planning, data collection and analysis; modifying their own verbal behavior in the conference so that it is clear, specific, and concrete; participating in problem solving about their own clinical performance rather expecting solutions from the supervisor; and a variety of other goals that will make the supervisory process more productive. The long-term goals can then be broken down and stated behaviorally in short-term objectives. Bartlett (1999) has developed a tool, the Supervisory Action Plan (Appendix 5C), which she uses to plan with supervisees and which includes the identification of specific objectives for both supervisor and supervisee in regard to increasing the participation and independence of the supervisee within the supervisory process. Such planning for and with supervisees should help decrease the domination of the supervisor by stating specifically what it is that supervisees will do as they move along the continuum to independence and self-supervision.

The Supervisor

Planning for the supervisor is the component of the proposal made in this book that is probably farthest from the traditional model of supervision. Such planning is based on the thesis that joint participation by supervisor and supervisee in the process produces not only independence in the clinician but satisfaction and growth in the supervisor as well. Planning for specific supervisory activity contributes to the process of continuous improvement (CI) and is consistent with the philosophy of lifelong learning for supervisors. In addition, with supervisors' need to adapt their strategies and styles of supervision to meet the specific needs of individual supervisees, the need for planning is increased to avoid the "one size (style) fits all" syndrome that has been identified by the descriptive supervisory style data in the literature and is clearly inconsistent with the new ASHA standards.

First, supervisors must be aware of their own behavior. The fundamental importance of self-knowledge and self-study for supervisors is discussed in other places in this book. Behaviors must be identified that make up patterns in the supervisor's behavior and that may be need to be modified or strengthened overall, and in relation to each supervisory interaction. A total plan for the supervisory process, then, should include objectives and procedures for the supervisor, as well as the client and the clinician/supervisee. Because procedures for the supervisor will be fully addressed later, this section focuses on the planning aspect of supervisor objectives.

Supervisor objectives, like those of other participants in the clinical and supervisory processes, may be long- or short-term; for example, overall broad objectives may be related to the supervisor's general patterns of behavior, or specific to certain interactions with specific supervisees. The setting of such goals assumes ongoing self-study by supervisors and supervisees of their interactions. This may come as a result of listening to audiotapes or viewing videotapes; from evaluations by supervisees; analysis with their own supervisors, program administrators, or their peers; and, in the best of all experiences, from open discussion with supervisees about whether what is happening is congruent with their perceived needs and expectations or objectives that have been set. The list of tasks and competencies adopted by ASHA (ASHA, 1985b) can provide a focus for both supervisors and supervisees in formulating objectives, especially for those who are just beginning to analyze the supervisory process and are attempting to modify it. Examples of objectives for supervisors might be such general ones as reducing verbal behavior in the conference, giving less information, encouraging problem solving by supervisees, or asking more questions that require synthesis and analysis of information by the supervisee.

Some supervisor objectives will be directly related to the objectives set for a specific supervisee. If an objective for the supervisee has been to engage in problem solving, then the supervisor may set an objective that directs him or her toward asking more questions that require divergent, critical thinking responses and eliminate the practice of providing strategies and solutions before the supervisee has an opportunity to problem solve. Participation by supervisees in planning the supervisor's objectives adds to the collaborative nature of not only the planning phase, but the entire supervisory process as well.

Planning for supervisors, which includes setting objectives and planning procedures for observation, data collection, and analysis, should provide direction for the supervisory process. If objectives are set appropriately, the domination and control of the process by the supervisor should be reduced and, along with them, supervisee anxiety. Activities should be planned so that supervisees know what to expect, and their needs will be reflected in the supervisor's objectives as well as their own. Just as important, their involvement in this planning adds to their understanding of the supervisory process and will help eliminate unknown and unpredictable supervisor activity.

REALITIES OF PLANNING

The immediate reaction of many supervisors and clinicians to this discussion of planning may well be "How can I find the time to do one more thing?" In a world where supervisors are assigned too many supervisees and clinicians too many clients, and where there are more and more demands for productivity, this is not an unreasonable question. Rather than thinking of this process as additional work, however, it seems more profitable to think of it instead as a different direction for supervisor/supervisee interaction. It would require for some a shift of emphasis and a more structured approach to supervision.

When the supervisory process is engaged, it is assumed that some time is spent in face-to-face interaction between supervisor and supervisee, usually a conference. **If not, it cannot be considered supervision,** and nothing that has been said applies. In educational programs, time is usually assigned for regular conferences, although occasionally there are reports of programs where conferences are arranged on an as-needed basis for assistance to the clinician. This is appropriate for the Consultative Stage of the continuum but cannot be considered adequate supervision, particularly for students who may not know how to identify their own needs in training. But, even when this is the case, the principles presented here are directly applicable for the times that they do meet.

How can the fourfold planning described here be implemented? The setting of clinician and supervisee objectives is basically a matter of broadening one's thinking about the nature of planning. Decisions about what the clinician will do to help the client attain the stated objectives are implied in any planning. Fourfold planning only suggests that objectives for the other participants be stated clearly and behaviorally at the same time and in the same way as client objectives. If this is done, clinician behaviors can be observed and analyzed and change measured. Supervisee objectives come naturally from clinician objectives: What will be done with the data about clinician and client from the clinical session? How will the supervisee participate in the supervisory process?

Studying the supervisor's behavior and setting subsequent objectives may be an additional activity. It can involve varying amounts of time, ranging from listening to an audiotape of a conference and targeting certain areas for change to extensive discourse analysis of ongoing interactions. People find time for those things that they are really motivated to do. Supervisors who are seriously interested in examining their behavior will find a way to do it and, hopefully, the content of this book will not only encourage them but also assist them in doing so.

Changes in one's supervisory practice will be accomplished more easily if taken one step at a time. Clients are not expected to change all behaviors simultaneously; supervisors and supervisees should have the same option.

SUMMARY

Planning for the client in speech-language pathology and audiology has always been considered an essential part of the responsibilities of the clinician and the supervisee. This chapter has extended that responsibility to include fourfold planning for all participants in the supervisory process. This fourfold approach to planning has the potential to meet the intent of the supervision requirements of the new ASHA standards (ASHA, 2000a) as well as provide a continuous improvement vehicle in the professional practice of supervisors who engage it.

RESEARCH ISSUES AND QUESTIONS

The literature suggests a lengthy list of factors that might be relevant for supervisors and supervisees to discuss in order to identify aspects of the supervisee's clinical and professional behavior, and an ability to participate in the supervisory process in preparation for planning for their work together. Are some factors more important than others in this discussion in that they are pertinent to every supervisory dyad regardless of clinician experience or setting? We may have intuitive thoughts about our own lists but there is not good data to substantiate our selections. Studies to identify a basic core of information about clinicians' entry-level behavior that is fundamental to every planning experience would be helpful to the practice of supervision; results would ensure that the most important information for planning is being shared and still allow for personalization of individual information through follow-up discussions between supervisor and supervisee.

For example:

■ Does writing detailed lesson plans enable a first-semester clinician to effect maximal responses at an acceptable rate of success?
■ Does writing detailed weekly lesson plans facilitate a clinician's ability to write effective semester plans?
■ Are written plans more effective for novice clinicians than verbal plans?
■ Are clinicians who write detailed plans better able to make modifications in therapy sessions when their clients are not understanding or performing the task?

Similarly, the literature in education and speech-language pathology is replete with discussion from both theoretical and applied contexts that the setting of goals and objectives and then the measurement of them is the most orderly and efficient way to change behavior and, most importantly, to document this change. This book suggests that the same is true of the continuum model of supervision and the stages of development that support it. However, there is no validation in the speech-language pathology and audiology literature that fully validates this model. Since the planning phase is the fulcrum of the process, a series of studies that would contrast the benefits of setting goals and objectives (and the action plans that are assumed by them) with the historical model of supervision along several dimensions (i.e., efficiency, efficacy, supervisee and supervisor satisfaction), would significantly contribute to the profession's ability to understand its own processes.

The Wisconsin Procedure for Appraisal of Clinical Competence (W-PACC)

In 1971, the clinical staff of the Department of Communicative Disorders, University of Wisconsin–Madison assigned themselves an in-house research project: to make explicit the processes by which students in clinical practicum are appraised and graded. In serial studies over three years, this research has yielded information in three areas: (1) a working conception of clinical supervision and the appraisal process, (2) a procedure for summative appraisal of clinical competence, and (3) an aggregate of descriptive information on correlates of supervisory processes and clinical competence.

The purpose of this Applications Manual is to train potential users in the summative appraisal procedure titled the Wisconsin Procedure for Appraisal of Clinical Competence (W-PACC). Information on both the conception of supervision underlying this procedure and reliability and validity data are presented in detail elsewhere. However, the following section is a brief summary of critical assumptions underlying the application of W-PACC.

ASSUMPTIONS ABOUT CLINICAL SUPERVISION AND APPRAISAL

Figure 5.1 is a conception of basic elements in the supervisory process and appraisal. Subsequent sections of this manual will clarify terms and concepts expressed in Figure 5.1 and those that are incompletely developed here. Essentially, W-PACC is based on the following three working assumptions:

1. In its fullest sense, clinical practicum competence is currently assessable only through the individual "filters" of a supervisor. This is comparable to the academic freedom given to faculty in the classroom situation. "Objective" competency criteria for the full range of clinical skills and professional behaviors have not been (and may never be) universally adopted by working professionals.
2. Assessment of clinical skills involves two types of judgments: Is the clinician effective in

a given skill? To what extent is effectiveness independent of the need for supervisory input?
3. Several factors may delimit the effective/independence scores achieved during any term of supervision; however, an adjustment for both entry characteristics and "process" characteristics (i.e., rate of clinician's learning and nature and quantity of a supervisor's input efforts) can be made when assigning a grade.

In W-PACC, each supervisor is given both the right and the responsibility to appraise the output "product" (e.g., clinician effectiveness during the last 20% of a semester, quarter, etc.) of his or her "supervisory-cycle" efforts. Summative product appraisal is based on the extent to which effectiveness is demonstrated to be independent of supervisory input, and grades can be assigned from normative or criterion-referenced product score tables, which adjust for the entrance characteristics of each trainee.

OVERVIEW OF THE WISCONSIN PROCEDURE FOR APPRAISAL OF CLINICAL COMPETENCE (W-PACC)

Subsequent pages of this manual are organized as a series of Guidelines that roughly correspond to the chronology of application of W-PACC. Following the assumptions just reviewed, W-PACC is a quantitative framework for appraisal of clinical trainees. Importantly, it allows the flexibility needed to accommodate individual differences across supervisors, practicums, and clinicians. Hence, the *Guidelines* to follow include choice points for the supervisor. The chronology of W-PACC administration is as follows:

STEP PROCEDURES

1. During the initial conference(s) the supervisor assigns the clinician to a Level.
   W-PACC Manual Reference:
   Figure 5.1 (Entry Considerations)
   Guideline 1

FIGURE 5.1   A Conception of Clinical Supervision and Appraisal

ENTRY CONSIDERATIONS	CYCLE OF SUPERVISION	SUMMATIVE APPRAISAL	GRADE ASSIGNMENT

Client
Type and extent of disorder
Other behavioral
  characteristics
 	
Clinician
Academic and clinical
  experience
■ General
■ With client's disorder
■ With supervisor's
  approach
 	
Supervisor
Experience with
  client's disorder
Management approach
Style of supervision
	Supervisory Input
	Conferences
	Demonstration
	Formative appraisal
	
	Supervisor's Standards
	Desired (output)
	Product
	
	Clinician Input
	Conduct of management
	Conference behavior
	Reports, etc.
		Product
		Interpersonal skills
		Professional-technical
		  skills
			Norm-referenced or
			Criterion-referenced
			
			Process
			Personal qualities
			Formative appraisal
			
			Entry Considerations
			Clinician qualifications
			Difficulty of task
			
			Grade

Initial Conference	Period of Client Contact Final 20% Report Writing	Final Conference

2. During the initial conference(s) with the clinician, the supervisor reviews all pertinent information in this manual, including item descriptors for the practicum. The clinician should be fully aware of the basis for appraisal and grading.
   W-PACC Manual Reference:
   Figure 5.1
   All Guidelines
   All Appendices

3. Supervision proceeds in the customary mode for the practicum, including use of formative appraisal instruments, observational analyses, and so on. Filling out a Clinician Appraisal Form (CAF) at mid-term is optional.
   W-PACC Manual Reference:
   Figure 5.1 (Cycle of Supervision)

4. At the completion of the term the supervisor fills out a CAF based on the clinician's performance during the last 20% of the term (i.e., appraisal of the "product" of supervision).
   W-PACC Manual Reference:
   Figure 5.1 (Appraisal)
   Guidelines II, III, IV, V

5. Supervisor calculates Interpersonal Skills, Professional-Technical Skills, and "Average" Scale scores on CAF.
   W-PACC Manual Reference:
   Figure 5.1
   Guideline VI

6. Supervisor assigns a grade.
   W-PACC Manual Reference:
   Guideline VII

GUIDELINE I: ASSIGNMENT OF CLINICIAN TO LEVEL

Rationale

As indicated in Figure 5.1, a clinician's entrance characteristics for a practicum experience should be taken into account at the end-of-term grade assignment. To accomplish this, entry considerations have been formalized to four clinician Levels (Level I, II, III, IV). Each level (see Figure 5.2, Criteria for Assignment of Clinician Level) accounts for (1) a clinician's academic and clinical background relative to the practicum needs and expectations (e.g., client, task, supervisor) and (2) the total number of supervised clinical clock hours the clinician has accumulated. On this latter criterion, the assumption is that basic principles of and experience in clinical management are summative and generalizable.

When to Assign Level

At the *beginning* of the practicum assignment, the clinician and the supervisor should review the clinician's previous experiences (as below) and circle the appropriate level on the Clinician Appraisal Form (CAF).

How to Assign Level (Refer to Figure 5.2)

1. In the row titled "Experience," find the Level at which the clinician meets the total number of supervised *therapy* clock hours criteria (do not include observation hours).
2. Inspect the other criteria at that Level:
   a. If the clinician meets all of the criteria for the Level as required in the row titled "Requirements," assign the clinician to that Level.
   b. If the clinician does not meet the required criteria, move back one level only and assign the clinician to this Level (even

FIGURE 5.2   Criteria for Assignment of Clinician Level

	LEVEL I	LEVEL II	LEVEL III	LEVEL IV
Requirements	Student clinician must meet two or more criteria	Student clinician must meet or exceed all criteria	Student clinician must meet or exceed all criteria	Student clinician must meet or exceed all criteria
Experience	Less than 20 clock hours of practicum	At least 30–40 clock hours of practicum	At least 90–100 clock hours of practicum	At least 150–200 clock hours of practicum
Number of Clients	None previously or first semester of practicum	At least 2 clients and/or the equivalent of a semester's therapy experience	At least 5–6 clients and/or a student teaching experience	At least 8–10 clients
Immediate Practicum	Past experiences, number of clients, or clinical preparation is insufficient in supervisor's judgment	First client with this problem	First client with this problem or first experience with this specific management approach	Approximately the same management approach used with at least one other client*
Academic or Equivalent Info	Is or is not prepared, in supervisor's judgment	Has or is currently receiving, in supervisor's judgment	Has or is currently receiving, in supervisor's judgment	Has or is currently receiving, in supervisor's judgment

* If the student clinician does not meet this criterion, move back only one level.

though some of the requirements will be exceeded). Note that if the clinician does not meet the "Academic or Equivalent Information" criteria listed for Level III and Level IV, move back *only one level.*

GUIDELINE II: STRUCTURE OF THE CLINICIAN APPRAISAL FORM

The Clinician Appraisal Form (pp. 134–140) consists of: (1) a face sheet for summarizing pertinent information; (2) an Interpersonal Skills Scale (10 items); (3) a Professional-Technical Skills Scale (28 items); (4) a Personal Qualities Scale (10 items). Completion of face sheet information (p. 134) is self-explanatory; calculation of scale scores is discussed in Guideline VI.

Interpersonal Skills Scale

The 10 items in this scale appraise the clinician's ability to relate to and interact with the client, the client's family, and other professionals in a manner that is conducive to effective management.

Professional-Technical Skills Scale

The 28 items in this scale are nominally divided into four subdomains:

Developing and Planning:
the clinician's approach to the task (8 items)

Teaching:
the clinician's ability to modify behavior (9 items)

Assessment:
the clinician's ability to assess behavior and make recommendations (7 items)

Reporting:
the clinician's ability to formulate oral and written reports (4 items)

Personal Qualities

The 10 items of this scale provide additional information about the clinicians' general responsibility in clinical tasks. Clinicians' scores on this scale have been found to be statistically unrelated to effectiveness decisions. However, this information is available for grading decisions (see Guideline VII).

GUIDELINE III: INTERPRETATION OF CAF ITEMS

Background

The following statements about interpretation of items on each Scale (Interpersonal Skills, Professional-Technical Skills) on the Clinician Appraisal Form (CAF) are important to an understanding of the appraisal procedure.

1. At first inspection, some items on the CAF may appear to be appraising similar behaviors. In part, this is due to the necessary brevity of description for each item. Each of the items is *meant* to tap a *different* subskill within a Scale domain or subskill domain.
2. In keeping with the conception of supervision described, some items are interpreted differently by different supervisors—or the same supervisor may need to interpret an item differently for different practicum sites. Hence, explicit "Item Descriptors" are needed.
3. Sample Item Descriptors are contained on page 133 and pages 141–145. These descriptors should both *clarify item wording* and indicate *item flexibility;* they are suggestive rather than exhaustive.

Recommendation

Each supervisor who uses the CAF should derive *his or her own* descriptors for CAF items, using the Sample Item Descriptors on page 133 and pages 141–145 *only* as possible guidelines. This suggestion is critical because:

1. Preparing descriptors for items will force an explicit understanding of how each item relates to the Scale domain (and for Professional-Technical Skills items, to subskill domains).

2. Items that initially seem similar can be differentiated.
3. Different practicums may warrant different descriptors for the same item.
4. Both test–retest stability and consistency in scoring items across students will be enhanced.
5. Supervisors have found such predetermined descriptors to be extremely helpful in conferencing with students, both as initial guidelines to appraisal domains and for end-of-term feedback (see Overview of W-PACC, Step 1, pp. 125–126).

GUIDELINE IV: MATCHING CLINICIAN BEHAVIORS TO NUMERICAL VALUES

Supervisors should adopt some explicit scheme for matching clinician behaviors to numerical values—i.e., the "decision" process. Scoring a CAF requires that a number from 1–10 be circled for each item (or "Does Not Apply" can be used for any of a number of reasons). Data (available elsewhere) indicate that supervisors can use this 10-point system reliably. Each of the following two schemes has been used successfully. *Scheme 2 may be particularly useful when a supervisee has more than one client.*

SCHEME 1: A DESCRIPTIVE/ QUANTITATIVE SCHEME

Figure 5.3 contains the information and the sequence of decisions used in application of this scheme. For *each* item on the CAF, essentially two sequential decisions are made:

First decision:
Referring to the column headings on the CAF (as reproduced in Figure 5.3), the supervisor first decides which of the four column headings best matches the clinician's behavior for *70% of the time or occasions.* Recall that this decision is made on the "product" of supervision (i.e., clinician behavior) during the last 20% of the supervisory term. If clinician behaviors appear to warrant placement *between* either of two column headings, select the number next to the boundary that best quantifies the level of assistance needed—and no second-level decision is necessary.

Second decision:
The decision as to which of the numbers within a column heading best matches clinician behavior is next made by applying the descriptors listed under each column heading (Figure 5.3).

SCHEME 2: A PROPORTIONAL/ QUANTITATIVE SCHEME

Figure 5.4 is an alternative scheme for matching clinician behaviors to a numerical value. This scheme accounts for the "proportion" of time or occurrences that a clinician needs assistance from the supervisor. It assumes that a clinician's need for assistance varies between only two categories of behavior (i.e., only in *adjacent* rows of Figure 5.4). To use this procedure:

1. For *each* CAF item, decide the proportion of time or occurrences for which a clinician requires the type of assistance described by the four rows.
2. Then, using the conversion values in Figure 5.4, circle the number on the CAF that corresponds to that proportion.

GUIDELINE V: MAXIMIZING RELIABLE SCORING

Completing a Clinician Appraisal Form should average 20 minutes per student. The following suggestions, which are based on experience and extensive discussion, are recommended for the "mechanics" of completing the forms at the conclusion of each semester:

1. Keep notes on supervisory observations, conferences, lesson plans, and formative appraisals. This is endorsed as the *most* important aid to making valid and reliable judgments for each item.
2. Complete the forms *as soon as possible* after the term of therapy has ended. Furthermore,

FIGURE 5.3   A Descriptive/Qualitative Scheme for Matching Clinician Behaviors to Numerical Values

FIRST DECISION

Which column heading describes clinician behavior for 70% of the time or occasions during final 20% of the supervisory term?

Specific direction from supervisor does not alter unsatisfactory performance and inability to make changes.	Needs *specific directions and/or demonstration* from supervisor to perform effectively.	Needs *general direction* from supervisor to perform effectively.	Demonstrates independence by taking initiative; makes changes when appropriate; and is effective
1	**2–3–4**	**5–6–7**	**8–9–10**

SECOND DECISION

Which number to circle?

	2 Needs specific direction *and* demonstration with the client.*	**5** Needs general direction consisting of direct discussion with repetition and further clarification of ideas immediately or in succeeding discussions.	**8** 80% of the time operates independently.
	3 Needs specific direction and role-played demonstration where supervisor and clinician verbalize client–clinician interaction.	**6** Needs general direction with no repetition or further clarification.	**9** 90% of the time operates independently.
	4 Needs specific direction but *no* demonstration.	**7** Via limited general direction the student can be led to problem solve.	**10** 100% of the time operates independently.

*Specific directions—step-by-step review of every aspect of the problem.

try to complete all appraisals within a relatively short space of time, i.e., try to avoid spacing the task over more than a few days.

3. Organize the total of clinicians to be appraised according to *some* subgroup commonality. The following organizing principles, listed here in decreasing order of endorsed value, have been employed:

■ *Group clinicians by practicum site.*
Comment: This is by far the most useful

principle; students from similar sites are grouped and scored sequentially.

■ *Group clinicians by similar client disorders.*
Comment: This may or may not result in a grouping similar to the above, e.g., group all clinicians who worked with stuttering, etc.

■ *Group clinicians with clinicians of similar Levels.*
Comment: Grouping by Level (e.g., all Level I then all Level II, etc.) may at first

FIGURE 5.4   A Proportional/Qualitative Scheme for Matching Clinician Behaviors to Numerical Values

What proportion of the time or occurrences does clinician behavior "match" each category?

	1	2	3	4	5	6	7	8	9	10
Specific direction from supervisor does not alter unsatisfactory performance and inability to make changes.	70%									
Needs specific *direction and/or demonstration* from supervisor to perform effectively.	30%	70%	60%	50%						
Needs *general direction* from supervisor to perform effectively.		30%	40%	50%	60%	50%	40%	30%	15%	0–5%
Demonstrates independence by taking initiative; makes changes when appropriate; and is effective.					40%	50%	60%	70%	85%	95–100%

appear logical. However, supervisors have found the two previous principles to be more useful, although for some supervisory situations this principle is preferred.

- *Group clinicians by similarity in overall clinical skills.*
  Comment: Some supervisors prefer to appraise their "best" clinicians first, regardless of Level, etc.

A *combination* of these grouping principles may be most useful, with one principle being used for the first organization into subgroups, and a second principle for further sequencing of clinicians for scoring within each group. The important recommendation is for supervisors to adopt *some* organizing principle for scoring a group of clinicians, rather than filling out CAFs in a non-specified or chance sequence.

GUIDELINE VI: COMPUTATIONAL PROCEDURES FOR DERIVING SKILL SCALE PERCENTAGES

After circling values for each item chosen for appraisal, the supervisor can calculate Scale scores on Interpersonal Skills, Professional-Technical Skills, and an "Average" of these two Scales. These values, expressed as percentages (to adjust for unscored items) are entered in the appropriate boxes on the face sheet of the CAF (see p. 134). For each Scale, completing the following procedure will yield the Scale percentage:

1. Add the values circled for each item used. This total becomes the NUMERATOR.

   Example: If a student received five 7s and three 8s on the Interpersonal Skills

Scale (two items were not scored) the total equals:

$$35 + 24 = 59$$

2. Multiply only the number of items actually used by 10. This product becomes the DENOMINATOR.

   Example: For the student above, only eight items were used, hence:

   $$8 \times 10 = 80$$

3. Divide the NUMERATOR by the DENOMINATOR; move decimal point two places to the right; round to a whole number (move any decimal .5 or above to the next highest *whole number*)

   Example: As above, $59/80 = .7375$
   $$= 73.75$$
   $$= 74\%$$

4. Record each of the percentages obtained for Interpersonal Skills and Professional Technical Skills in the appropriate boxes on the face sheet. An "Average" of these two scores (i.e., the sum of the two scores divided by two) is also entered in the appropriate box on the face sheet.

GUIDELINE VII: SUGGESTIONS FOR GRADE ASSIGNMENTS

Discussion

A conception of the elements of grade assignment is presented in Figure 5.1 (see Summative Appraisal and Grade Assignment). The working assumption is that a grade can be derived from a three-way weighting of "product" information, "process" information, and "entry characteristics" considerations. Both the function of "clinical" grades and the contingencies for receiving a specific grade in a particular setting should influence weighting and grading decisions. For example, grades can be used (1) to certify skill, (2) to predict success, (3) to suggest entry points for subsequent practicums, (4) as feedback to clinicians, (5) to compare the outcomes of different groups, and (6) to allow continuation in a clinical program (the customary academic contingency). Functional differences among grades of A, AB,

B, BC, C, or D, for example, might vary according to the purpose(s) above for which a set of grades is used. As with previous Guidelines, the suggestion is that *some* explicit framework for grade assignment must be developed by a supervisory team. Three suggestions for grade assignment are presented here.

SUGGESTIONS FOR GRADE ASSIGNMENT

Procedure 1: Non-Specified

Some supervisors or supervisory groups may prefer to use the CAF skill scores (Interpersonal, Professional-Technical, "Average") and Personal Qualities Summary solely as advisory input to grading decisions. Some supervisors prefer to avoid unwarranted use of "numbers" to characterize clinician competence. Following this procedure, which might be *closest to a subjective approach to grading,* the supervisor weighs (1) the CAF skill scores, (2) the "process" information, and (3) the student's level and difficulty of the client—and in some non-specified fashion, determines an appropriate grade. Such procedures are defensible to the extent that grading decisions obtain the same validity, on any of the six purposes for grading listed above, as that obtained by supervisors using more explicit quantitative procedures.

Procedure 2: Individual-Supervisory Norms

Procedures 2 and 3 are each in turn subdivided into two options. These options refer to two possible ways of converting Interpersonal Skills or Professional-Technical Skills scores (or the "Average") to tentative letter grades.

OPTION A—NORMATIVE-REFERENCED
Step 1.

Each supervisor plots the distributions of scale scores[1] obtained by his or her supervisees at

[1]Sample Grade Assignments, aggregated over several supervisors, are presented on page 146. As evident in the assumptions about supervision and appraisal reviewed (pp. 1–25), Option B has been of greatest interest to the authors of this manual.

each Level (or each Level by Practicum Site), for the current term and cumulatively over several terms.

Step 2.
A tentative letter grade is assigned based on a clinician's performance in comparison with peers. Either natural "breaks" in the distribution or frequency percentages can be used, similar to grading practices in some large academic courses.

Step 3.
The final grade assignment may be derived by weighting the tentative letter grade derived above against information on "process" characteristics, personal qualities, and difficulty of task (other than as already adjusted for by Level assignment—see Figure 5.1, Grade Assignment).

Comment: Such norm-referenced grading generally promotes competition rather than cooperation among clinicians and is counter to the objectives of skills competency training.

OPTION B—CRITERION-REFERENCED[2]
Step 1.
In criterion-referencing grading, the distribution of scores is *not* used for grade assignments. Rather, each supervisor has a particular CAF score in mind which corresponds to a specific letter grade. (For example, in one practicum a supervisor may decide that a Level II clinician will need to obtain a CAF Professional-Technical Skills score of 88 or above to be considered for an "A." In normative-referenced grading, a clinician's grade depends on how well the other clinicians in the practicum performed; in criterion-referenced grading such comparisons are *not* relevant.) These decisions may not be possible to make until a supervisor has had several terms of experience with W-PACC and CAF data.

Step 2.
Grades may again be weighed against "process" information, personal qualities sum-

mary, and difficulty of task—final grading may be adjusted up or down accordingly.

Procedure 3: Group Supervisory Norms

The steps to apply each of the two options in Procedure 3 are essentially the same as those reviewed for Procedure 2 above. However, In Procedure 3, *grouped* supervisory CAF scores are used for all clinicians, rather than each supervisor's individual distribution of scores.

OPTION A—NORMATIVE REFERENCED
Step 1.
The CAF skill scores (Interpersonal, Professional-Technical, and "Average") from *all* clinicians in a training program are arranged in distributions for each Level or Level by Practicum Site.

Step 2.
Based on this frequency distribution, the supervisory *group* determines which scores will be considered for "As", which scores will be considered for "Bs, and so on.

Step 3.
Each supervisor may adjust these tentative grades of the clinician she or he supervised up or down according to "process" information, personal qualities summary, and difficulty of task considerations.

OPTION B—CRITERION-REFERENCED
Step 1.
The supervisory *group* determines the CAF score that is required for each tentative letter grade at each Level or Level by Practicum site.

Step 2.
Each clinician is assigned a tentative letter grade according to the CAF skill scores obtained.

Step 3.
Each supervisor adjusts grades by the other three considerations as above.

SAMPLE ITEM DESCRIPTORS

(See Guideline III for perspective on these descriptors.)

---

[2]Of the three scores, Interpersonal, Professional-Technicsal, and "Average," Professional-Technical appears to correlate highest with subjective grades.

(Continued on page 141)

CLINICIAN APPRAISAL FORM (CAF)

Clinician's Name _____ Date _____

Circle: Clinician Level 1 2 3 4

Class Standing: JR. 1st. Sem. JR. 2nd Sem. SR. 1st Sem. SR. 2nd Sem.

GRAD. 1st Sem. GRAD. 2nd Sem. GRAD. 3rd Sem. Other _____

Practicum Site _____

Type(s) of Problem(s) _____

_____

Problems in Addition to Communication _____

Age(s) of Clients(s) _____

Total Number of Therapy Sessions _____

Supervisor _____

_____

_____

Comments:

Interpersonal Skills Scale . . . . /___/

Professional-Technical Skills Scale . . . . /___/

Average $\dfrac{IS + PTS}{2}$ = ... /___/

PERSONAL QUALITIES SUMMARY

No. of "Satisfactory" items . . . . /___/

No. of "Inconsistent" items . . . . /___/

No. of "Unsatisfactory" items . . . . /___/

No. of "Lack Information" items . . . . /___/

No. of "Does not Apply" items . . . . /___/

(total should = 10)

% SCORE = $\dfrac{\text{Sum of Scored Items}}{\text{Number of Items Scored} \times 10}$

INTERPERSONAL SKILLS	Does Not Apply	Specific direction from supervisor does not alter unsatisfactory performance and inability to make changes.	Needs specific direction and/or demonstration from supervisor to perform effectively.	Needs general direction from supervisor to perform effectively.	Demonstrates independence by taking initiative; makes changes when appropriate; and is effective.
1. Accepts, empathizes, shows genuine concern for the client as a person and understands the client's problems, needs, and stresses		1	2–3–4	5–6–7	8–9–10
2. Perceives verbal and nonverbal cues that indicate the client is not understanding the task; is unable to perform all or part of the task; or when emotional stress interferes with performance of the task		1	2–3–4	5–6–7	8–9–10
3. Creates an atmosphere based on honesty and trust; enables client to express his or her feelings and concerns		1	2–3–4	5–6–7	8–9–10
4. Conveys to the client in a nonthreatening manner what the standards of behavior and performance are		1	2–3–4	5–6–7	8–9–10
5. Develops understanding of teaching goals and procedures with client		1	2–3–4	5–6–7	8–9–10
6. Listens, asks questions, participates *with* supervisor in therapy and/or client-related discussions; is not defensive		1	2–3–4	5–6–7	8–9–10
7. Requests assistance from supervisor and/or other professionals when appropriate		1	2–3–4	5–6–7	8–9–10

(continued)

INTERPERSONAL SKILLS

	Does Not Apply	Specific direction from supervisor does not alter unsatisfactory performance and inability to make changes.	Needs specific *direction and/or demonstration* from supervisor to perform effectively	Needs *general direction* from supervisor to perform effectively.	Demonstrates independence by taking initiative; makes changes when appropriate; and is effective.
8. Creates an atmosphere based on honesty and trust, enabling family members to express their feelings and concerns		1	2–3–4	5–6–7	8–9–10
9. Develops understanding of teaching goals and procedures with family members		1	2–3–4	5–6–7	8–9–10
10. Communicates with other disciplines on a professional level		1	2–3–4	5–6–7	8–9–10

PROFESSIONAL-TECHNICAL SKILLS

	Does Not Apply	Specific direction from supervisor does not alter unsatisfactory performance and inability to make changes	Needs specific *direction and/or demonstration* from supervisor to perform effectively	Needs *general direction* from supervisor to perform effectively.	Demonstrates independence by taking initiative; makes changes when appropriate; and is effective.
Developing and Planning					
1. Applies academic information to the clinical process		1	2–3–4	5–6–7	8–9–10
2. Researches problems and obtains pertinent information from supplemental reading and/or observing other clients with similar problems		1	2–3–4	5–6–7	8–9–10

		1	2–3–4	5–6–7	8–9–10
3.	Develops a semester management program (conceptualized or written) appropriate to the client's needs	1	2–3–4	5–6–7	8–9–10
4.	On the basis of assessment and measurement can appropriately determine measurable teaching objectives	1	2–3–4	5–6–7	8–9–10
5.	Plans appropriate teaching procedures	1	2–3–4	5–6–7	8–9–10
6.	Selects appropriate stimulus materials (age and ability level of client)	1	2–3–4	5–6–7	8–9–10
7.	Sequences teaching tasks to implement designated program objectives	1	2–3–4	5–6–7	8–9–10
8.	Plans strategies for maintaining on-task behavior (including structuring the teaching environment and setting behavioral limits)	1	2–3–4	5–6–7	8–9–10

Teaching

		1	2–3–4	5–6–7	8–9–10
9.	Gives clear, concise instructions in presenting materials and/or techniques in management and assessments	1	2–3–4	5–6–7	8–9–10
10.	Modifies level of language according to the needs of the client	1	2–3–4	5–6–7	8–9–10
11.	Utilizes planned teaching procedures	1	2–3–4	5–6–7	8–9–10
12.	Adaptability—makes modifications in the teaching strategy such as shifting materials and/or techniques when the client is not understanding or performing the task	1	2–3–4	5–6–7	8–9–10

(continued)

PROFESSIONAL-TECHNICAL SKILLS	Does Not Apply	Specific direction from supervisor does not alter unsatisfactory performance and inability to make changes	Needs specific direction and/or demonstration from supervisor to perform effectively	Needs general direction from supervisor to perform effectively	Demonstrates independence by taking initiative; makes changes when appropriate; and is effective.
Teaching					
13. Uses feedback and/or reinforcement that is consistent, discriminating, and meaningful to the client		1	2–3–4	5–6–7	8–9–10
14. Selects pertinent information to convey to the client		1	2–3–4	5–6–7	8–9–10
15. Maintains on-task behavior		1	2–3–4	5–6–7	8–9–10
16. Prepares clinical setting to meet individual client and observer needs		1	2–3–4	5–6–7	8–9–10
17. If mistakes are made in the therapy situation, is able to generate ideas of what might have improved the situation		1	2–3–4	5–6–7	8–9–10
Assessment					
18. Continues to assess client throughout the course of therapy using observational recording and standardized and nonstandardized measurement procedures and techniques		1	2–3–4	5–6–7	8–9–10
19. Administers diagnostic tests according to standardization criterion		1	2–3–4	5–6–7	8–9–10

	1	2–3–4	5–6–7	8–9–10
20. Prepares prior to administering diagnostic tests by: (a) having appropriate materials available and (b) familiarity with testing procedures	1	2–3–4	5–6–7	8–9–10
21. Scores diagnostic tests accurately	1	2–3–4	5–6–7	8–9–10
22. Interprets results of diagnostic testing accurately	1	2–3–4	5–6–7	8–9–10
23. Interprets accurately results of diagnostic testing in light of other available information to form an impression	1	2–3–4	5–6–7	8–9–10
24. Makes appropriate recommendations and/or referrals based on information obtained from the assessment or teaching process	1	2–3–4	5–6–7	8–9–10

Reporting

	1	2–3–4	5–6–7	8–9–10
25. Reports information in written form that is pertinent and accurate	1	2–3–4	5–6–7	8–9–10
26. Writes in an organized, concise, clear, and grammatically correct style	1	2–3–4	5–6–7	8–9–10
27. Selects pertinent information to convey to family members	1	2–3–4	5–6–7	8–9–10
28. Selects pertinent information to convey to other professionals (including all nonwritten communications such as phone calls and conferences)	1	2–3–4	5–6–7	8–9–10

(*continued*)

PERSONAL QUALITIES	Does Not Apply	Lack Information	Unsatisfactory	Inconsistent	Satisfactory
1. Is punctual for client appointments					
2. Cancels client appointments when necessary					
3. Keeps appointments with supervisor or cancels appointments when necessary					
4. Turns in lesson plans on time					
5. Meets deadlines for reports					
6. Turns in attendance sheets on time					
7. Respects confidentiality of all professional activities					
8. Uses socially acceptable voice, speech, and language					
9. Personal appearance is appropriate for clinical setting and maintaining credibility					
10. Appears to recognize own professional limitations and stays within boundaries of training					

(Continued from page 133)

Interpersonal Items

1. Accepts, empathizes, shows genuine concern for the client as a person and understands the client's problems, needs, and stresses.

   The clinician demonstrates openness, acceptance, supportiveness, and honesty through verbal and nonverbal language. The clinician does not make parent-like statements or reassurances such as "Don't feel that way; don't worry; Everything will be all right; You should…; You shouldn't…," etc.
   During the session, the clinician demonstrates acceptance, empathy, and concern for the client. During conferences with the supervisor the clinician discusses the client and reflects these feelings and understanding of the client; thoughtful preparation for session is one indication of concern.

2. Perceives verbal and nonverbal cues that indicate the client is not understanding the task; is unable to perform all or part of the task; or when emotional stress interferes with performance of the task.

   The clinician demonstrates this by (1) making attempts to alter the task or terminating the task, (2) using language that indicates that he or she is aware the client is unable to perform the task. (This statement is made either to the client or to the supervisor, or to both.)
   The clinician's behavior indicates an *awareness* of the client's difficulty although he or she may not have the Professional-Technical Skills to make the most appropriate and effective changes during the session.

3. Creates an atmosphere based on honesty and trust; enables client to express his feelings and concerns.

   Verbal and nonverbal responses of the client are included. The clinician does not "turn off" client questions, knows limits of knowledge, can say "I don't know," and listens to client.
   Look to the behavior of the client to measure the clinician's interpersonal skill. Does the client feel the clinician is accepting, interested, concerned for the client as a person, and understanding of the client's needs, problems, and stresses?
   The client's behavior is interpreted as a reflection of the atmosphere created by the clinician.

4. Conveys to the client in a nonthreatening manner what the standards of behavior and performance are.

   In a positive manner the clinician indicates acceptable behavioral limits, verbally and nonverbally by manner and facial expression.
   The language of the clinician reflects a willingness to confront undesirable behavior and talk about it objectively and constructively.
   The clinician is able to state expectations in a positive manner and to handle unacceptable behaviors in such a way that the client feels that a positive relationship with the clinician is not in jeopardy.
   Applies only to interactions that occur *after* the client has performed inappropriately.

5. Develops understanding of teaching goals and procedures with client.

   The clinician informs the client of immediate and long-range goals, explains the sequencing of tasks and procedures, and questions the client for her or his ideas regarding teaching objectives and therapy procedures.
   The client is made aware of his purpose in therapy to the extent to which it is appropriate at any point in time. He is led to understand the goals and procedures and recognize them as something he can accomplish.

6. Listens, asks questions, participates *with* supervisor in therapy and/or client-related discussions; is not defensive.

   The clinician contributes to discussion at a level commensurate with academic background and clinical experience and "teams" for problem solving with the supervisor.
   The clinician is candid with the supervisor. The clinician discusses successes and failures and attempts to look for alternatives to deal with problems about teaching objectives and related clinical issues.

7. Requests assistance from supervisor and/or other professionals when appropriate.

    The clinician recognizes when he or she needs assistance. The clinician indicates when he or she is unsure about teaching tasks or behavioral expectations and checks with the supervisor regarding any changes made on the lesson plans.

    The clinician is willing to ask for assistance as soon as possible to ensure that teaching is continuously effective.

8. Creates an atmosphere based on honesty and trust, enabling family members to express their feelings and concerns.

    Look to the behavior of the parents to measure the clinician's interpersonal skills. Do the parents feel that the clinician is accepting of and concerned for their child and for them? Can the parents openly discuss their feelings and concerns without feeling defensive?

9. Develops understanding of teaching goals and procedures with family members.

    The clinician's manner is straightforward and self-assured. The clinician respects the desire of family members "to know."

    The clinician clarifies goals and procedures without being judgmental. The clinician encourages and rewards parent involvement.

10. Communicates with specialists in other disciplines on a professional level.

    The clinician exhibits professional self-confidence. The clinician attempts to understand the background of other professionals involved and adapts his or her language accordingly.

    The clinician respects the integrity of specialists in other disciplines when there is an exchange of information.

Professional–Technical Items

1. Applies academic information to the clinical process.

    This item includes the application of classroom information as well as supervisory information given during the current assignment.

    As a result of attending class, group meetings, and discussions with supervisors, the cli-

nician demonstrates an understanding of (1) the psychology of fear, (2) use of the DAF, (3) use of problem solving, and (4) stuttering behavior (these are only *some* examples.)

2. Researches problems and obtains pertinent information from supplemental reading and/or observing other clients with similar problems.

    The clinician actively seeks additional information. The clinician reads and evaluates materials recommended by other sources including the clinical supervisor.

3. Develops a semester therapy program (conceptualized or written) appropriate to the client's needs.

    The development of a therapy program is an ongoing procedure that extends throughout the clinicians' assignment with the client.

    Within the first half of the semester the clinician defines long- and short-range goals.

4. On the basis of assessment and measurement can determine measurable teaching objectives.

    The clinician uses information obtained through formal and informal assessment procedures to determine appropriate teaching objectives.

    As a result of analyzing the client's speaking behavior and expressed feelings and attitudes, the clinician can identify the problems and determine appropriate objectives to alleviate these problems.

    The clinician can delineate which aspects of behavior on which to keep data.

5. Plans appropriate teaching procedures.

    Teaching procedures reflect knowledge of what the client might be able to do and at what level he or she is functioning.

6. Selects appropriate stimulus materials (age and ability level of client).

    The clinician makes good use of commercial materials, altering them if necessary to meet the client's needs, and/or creatively devises his or her own materials.

    The clinician respects limits imposed by motor development and interest.

7. Sequences teaching tasks to implement designated program objectives.

   The clinician knows baseline behaviors for task requirements and places the client's ability along the continuum.
   The clinician teaches various tasks using a hierarchy of difficulty format. He or she does not start with a difficult level of performance before client demonstrates ability to perform at a lower level.

8. Plans strategies for maintaining on-task behavior (including structuring the teaching environment and setting behavioral limits).

   The clinician explores alternative teaching environments and strategies for maintaining on-task behavior in order to provide structure for the client's progress.
   The clinician knows when it is important to keep the client on task and when it is important to deal with something else. The clinician helps define criteria for acceptable or successful speech behavior at a particular stage.
   The clinician can deal effectively with client behaviors such as inattentiveness, hyperactivity, or distractibility.

9. Gives clear concise instructions in presenting materials and/or techniques in therapy and assessment.

   The clinician demonstrates adequate preparation, which eliminates the need to reword instructions or redesign materials during the session.
   The clinician uses language that is clear, specific, and concise and is not redundant when giving direction or explanations.

10. Modifies level of language according to the needs of the client.

   The clinician uses active rather than passive language. The clinician uses "doer" language ("You are pressing your lips together") and descriptive language rather than labels such as pullouts, cancellations, and so on.
   By use of his or her words, the clinician indicates his or her understanding of the concept of the "total child" (i.e., does not talk down to the child yet uses words that can be understood).
   The clinician provides a verbal model that is within the client's comprehension and/or modifies his or her speaking behavior so that the client's fluency is not adversely affected.

11. Utilizes planned teaching procedures.

   The clinician knows in advance the planned teaching procedures. He or she does not have to refer extensively to written lesson plan.
   The clinician demonstrates knowledge and purpose of the teaching procedure. The clinician uses this knowledge to (a) identify and describe those behaviors which facilitate the client's use of the procedure and (b) monitor the client's behavior as it relates to achieving the objective.

12. Adaptability—makes modifications in the teaching strategy such as shifting materials and/or techniques when the client is not understanding or performing the task.

   The clinician overplans by having alternative procedures and materials available in case they may be needed. He or she knows baseline behaviors and can spontaneously return to these or to more advanced behaviors as appropriate with the session.
   This item deals with how the clinician reacts in *one particular session;* for example, ability to see that, for that particular day, the material is too complex and is therefore able to modify the material; ability to modify a particular technique that is not effective (change from pullouts to cancellations, change from modifying real blocks to faked blocks, etc.).

13. Uses feedback and/or reinforcement that is consistent, discriminating, and meaningful to the client.

   The clinician's own verbal and nonverbal behaviors are used as reinforcement for desired verbal and nonverbal client behaviors.
   The clinician positively reinforces *on-target* behavior. The clinician positively reinforces attitudes and feelings that the client verbalizes that are conducive to progress.

14. Selects pertinent information to convey to the client.

   The clinician includes information related to the client's problems with communication and knows when to extend the information. The clinician keeps the client informed of progress during each session.

The clinician demonstrates the ability to give information that is relevant to the client's problems, questions, and so on.

The clinician explains teaching strategies and expectations for progress to the client; this item may be particularly applicable to school-age and adult clients.

15. Maintains on-task behavior.

The clinician is consistent in maintaining set behavioral standards.

The clinician facilitates client concentration or attentiveness to task.

16. Prepares clinical setting to meet individual client and observer needs.

The clinician uses appropriate furniture for the client and places chairs so observers can see the client's face; arranges supplies including personal notes and books so they are available but not cluttered; and respects the client's wishes regarding observers.

Setting is interpreted to include not only physical elements (furniture, materials) but people as well. When teaching in a group situation, the clinician prepares seating arrangements that recognize the needs of individual children in relation to the needs and behavior of other children.

17. If mistakes are made in the therapy situation, is able to generate ideas of what might have improved the situation.

In conferences with the supervisor the clinician indicates an understanding of his or her mistakes and can creatively plan alternative procedures to meet problems that were unsuccessfully dealt with during the session.

The clinician can independently verbalize future modifications in the therapy format.

18. Continues to assess client throughout the course of therapy using observational recording and standardized and nonstandardized measurement procedures and techniques.

The clinician recognizes goal achievement and moves the client through a systematic progression of designated objectives.

The clinician recognizes when the client should add another goal, or when a particular goal needs to be emphasized (for example, desensitization procedures; identification of stresses, etc.).

The clinician keeps systematic data on measurable aspects of behavior.

19. Administers diagnostic tests according to standardization criterion.

(no descriptors)

20. Prepares prior to administering diagnostic tests by: (a) having appropriate materials available; (b) becoming familiar with testing procedures.

The clinician knows how to administer various diagnostic tests. He or she does not become overly absorbed in test materials and procedures and so misses interpersonal contact with the client.

21. Scores diagnostic tests accurately.

(no descriptors)

22. Interprets results of diagnostic testing accurately.

(no descriptors)

23. Interprets results of diagnostic testing accurately in light of other available information to form an impression.

(no descriptors)

24. Makes appropriate recommendations and/or referrals based on information obtained from the assessment or teaching process.

(no descriptors)

25. Reports information in written form that is pertinent and accurate.

The clinician includes information that enables the reader to understand goals and procedures. The clinician effectively summarizes the information rather than detailing it.

The clinician's first draft of the final report reflects a knowledge of client's behavior, teaching objectives, and clinical procedures.

26. Writes in an organized, concise, clear, and grammatically correct style.

The clinician is able to write, using language that will be meaningful and useful to people outside the speech and hearing clinic.

27. Selects pertinent information to convey to family members.

    The clinician selects relevant facts from therapy sessions or other observable aspects of behavior to share with family members.

28. Selects pertinent information to convey to other professionals (including all nonwritten communications such as phone calls and conferences).

    The clinician selects relevant facts from therapy sessions or other observable aspects of behavior to share with allied professionals. The clinician knows when to initiate contact with these professionals.

Sample Grade Assignments

The table that follows summarizes the correspondence between the "product" scores and grade assignments obtained over one group of supervisors ($n = > 400$ appraisals). Briefly, the values for each scale represent the *mean* value obtained by clinicians who would "subjectively" have been given the corresponding letter grade. Obviously, no claim is intended or should be inferred that these values are the recommended "norms" for grade assignments. Recall that the authors of this manual have been most interested in developing criterion-referenced norms at the *individual* supervisory level (again, the values that follow have been aggregated over several supervisors solely for the purposes of summary inspection). Moreover, in addition to reflecting "product" or scale scores, an individual grade can be adjusted *upward* or *downward* by a supervisor in consideration of (1) "process" information (up or down), (2) Personal Qualities Summary information (usually down), or (3) "Difficulty of task" information (usually up).

LEVEL	GRADE	INTERPERSONAL SKILLS	PROFESSIONAL-TECHNICAL SKILLS	"AVERAGE"
1	A	92	85	88
	AB	81	72	76
	B	78	65	72
	BC	–	–	–
	C	48	41	45
2	A	94	88	90
	AB	88	81	84
	B	76	67	72
	BC	–	–	–
	C	–	–	–
3	A	96	93	95
	AB	92	86	89
	B	80	76	78
	BC	–	–	–
	C	81	61	71
4	A	98	96	97
	AB	96	89	93
	B	92	87	89
	BC	98	66	82
	C	–	–	–

Reprinted with permission from Shriberg, L., Filley, F., Hayes, D., Kwiatkowski, J., Schatz, J., Simmons, K., & Smith, M. (1974). *The Wisconsin procedure for appraisal of clinical competence (W-PACC)*. Madison, WI: Department of Communicative Disorders, University of Wisconsin–Madison.

Indiana University Evaluation of Speech-Language Pathology Student Practicum

Student: _____ Midterm Date: _____ Final Date: _____

Clock hours this report: _____ Client initials/disorder: _____

7 — Independent/Excellent
6 — Minimal or occasional assistance/Very good
5 — Performed well with guidance/Good
4 — Attempted, required specific guidance, some demonstration, or modeling/Average
3 — Attempted, but frequently required specific direction or modeling/Below average
2 — Relied on supervisor to direct each aspect
1 — Performance unacceptable

First & Second Semester Clinician:
A+ = 6.0–5.8 A = 5.7–5.4 A– = 5.3–5.0
B+ = 4.9–4.5 B = 4.4–3.5 B– = 3.4–3.1 C = 2.6–3.0

Third Semester Clinician:
A+ = 6.5–6.3 A = 6.2–5.9 A– = 5.8–5.5
B+ = 5.4–5.0 B = 4.9–4.1 B– = 4.0–3.6 C = 3.1–3.5

Fourth Semester Clinician:
A+ = 7.0–6.8 A = 6.7–6.4 A– = 6.3–6.0
B+ = 5.4–5.0 B = 4.9–4.1 B– = 4.0–3.6 C = 3.6–4.0

SECTION	TOTAL SCORE M	TOTAL SCORE F	GRADE EQUIV. M	GRADE EQUIV. F	CONTRACT REQUIRED M	CONTRACT REQUIRED F
I. Beginning Program Preparation						
II. Initial Documentation						
III. Program Development						
IV. Documentation/Lesson Plan						
V. Documentation/SOAP						
VI. Program Implementation						
VII. Treatment Process—Feedback/Reinforcement						
VIII. Treatment Process—Data						
IX. Treatment Process—Interaction Skills						
X. Documentation/Report Writing						
XI. Response to Supervision						
XII. Professional Behavior						

(M = Midterm grade / F = Final grade)

(Any section with grade below B average will be identified as requiring clinical contract)

Mean Score _____ _____   Clinical Practicum Total Grade _____ _____
              M   F   M   F

Supervisor _____ Date _____

_____ Date _____

Graduate Clinician _____ Date _____

_____ Date _____

INDIANA UNIVERSITY EVALUATION OF STUDENT PRACTICUM

Student: _____   **Date:** _____

I. BEGINNING OF SEMESTER TREATMENT PROGRAM PREPARATION

___ ___   Researched client disorder (class notes, textbooks, articles)

___ ___   Demonstrated ability to read file and gather critical information regarding client's communication

___ ___   Extracted pertinent information from client file

___ ___   Demonstrated understanding of client's communication level and disorder

___ ___   Demonstrated ability to analyze client's program/communication for appropriateness/additional need area(s)

___ ___   Attended and participated in supervision meetings/conferences

___ ___   **Total score for section/Grade equivalent**

___ ___   **Clinical contract required**

II. INITIAL DOCUMENTATION

___ ___   Developed appropriate initial session plan to obtain pertinent information (tests, probes)

___ ___   Administered and scored standardized tests accurately

___ ___   Interpretation and analysis of standardized tests done appropriately

___ ___   Reported test data accurately

___ ___   Administered appropriate probes/baseline

___ ___   Obtained accurate initial baseline data

___ ___   Interpreted/analyzed baseline data appropriately

___ ___   Observed timelines to submit initial plans/revisions

___ ___   **Total score for section/Grade equivalent**

___ ___   **Clinical contract required**

III. PROGRAM DEVELOPMENT

___ ___   Clinician demonstrated adequate application of clinical knowledge/theory to develop appropriate treatment program

___ ___   Developed goals and objectives that were a logical outgrowth of gathered information and testing

___ ___   Lesson activities planned that supported client treatment goals

___ ___   Materials and activities were appropriate to client's age, needs, abilities

___ ___   Demonstrated appropriate modifications for treatment materials and activities

___ ___ Clinician demonstrated the ability to appropriately modify the program for the client as necessary

___ ___ **Total score for section/Grade equivalent**

___ ___ **Clinical contract required**

IV. DOCUMENTATION/LESSON PLAN

___ ___ Goals and objectives were written in behavioral terms

___ ___ Goals and objectives encompassed appropriate treatment areas

___ ___ Demonstrated ability to break down goals into appropriate steps (task analysis skills)

___ ___ Lesson plan written with appropriate teaching techniques/materials

___ ___ Lesson plan written with appropriate verbal script

___ ___ Lesson plan written with appropriate criteria

___ ___ Lesson plan written with appropriate cueing levels

___ ___ Lesson plan written with appropriate reinforcement and feedback

___ ___ Clinician made appropriate edits based on supervisor comments in a timely manner

___ ___ Observed timelines to submit initial plans, lessons, and revisions

___ ___ **Total score for section/Grade equivalent**

___ ___ **Clinical contract required**

V. DOCUMENTATION/ SOAP

___ ___ Accurately completed SOAP with information in appropriate sections

___ ___ Accurately and appropriately reported data in session notes

___ ___ Interpreted data and session appropriately

___ ___ Note writing was clear, well-organized

___ ___ Indicated when objective had been met with revision of plan timely and appropriately

___ ___ SOAPs were edited with attention to supervisory comments

___ ___ Observed timelines to submit notes/revisions and utilized suggestions to modify notes

___ ___ **Total for section/Grade equivalent**

___ ___ **Clinical contract required**

VI. PROGRAM IMPLEMENTATION

___ ___ Level of treatment was appropriate for the client

___ ___ Clinician implemented treatment activities that supported client treatment goals

___ ___ Clinician used materials and activities appropriately for client's age, needs, abilities

___ ___ Clinician used teaching techniques to maximize client performance

___ ___ Clinician used teaching techniques to maximize client cooperation and motivation

___ ___ Clinician effectively used instruction to support the client's success

___ ___ Clinician effectively used demonstration with instruction to support the client's success

___ ___ Clinician demonstrated ability to modify session during treatment to meet client's needs

___ ___ Clinician effectively modeled/shaped the desired response

___ ___ Clinician effectively obtained responses with a variety of stimuli

___ ___ Clinician efficiently obtained adequate number (N) of responses

___ ___ Clinician followed through on supervisor suggestions

___ ___ **Total score for section/Grade required**

___ ___ **Clinical contract required**

VII. TREATMENT PROCESS—FEEDBACK/REINFORCEMENT

A. Feedback

___ ___ Accurate, corrective feedback was used to support client progress

___ ___ Feedback was contingent upon client responses

___ ___ Schedule of feedback was planned and consistently observed

___ ___ Type of feedback was appropriate for the client

___ ___ Feedback produced continued effort on the part of the client

B. Reinforcement

___ ___ Reinforcement was used appropriately

___ ___ Reinforcement was contingent upon client responses

___ ___ Schedule of reinforcement was planned and consistently observed

___ ___ Type of reinforcement was appropriate for the client

___ ___ Reinforcement produced continued effort on the part of the client

___ ___ **Total score for section/Grade required**

___ ___ **Clinical contract equivalent**

VIII. TREATMENT PROCESS—DATA COLLECTION/ ANALYSIS

___ ___ Data were consistently taken

___ ___ Data were accurate and reliable

___ ___ Data were collected online quickly and discreetly

___ ___ Analysis and evaluation of data was accurate and comprehensive

___ ___ Data were used for ongoing case management (changes in program)

___ ___ Data were accurately reported in the SOAP

___ ___ **Total score for section/Grade required**

___ ___ **Clinical contract equivalent**

IX. TREATMENT PROCESS—INTERACTION SKILLS WITH CLIENT AND FAMILY

___ ___   Clinician clearly set and consistently enforced behavioral limits

___ ___   Clinician employed behavior management techniques that were appropriate for client

___ ___   Clinician's pace of session allowed for maximum use of time

___ ___   Clinician recognized communicative intent of nonverbal/challenging behaviors and responded appropriately

___ ___   Clinician conducted session in an organized and sequenced manner that reflected preplanning

___ ___   Clinician demonstrated warmth, ease, and sensitivity to the client's or family's feelings

___ ___   Clinician recognized the impact of communication style/speaking style on success of client and made appropriate adjustment

___ ___   Clinician recognized impact of eye contact/other nonverbal behaviors on the performance of client

___ ___   Clinician employed appropriate conference/counseling skills with client/family

___ ___   Clinician conducted appropriate parent in-service on an ongoing basis

___ ___   Clinician encouraged client and/or family responsibility in management

___ ___   **Total score for section/Grade equivalent**

___ ___   **Clinical contract required**

X. DOCUMENTATION/ REPORT WRITING

___ ___   Included all pertinent information in client report

___ ___   Reported information accurately

___ ___   Demonstrated appropriate writing skills (spelling, grammar, sentence construction)

___ ___   Used professional writing style

___ ___   Report was understandable for client or parent/caregiver

___ ___   Report was well organized

___ ___   Test, results, interpretation written accurately and appropriately

___ ___   Report discussion of procedures and progress written accurately

___ ___   Report summary written comprehensively with synthesis and integration of information

___ ___   Made appropriate recommendations

___ ___   Observed timelines to submit drafts, revisions

___ ___   **Total score for section/Grade equivalent**

___ ___   **Clinical contract required**

XI. RESPONSE TO SUPERVISION

___ ___   Considered supervisory suggestions and openly discussed differences in ideas

___ ___   Demonstrated reflective practice and engaged in self-supervision to discover areas of strength and those that needed improvement

___ ___ Suggested ways to enhance clinical performance

___ ___ Developed increasing confidence about own performance and professional growth

___ ___ Positively dealt with own frustrations in treatment and/or supervision

___ ___ Discussed supervisory analysis and evaluation in a positive manner

___ ___ **Total score for section/Grade equivalent**

___ ___ **Clinical contract required**

XII. **PROFESSIONAL BEHAVIOR (+/–)**

A. General

___ ___ Demonstrated cooperation and teamwork

___ ___ Kept verbal commitments

___ ___ Never had an unexcused clinical or supervisory absence

___ ___ Observed legal mandates, most especially client privacy and confidentiality policies

___ ___ Dressed for activities with respect for observers, clients, and the professional setting

___ ___ Was punctual in beginning and ending clinical sessions

___ ___ Encouraged client and/or family responsibility in management

___ ___ Written and/or verbal communication is free from judgmental statements

B. Public Health Precautions (+/–)

___ ___ Demonstrated care and concern for general well-being of client

___ ___ Adhered to standards of health practices for clinical materials

___ ___ Adhered to standards of sanitary conditions for room space and equipment

___ ___ Understood and observed the health precaution information provided by the setting

___ ___ Other (_____)

___ ___ **Clinical contract required**

MIDTERM COMMENTS:

RECOMMENDATIONS FOR CONTINUED CLINICAL AND PROFESSIONAL GROWTH:

FINAL COMMENTS:

RECOMMENDATIONS FOR CONTINUED CLINICAL AND PROFESSIONAL GROWTH:

APPENDIX 5C

Bartlett's Supervisory Action Plan

SUPERVISORY ACTION PLAN

Date of Plan _____

Supervisee _____

Site/Setting _____

Supervisor _____

Assignment Period _____

ANALYSIS AND EVALUATION			SUPERVISOR/SEE RELATIONSHIP	ACTION PLAN	
Supervisee's Strengths/ Weaknesses	*Effect(s) on Supervision*	*Expected Outcome*	*Behaviors/Skills to Modify*	*Techniques and Strategies*	*Results*
Should include documented evidence of supervisee's skills and behaviors	Is the effect positive or negative? Is there a problem?	What is the desired end result? What will happen with planned change?	What changes need to be made by supervisee/sor?	Who will do what?	Date and document what occurred

Action Plan Case Study

Jessica is a third-semester graduate student in speech-language pathology assigned to a practicum in an elementary school that uses a collaborative approach to service delivery. Her caseload consists of preschool and K–3 students with moderate to severe communication disorders who are enrolled in inclusive classrooms. Several of the children also receive special education and related services in the context of daily school activities.

Jessica has previously completed 175 hours of clinical practicum in the university's clinic and in an acute care facility; in both places she worked with clients individually. The assignment to the school is her fourth practicum experience after having completed a full academic year and an eight-week intensive summer experience. She has a strong academic background for normal and disordered communication and a solid grasp of theoretical concepts to support her assessment and intervention activities. Previous supervisors have rated her clinical skills as good to excellent. She is skilled in using computers for clinical and search applications and she routinely familiarizes herself with resources that are available for clinical implementation. Using the university's checklist for clinical skills—a formative tool for assessing progress in developing skills and competencies—at the conclusion of her third practicum assignment, Jessica's strengths were in the areas of behavior management, data collection, preparation for treatment and assessment, and professionalism. She independently seeks out opportunities to solicit and share relevant information with families, teachers, and others for the purpose of identifying functional outcomes. She is conscientious about submitting lesson plans, progress summaries, and evaluation reports on time. In the school setting, she has used spare time to conduct classroom observations, meet with teachers, and review records.

Skills in self-evaluation and modifying objectives are rated as emerging. One supervisor reported that if an objective or procedure is not successful, Jessica is likely to omit it from her plans, rather than to analyze the session and to alter it for a future session. She remains dependent on the supervisor for support in this area. Although Jessica's observation and evaluation of the client's behaviors are usually accurate and insightful, she has expressed her lack of confidence at evaluating her own clinical performance. Her written and verbal summaries of test findings and of clients' progress are areas that have been identified as weak. A sample from a recent conference with a parent illustrates this observation:

> "Max's speech is problematic. At this point in time, it is apparent that there is some evidence of residual phonological processes, coalescence, voicing of unvoiced consonants, devoicing consonants that should be voiced, syllable reduction, metathesis, and syllable reduction. Vowel distortions are present in nasalized contexts."

Post-session entries in the chart notes are usually ½ to ¼ of a page and Jessica has difficulty separating subjective from objective data in reporting the outcomes of her sessions. She needs to refine her skills in presenting information succinctly.

The supervisor reviews Jessica's lesson plans and other written work pertaining to her client and to her own clinical growth on a weekly basis. Direct observation of her management sessions occurs 75% of the time and verbal and written feedback are provided following each observation. Jessica has not consistently negotiated the focus of subsequent supervision or evaluated her own progress over time, and she has not proposed changes to the frequency or type of feedback. She has been asked to complete a questionnaire that will assist her with developing a supervisory plan.

SUPERVISORY ACTION PLAN

Supervisee _____

Site/Setting _____

Date of Plan _____

Supervisor _____

Assignment Period _____

ANALYSIS AND EVALUATION		SUPERVISOR/SEE RELATIONSHIP		ACTION PLAN	
Supervisee's Strengths/ Weaknesses	*Effect(s) on Supervision*	*Expected Outcome*	*Behaviors/Skills to Modify*	*Techniques and Strategies*	*Results*
Should include documented evidence of supervisee's skills and behaviors	Is the effect positive or negative? Is there a problem?	What is the desired end result? What will happen with planned change?	What changes need to be made by supervisee/sor?	Who will do what?	Date and document what occurred
e.g., *Strengths* ■ Thorough preparation ■ Accurate data collection ■ Initiates contact with family and education team ■ Solid theory ■ Meets deadlines ■ Uses time efficiently *Weaknesses* ■ Overuse of professional jargon ■ Lengthy documentation	■ Alter use of supervisory time for direct observation ■ Supervisee is a reliable and valued resource ■ Moving toward collaboration model on continuum ■ Not considered a problem to supervision	*Supervisor:* ↑ Collaborative role *Supervisee:* ↑ Self-evaluation ↑ Independence	*Supervisor:* → Amount of feedback → Direct feedback → Daily review of lesson plans *Supervisee:* ↑ Initiate focus of supervision ↑ Propose changes to supervision ↑ Efficiency of documentation	*Supervisor:* ■ Conference 1x/wk and reduce frequency to biweekly ■ Audiotape analysis of conference ■ 25% direct observation of treatment *Supervisee:* ■ Self-evaluation with videotape ■ Use of analysis tool ■ Use of personal journal for self-reflection ■ Set personal goals ■ Review a variety of documentation formats	

Original materials developed by Bartlett, S. Presented in Supervision 102: Short Course conducted with Brasseur, J., McCrea, E., Newman, W., Rassi, J., Solomon, B., and Weinrich, B., at the annual convention of the American Speech-Language-Hearing Association, Washington, DC, November 16, 2001. Reprinted with permission from S. Bartlett.

CHAPTER SIX

OBSERVING IN THE SUPERVISORY PROCESS

A supervisor can waste a professional lifetime trying to reconstruct a teacher's performance with him by talking about it from recollections.
—Cogan (1973, p. 136)

Task 6: Assisting the supervisee in observing and analyzing assessment and treatment sessions. Competencies required:

6.1 Ability to assist the supervisee in learning a variety of data collection procedures

6.2 Ability to assist the supervisee in selecting and executing data collection procedures

6.3 Ability to assist the supervisee in accurately recording data

6.4 Ability to assist the supervisee in analyzing and interpreting data objectively

6.5 Ability to assist the supervisee in revising plans for client management based on data obtained

Part of Task 6 and the first three associated competencies listed above are directly related to Observing, the third component of the supervisory process. As with the other components of the supervisory process, observation is a fourfold activity; each participant becomes the object of some type of observation at various times during the process. Further, the assumption in the Collaborative and the Consultative Styles is that clinicians, supervisees, and supervisors will all be involved in self-observation followed by self-analysis. This chapter will concentrate on general principles of observation and observation of the clinician and the clinical process, leaving the discussion of observation of the supervisory process for Chapter 9.

Before talking about what observation is, it seems essential to clarify what it is not. Some common misconceptions about observation are:

- Observation is supervision
- Observation is evaluation
- Observing and watching are synonymous terms
- The segment of the session observed by the supervisor was sufficient
- The segment of the session observed by the supervisor was accurately perceived
- The treatment or assessment session is the sole focus of observation

Although these misconceptions may be evident in a variety of behaviors, the following examples illustrate some of the more frequent ones we have observed.

Misconception: Observation is supervision
Example: "I'm supervising between two and five o'clock today"—meaning, I'm observing between two and five o'clock today.

Misconception: Observation is evaluation
Example: Immediately after an observation, the supervisor says to the supervisee, "You did a great job of discriminating correct–incorrect responses. Now you need to work on eliciting more responses."

Misconception: Observing and watching are synonymous terms
Example: Supervisor looks at interaction but no writing or taping takes place during the time she or he is attending.

Misconception: The segment observed was sufficient
Example: During an hour, the supervisor is observing two supervisees. After the session, one supervisee sees the supervisor and asks, "Were you watching when…?"

Misconception: The segment observed was accurately perceived
Example: The supervisor records only those client–clinician behaviors that she feels characterize "good" therapy. Client and clinician goals are minimally included.

Misconception: The treatment or assessment session is the sole focus of observation
Example: No data on written reports and records, or verbal and written communication with families and other professionals are collected throughout the term.

PURPOSES OF OBSERVATION

Before delving into the "How Tos," it seems pertinent to address first the purposes of observation. In educational programs, one obvious purpose is to meet the requirements stipulated by ASHA's Council on Academic Accreditation (ASHA, 1997) that one-fourth of treatment sessions and one-half of each diagnostic session be directly observed. Even though the former Council on Professional Standards (COPS), which is now the Council for Clinical Certification (CFCC), proposed a less prescriptive requirement for the new accreditation standards that become effective January 2005, member response overwhelmingly supported prescribing and maintaining a minimum of 25% for any clinical activity. Requirements are apparent in other settings. In some service delivery programs, supervisors are required to perform a certain number of observations before a formal evaluation of an employee is written.

In examining the competencies associated with Task 6, it is obvious that another purpose is to collect data. Goldhammer and colleagues (1980) considered observation synonymous with data gathering and stated, "Observation is the activity through which a supervisor becomes aware of the events, interactions, physical elements, and other phenomena in a particular place…during a particular time" (p. 70). Anderson (1988) stressed that "observation without data collection is a waste of time" (p. 123). According to Goldhammer (1969), the principal purpose of observation is to collect objective and comprehensive data in such a way that each session can be reconstructed validly enough to analyze it. He emphasized that **the observer should write what he sees, not how he feels about what he sees.** That instruction along with the following straightforward guideline should be posted in every room where observation takes place and on the front of every supervisor's notebook: *Perceptions—not inferences; description—not commentary!!*

Specific purposes will be related to the goals established for the clinical and supervisory processes. Content and procedures will depend on the exact purpose. Harris (1975) noted that an observation will focus on the learner when our purpose is to gather evidence on learning; will focus on the instructor when our purpose is to gather evidence about the instructor's behaviors and competencies; and will focus on the interaction among the learner, instructor, and environmental factors when we attempt to gather evidence about the teaching–learning process. Observers need to have a clear concept of their purpose, a focus, before they begin an observation. For example, are they attempting to collect baseline data? Monitor to assure quality services? Measure progress toward therapy objectives? Or to identify patterns of clinician behaviors that facilitate or impede the clinical process?

In reality, there may be multiple purposes. Surely, the subsequent analysis of the clinical or diagnostic process will be more productive and the conference more meaningful if it is assumed that the fundamental purpose of the observation is to collect data. Further, the data should be collected in a manner that will enable the observer, or someone else, to relate the behavior of the clinician to the consequences of that behavior in the client. Later, in the case of the observation of the conference, the importance of relating the behavior of the supervisor to consequences of that behavior on the supervisee will be considered. In other words, does the action of the clinician or supervisor appear to make a difference, positive or negative, in what the client or supervisee achieves? Can inferences or assumptions be made about the situation that has been observed? What data have been collected to support the inferences or assumptions about those behaviors?

CHARACTERISTICS OF OBSERVATION

Two main characteristics of observation are of importance. One is its scientific nature; the other is the fact that, to be of value, observation must be an active process.

Observation Is Scientific

Anderson (1988) stressed that the observation component is the point at which supervision begins to move from the realm of a somewhat undefined art to a scientific endeavor. It is the objective collection of data in the observation that changes supervision from being solely an art to more closely approximating science. Principles can be borrowed from the behavioral sciences, as Cogan (1973) suggested. "Supervisors need to apply the intellectual

rigor and discipline of science" and "to internalize the standards of evidence and proof that are characteristic of science" (pp. 18–19). In regard to assessment, Emerich and Hatten (1979) noted that the scientific approach leads to, among other factors, "more rigorous adherence to standardized procedures" and "objectivity, quantifiability and structure." The artistic approach, on the other hand, depends more on "casual and non-structured scrutiny…the hunch, or clinical intuition." Emerich and Hatten (1979) stated further that "Diagnosis is a unique blending of science and art" (pp. 12–13). Blending science and art in supervision is precisely what Anderson (1988) advocated.

It is in the observation component that supervision assumes an objective approach, where quantifying procedures begin to be utilized, where data are collected that will be submitted to much the same type of analysis required for research projects. Researchers describe data as numerical and verbal descriptions of attributes and events (Silverman, 1998), not a new concept to supervisors. Data from the observation provide the raw material for the conference. If they are not accurate, objective, and reliable, all subsequent stages of the process will be distorted or ineffectual. Without behavioral data as a foundation, the conference will become a potpourri of supervisee reports about what happened in the assessment or treatment session, supervisor attempts to recall the events, general discussion of treatment or assessment principles, guesses about the direction to take in future sessions, and subjective evaluations by the supervisor.

A clear distinction must be made between *data collection, analysis,* and *evaluation.* The purpose of the observation in the Collaborative and Consultative Styles is not "instant evaluation," but rather, to collect data. Inferences will be made from these data that will lead to interpretation, to further planning, and eventually to evaluation. The inferences are determined jointly to provide an opportunity for learning by the supervisee.

Many supervisors may find it difficult to resist writing instant evaluations during the observation. The fallacy of instant evaluations can be recognized by supervisors who recall how many times, in the darkness of the observation room or in the corner of the room where they were observing, have written an evaluative statement on the basis of one event or a few behaviors, only to erase the statement later, when subsequent events invalidated the previously written evaluation. In teaching courses or conducting workshops on supervision, it is obvious that eliminating instant evaluations from observation reports is a difficult habit to eliminate for many supervisors. Research substantiates that written comments tend to be highly evaluative. For example, Runyan and Seal (1985) reported that 46% of comments written by supervisors during an observation were evaluative. Peaper and Mercaitis (1987) reported a 40% rate in their investigation of written feedback provided to students. This propensity toward evaluation suggests that many supervisors perceive evaluation as their primary role. Although this supervisor-as-evaluator role is consistent with the Direct-Active Style, it is *incongruent* with the Collaborative and Consultative styles.

Observation Is Active

Observation is more than just looking at what is occurring, and to be done well, it demands attention, practice, and precision. Observation is an *active, systematic process*. It may be done by supervisors during the actual assessment or treatment session within the room, through an observation window, via a closed circuit system, or after the session by listening to an audiotape or viewing a videotape. Data may also be recorded by clinicians themselves during sessions or subsequently by audio- or videotaped observations. Observation may include data gathering by colleagues in the case of team therapy (Wegner, 1999), the teaching clinic (Dowling, 1983a, 1983b, 2001), or peer review. Whatever the circumstances, the observer will be actively involved in careful recording of events. As indicated in the planning session, the data to be collected will have been identified based on the objectives that have been set, and the method of data collection will have been determined. Planning provides guidance for the activities of the supervisor during the observation, or for

the supervisee during self-observation. The end product, then, is a set of carefully recorded data that can be utilized for a variety of purposes during the analysis and evaluation processes.

IMPORTANCE OF OBSERVATION

Systematic observation of supervisees is crucial in the process of supervision. Observational techniques formulate the data that provide the foundation for feedback that leads to change in the supervisee. It is an essential activity, on which the effectiveness and accuracy of the remainder of the supervisory process are dependent.

In speech-language pathology and audiology, the clinician's ability to observe the client has always been of concern, as evidenced by the inclusion of items related to observation on evaluation forms. Probably no existing evaluation forms are without items that assess observation and data collection skills in clinicians. Teaching these skills has been one of the responsibilities of supervisors, a fact substantiated by ASHA competencies such as: "(2.3) Ability to assist the supervisee in using observation and assessment in preparation of client goals and objectives" and "(3.5) Ability to assist the supervisee in integrating findings and observations to make appropriate recommendations" (ASHA, 1985b, p. 58).

Skills related to the observation of the client have received greater emphasis than has observation of the clinician in the literature in speech-language pathology and audiology. Discussion of the techniques and skills of observation of clients have long been available in various texts on evaluation of communication disorders (Darley & Spriestersbach, 1978; Emerich & Hatten, 1979; Johnson, Darley, & Spriestersbach, 1963; Shipley & McAfee, 1998).

Mowrer (1977) devoted several chapters to an in-depth treatment of observation and behavioral assessment of speech behaviors and stated, "*How* we observe, *what* we observe, *where* we observe, and *when* we observe, and what we do with the observations is, as you will discover, a very complex process" (p. 46).

Skilled observation of communicative behavior is the basis of all effective efforts in evaluation and treatment of disorders, according to Kunze (1967), who stated that "techniques in the observation of communicative behavior should be systematically taught as the first step in our clinical training programs and the student should have obtained observational skill before he faces his first practicum assignment" (p. 4). As supervisors in university settings know, completing 25 hours of observation prior to enrollment in practicum has been an accreditation standard for a number of years (ASHA, 1997). However, with the new standards for CCC in SLP (effective 2005), the 25 hours of observation are no longer a *prerequisite* to beginning direct patient/client contact. In off-campus practicum, students typically complete a period of observation, shadowing their master clinician, before beginning any service delivery to clients.

The scientific approach to case management, the need to validate techniques and strategies for learning, and the current emphasis on National Outcomes Measurements (i.e., ASHA NOMS) and accountability actually mandate the systematic collection of data. The need for the supervisor to teach the supervisee techniques of scientific observation and data collection is apparent. In addition, supervisors have a responsibility to model this kind of approach in their observations of the clinical process.

There are many sources of information about collecting and utilizing data on client behavior that the supervisor can use in assisting supervisees and themselves to attain or improve observational skills. These sources also provide a basis for competent evaluation and treatment (Hegde & Davis, 1995; Lund & Duchan, 1993; Moon Meyer, 1998; Mowrer, 1969, 1977; Shipley, 1997; Shipley & McAfee, 1998). Supervision research substantiates the need to "calibrate" observers in order to effect reliable, valid data (Filter, Brandell, Smith, & Kopin, 1989; Runyan & Seal, 1985; Sbaschnig & Williams, 1983). Further, the similarity between the research and supervisory processes should be clear here. That is, training for researchers has always emphasized the importance of precise data collection, which is achieved by training prior to

and monitoring during an experiment (McReynolds & Kearns, 1983; Schiavetti & Metz, 1997; Silverman, 1998). There are some innovative strategies such as the use of interactive computer programs (Shadden & Aslin, 1993), using student-directed training (Schill, 1992), and using computers to manage client databases (Rushakoff & Farmer, 1989) that supervisors may want to use and implement.

Objectivity. An individual's perceptual sets, biases, and predispositions about what is seen pose a threat to objectivity. Total objectivity is a myth (Goldhammer et al., 1980). Perceivers attend to different aspect of situations and behavior. Their needs, values, purposes, and past experiences affect their categorization and coding of events or the way they describe them. Additionally, physical, cultural, and social contexts influence the perceiver's interpretation of behaviors and determine the kinds of inferences drawn from their observations (Schneider, Hastorf, & Ellsworth, 1979). Andersen (1981) found biases in supervisor ratings based on prior information about the supervisee. Familiarity with the supervisee was hypothesized to be a source of bias in Blodgett and colleagues' (1987) study of supervisor ratings. Hatten, Bell, and Strand (1983) and Runyan and Seal (1985) found lack of agreement among speech-language pathologists viewing the same clinical session. That perceptions, biases, and preconceived notions affect observations is readily apparent when witnesses report differently at an accident scene or when jurors render different decisions after hearing the same testimonies and seeing the same pieces of evidence in a trial.

Another problem in relation to objectivity and accuracy of data collection is that of reactivity. In research, subjects may behave differently simply because they know they are participants in a study (*Hawthorne Effect*). The very presence of observers, change in routine, the setting itself, or attention the subject receives may change a subject's behaviors (Campbell & Stanley, 1963; Schiavetti & Metz, 1997). In addition, certain measures may yield reactive effects; tests, inventories, rating scales, videotapes, computers, or other equipment may produce changes in the phenomenon being studied. "The more novel and motivating the test device, the more reactive one can expect it to be" (Campbell & Stanley, 1963, p. 9). In attempting to become more scientific in their techniques, supervisors should assume that the risks to objectivity and the basic facts on reactivity are as valid for supervision as they are for research.

One way to manage problems associated with reactivity is to apply the principles of desensitization. Anyone who has observed a new client's initial attention to a tape recorder on a table and watched it become as unobtrusive as piece of paper or a picture card over time knows that reactivity can be diminished.

There are several ways to manage the risks to objectivity. One is training. In addition to some of the training resources cited previously, self-knowledge is an integral part of training to enhance objectivity. Awareness is the first step in the change process. All individuals have what Cogan (1973) termed "square boxes" or "inferential sets," our biases and preconceived notions of "the way things ought to be." Not all of these may be bad. The important thing is to bring them to a level of consciousness, to understand them and test their validity. One technique to identify inferential sets is to pay attention to "gut feelings." If an urge to make an instant evaluation or to intervene in a session being observed is experienced, the supervisor should pause, write the feeling down and carefully examine it after the observation.

Consider this example from the second author. Early in her career as an untrained supervisor she felt that enthusiasm was an important variable for the clinical process and thought that it was manifested by exuberant, "peppy," lively clinician behavior. If a clinician's style was more subdued, calm, and quiet than she thought it ought to be, she'd pop into a session and demonstrate and instruct the clinician to follow her model. After being introduced to the concept of "square boxes," she refrained from commenting or interrupting the session of a calm clinician working with an active preschooler. Over the period of a few weeks, the data collected substantiated that the clinician's style was equally as effective as hers, as evidenced by client response rate, success, time on task, and so on. She learned the first of many valuable lessons.

PLANNING THE OBSERVATION

Observation should not "just happen." Given the vast amount of behavior available to supervisor and supervisee in the clinical session, and the variability in recording methods, some selection must be made to make the observation manageable and the subsequent analysis meaningful. Like all other activities, the planning should be done jointly by the participants. At the Evaluation-Feedback Stage, the bulk of decision-making about observation will probably be done by the supervisor. As the participants move away from this stage, there will be more participation by the supervisee in deciding what behaviors are important enough for data collection. This moves the interaction away from the traditional style, where behaviors to be observed are selected by the supervisor, possibly after entering the observation situation. It is essential to limit the extent of data collection by deciding which behaviors will be the focus of the observation, how the observation will be conducted, and how and by whom the data will be recorded.

Planning for observation will take place at different times during the term of supervision. It certainly will occur at the beginning when long-range plans are being worked out and also throughout the supervision sequence as plans are being made for subsequent therapy sessions or conferences.

Early Planning for the Observation. When supervisees begin their clinical experiences, they may need specific assistance from the supervisor in data collection methods not only for their clients but also for themselves. Although novice supervisees will have had limited experience with data collection as part of their experience in observing all or part of the 25 hours of therapy, it's different when you're on the inside looking out versus the outside looking in. Assisting the supervisee in learning a variety of data collection procedures (6.1) and in selecting data collection procedures to be used in sessions (6.2) is likely to be one of the first tasks the supervisor performs. Variety is important. Although clinicians need to learn that certain observation tools exist for their use, they should not view such tools as the exclusive approach to data collection.

At the beginning planning stages, certain general principles about observation should be discussed as required by each supervisee. This discussion will cover such topics as the purpose and importance of data collection; the supervisee's past experiences and skills in recording data; potential methodologies for recording both client and clinician data and the possible reasons for selecting one or another of those methodologies; the responsibilities of the supervisor for observation; the responsibility of clinicians for data collection on the client and on themselves; and the preferences, biases, or feelings of each participant about observation. A thorough, rational, objective discussion of the purposes of observation at this point will encourage efficient and effective data collection; it may also relieve some of the anxieties of the supervisees if they know what is to be recorded.

Clinicians must be helped to see at a very early point in their education that without complete, accurate, ongoing data collection on their clients, as well as their own behaviors, there is no measurement, no accountability. They must learn that they, as well as the supervisor, have responsibilities for data collection that will benefit them *and* the client.

Data collection may seem to be a given, but supervisors often have to be vigilant in determining that it is actually done. Many clinicians, and indeed supervisors, resist data collection. It is sometimes hard work, and often tedious. It requires concentration and purpose. Clinicians often take great pains to collect objective data on the client during the diagnostic period but then do not continue the collection of the same kind of objective data to measure progress during therapy. Rather, comments about therapy may be subjective and evaluative (Turton, 1973). For this reason, some supervisors instruct supervisees to take the "s" out of SOAP notes. Long-range planning for observation of the clinical session makes it more meaningful to clinicians and results in a greater commitment to the task. A clear, specific intent to collect certain data will make the clinical process not only more purposeful, but also more interesting. Tangible evidence of change is much more reinforcing than subjective guesses about results of therapy. Clinicians also need to understand that responsibility for data collection does not end with the receipt of their degree—it continues into the job setting, wherever it may be.

There are advantages for the supervisor, too, in planning the data collection. Tangible evidence of progress in their supervisees is rewarding. Definite goals for data collection keep the observation more interesting. Any supervisor who has ever nodded off momentarily in the dark shadows of the observation room will probably welcome structure and direction in the data collection task. Supervisors also report that data collection makes them feel more fair and impartial later, when they evaluate the supervisee's clinical performance.

Who Does the Data Collection?   Supervisors and supervisees will have different responsibilities for data collection, depending on the situation. Basically, there is a natural division of labor between them. The supervisee collects client data as a part of treatment or assessment session or later via audio- or videotape. The supervisor usually collects data on the clinician or the interaction between clinician and client. There will be times when supervisors, to be truly collaborative, also will collect data on clients for certain purposes— for example, to check the reliability of the clinician's observation, to gather data about behaviors that cannot be collected by the clinician during the session, to identify behaviors not perceived by the clinician, or to record the unexpected. Particularly at the beginning of the interaction, both will want to collect baseline data on the clinician for purposes of establishing objectives, parallel to the process used for clients.

At some point, clinicians will need to be responsible for collecting data on their own behavior as well as that of the client. For some time we have known that clinicians can develop an awareness of their own abilities through analysis of their own audio- or videotape recordings (Boone & Stech, 1970). Some clinicians may reach the stage where they can collect data on their behaviors *during* rather than after the clinical session. This is one of the areas where supervisees must be involved if a true collaborative relationship is to develop and if they are going to learn the process of self-analysis and self-evaluation.

Ongoing Planning of Observation. A portion of every conference should be used for dual planning of the details of the observation of the next clinical session. Just as selection of client data to be collected depends on the stated objectives, so does the collection of clinician data. Progress of *clinicians* toward their objectives must be measured just as client behavior is measured. Once again there is blending of one component of the supervisory process into another. Establishing the relationship and determining needs lead to planning and setting of objectives. Data collections planning comes directly out of those objectives—with space left for serendipity! (Goldhammer et al., 1980).

Leaving space for serendipity is an important point. Despite the stress placed here on planning the observation, supervisors and supervisees must allow for the unexpected. Cogan (1973) described the importance of capturing "critical incidents," those unanticipated events that have a profound impact on learning. The impact may be positive or negative. For example, a child who volunteers to answer a question in class and whose answer is followed by laughter may quickly learn not to answer questions.

Observation that is not planned but left to the supervisor's choice, however, is subject to bias. What supervisors will see and choose to record as they observe without planning will depend to a great extent on their theoretical base, their own mood or feelings at the time, and the importance that their own professional experience or expertise places on certain aspects of the clinical session such as direction giving, stimulation, reinforcement, modeling, client participation, expansion, and feed-

back (Roberts & Naremore, 1983). Unplanned, subjective observations also make it difficult to document change or to provide feedback other than evaluative judgments based on impressions.

Ongoing, joint planning includes planning what behaviors will be observed, how they will be operationalized, what kinds of data will be collected, how it will be recorded (tallies, observations systems, verbatim written notes, etc.), the physical aspects of the observation (in-room, observation room, videotape, etc.), who will collect what behaviors, and when the data will be collected. Comparable planning for observations of the supervisory process will need to be completed and will be discussed in Chapter 9.

CHECKLIST FOR OBSERVATION PLANNING
- Observation and data collection have been jointly planned
- There is a rationale for data collection
- Data to be collected are consistent with long and short term goals for the client *and* clinician
- Data come out of the needs, concerns, or self-identified strengths or weaknesses of the supervisee, and from the experience and impressions of the supervisor
- Options for supervisor selection of behaviors not in the plan have been discussed
- Plans are detailed sufficiently and mutually understood
- Data collection methods will facilitate effective analysis
- The plan allows for variance such as interruptions, mood of the client, unexpected client learning, and so on
- The amount of data to be collected is sufficient for drawing inferences
- The plan includes data collection by the clinician of his or her own behavior
- The plan has accounted for changes necessitated from previous observation plans and outcomes

All supervisors have experienced the frustration of losing some important observation while madly trying to synthesize previous observations to support a point. Or at times not being able to substantiate a point because of insufficient data. Data collection on clinician behavior is so important that supervisors must make a great effort to perfect systems for recording that they can use easily and efficiently. Anyone who has had a problem supervisee understands this even more. A word of caution seems warranted here. To avoid litigation, it is essential to be able to demonstrate that all supervisees are being treated the same and being treated fairly. Thus, a supervisor must use the same general procedures for planning, observing, collecting data, and keeping records for all of his or her supervisees. That is, although individual variation between supervisors is to be expected, individuals should strive for a reasonable degree of internal consistency.

STRATEGIES FOR OBSERVATION

Selection of the method of observation depends on a number of variables, including:

- the setting
- the philosophy or personal preference of the participants
- the objectives for the observation
- the availability of equipment
- time
- the training and experience of the supervisor and supervisee

Concurrent Observation

Probably the most frequently used form of observation is online recording, in which the supervisor is observing at the same time that the treatment or assessment session is being conducted. Observations may be done with the clinician and the client in the room or in an adjacent observation room.

Based on the previous discussion of reactivity, it is apparent that observers in the same room with the clinician and client will have some effect on them. At the same time, clinicians and clients are usually conscious of the ever-present possibility of a live body on the other side of the window or at the closed-circuit video monitor. The self-consciousness of being observed may influence the behaviors of the individuals being observed, and it is important for observers to be sensitive to this possibility.

Videotape or Audiotape Recording. Speech-language pathologists and audiologists have used audio- and videotaping equipment to enhance the learning process with clients and clinicians for decades, but there is a paucity of research to demonstrate the usefulness of taping to support any specific methodology.

The most extensive study of the use of videotape in the preparation of speech-language pathologists was conducted by Boone and Stech (1970). They reported that both audio- and videotape confrontation, listening or viewing, were useful in changing the behavior of clinicians. They also indicated that mere listening or viewing was not as powerful as when accompanied by the use of an analysis matrix on which clinicians recorded their behavior. Further, Boone and Stech found audiotape and behavioral scoring to be as effective in changing *verbal* behaviors as videotape confrontation because 80 to 95% of the therapy process occurs at the verbal level. They added that this does not imply that videotape confrontation is not more effective in studying therapy. Rather, viewers of videotape should concentrate more on the nonverbal level—facial expressions and gestural cues, attending to the client, and behaviors used to punctuate therapy interaction.

Videotape recording as a teaching device in speech-language pathology was investigated by Hall (1971), Irwin (1972, 1975, 1981a, 1981b), Irwin and Hall (1973), and Schubert and Gudmundson (1976). Most of their studies incorporated the microteaching techniques developed in education by Ivey (1971) and used in preparing teachers and counselors (Kagan, 1970). This technique varies in its use but essentially follows this pattern: a short microlesson is conducted and videotaped, the tape is observed by the clinician and supervisor, behaviors to be modified are identified, the lesson is redone and videotaped, and another observation and analysis by supervisor and clinician is conducted to determine if behaviors have changed. Irwin (1981a) recommended this method for speech-language pathology and audiology education and made a case for further study of its use.

Schubert (1978) advocated the use of videotape recording for teaching, demonstration, and self-analysis. He stated clearly that the videotape recording should not become a substitute for online observation. The quantification of behaviors from videotape provides an invaluable method of analyzing change in the clinical process.

The use of audio- or videotaping in observation and self-observation provide a powerful teaching tool. As with any type of observation, these techniques are only as useful as the data that are collected and analyzed. To maximize the effectiveness of taping, users have to learn methods for collecting and analyzing data (Camarata, 1992; Farmer, 1987b; Farmer & Farmer, 1989; Schill, 1992). Merely listening or watching is likely a waste of time. Formerly, video equipment was available primarily in university programs, but today it is readily available in most service delivery settings in the United States.

Live Supervision. The term *live supervision* appears to have its origin in counseling and psychotherapy. As practiced in those disciplines, it involves both observation and feedback. The supervisor is in the room and participates with the supervisee in the session. Rassi (2001) reports this type of supervision in audiology practica. Speech-language pathology programs that use an apprenticeship model to train their students also use live supervision (Gillam, 1999; Messick, 1999). Another form of live supervision is the "bug-in-the-ear" technique, an electronic device that allows the supervisor to communicate directly with the supervisee. Used in the early 1950s in training counselors (Korner & Brown, 1952), it has also been used in speech-language pathology (Brooks & Hannah, 1966; Engnoth, 1974; Hagler, 1986; Hagler & Holdgrafer, 1987). This will be discussed further in Chapter 8 in section on Feedback.

DEVELOPMENT OF OBSERVATIONAL TECHNIQUES

The techniques of observation are a part of scientific heritage and have long been the tools of scientists who have studied behavior in a variety of disciplines. The behavior modification movement of the 1960s had a strong influence on approaches to observation in education and in our professions. Structured observation systems proliferated in the 1970s (Simon and Boyer, 1970a, 1970b, 1974) and had a powerful impact on the study of many types of interactions. Naturalistic or qualitative research suggests other strategies for observation (Lincoln & Guba, 1985; Pickering, 1980). In the 1980s, the explosion in technology, and the advent of the personal computer in particular, have further expanded approaches to observation and data collection.

Methods of Data Collection

The understanding and appropriate use of systematic observation and data collection methods by supervisors is important for establishing supervision as a thoughtful, scientific, and validated process. Supervisors need to be skilled observers, but more than that, they must also develop efficient, practical procedures for recording their observations for later use. The following methods have been used in our professions, some more than others. Readers are encouraged to try some they have not used to expand their personal repertoire and to become proficient in using a *variety* of procedures (6.1).

Recording Evaluative Statements. The most traditional procedure, and perhaps the method of least effort or the most expediency for supervisors is to simply write evaluative statements reflecting their perceptions of the appropriateness of the behaviors in the treatment or assessment session as they view it; for example, "Your directions were too difficult for the client" or "you did a good job of motivating him today." Such action is consistent with the Direct-Active Style of the Evaluation-

Feedback Stage. This procedure may be expanded slightly as supervisors record behavioral data selected to support their judgments or to illustrate to the clinician what they perceived as good or poor clinical practice. This methodology is neither appropriate nor inappropriate *per se*. It may be decided during the planning component that there is a need for such direct evaluative procedures, if not in the entire session, at least in certain parts of it.

If it has been determined that there is a need for such judgments at certain times, however, the aim of supervisors and supervisees should be to reduce their numbers as rapidly as possible and to involve the supervisee in more self-evaluation. The caution here should not be against occasional, but rather against habitual, use of the instant evaluation without rationale. Furthermore, regardless of intent, supervisors' written comments tend to be highly evaluative (Peaper & Mercaitis, 1987; Runyan & Seal, 1985). As stated previously, it is these active, direct behaviors of the supervisor that do not *en*courage, in fact probably *dis*courage, self-analysis and creative thinking on the part of supervisees.

Tallies of Behaviors. Collection of baseline data or recording of data on clinician behaviors selected during the joint planning session may be done by a simple tallying by supervisor and/or supervisee—exactly the type of tallying and charting completed for clients. For example, if the clinician is working on a simple, straightforward goal such as decreasing the number of utterances of "OK," a simple tally by the supervisor over a period of time will measure progress toward that goal. Certain reinforcement techniques, accurately or inaccurately evaluated target sounds, responses to clients, or other specific behaviors can be tallied in this manner. As clinicians gain more experience, they can tally their own behavior. Dowling (2001) provided a number of innovative examples for collecting data using a tally technique. Further, she demonstrated a profile format and several other informal techniques that are easy to use and provide an excellent means for supervisors and supervisees to measure change over time. The Kansas Inventory of Self-Supervision (KISS) developed by Mawdsley (1985b) contains seven clinician behaviors: overuse of "OK," corrective feedback, response rate, group management rotation rates, positive reinforcement, clinician response to client social comments, and clinician versus client talk time. The system provides an easy way to introduce clinicians to data collection, analysis, and data interpretation. It also provides an easy technique for supervisors to tally one of the target behaviors during observations (see Appendix 6A).

In developing this skill, it is usually easier to tally behaviors from an audio- or videotape before attempting to do so in an actual session. It may appear gratuitous to discuss this method because most supervisors and supervisees do this at some time. The important point for the Collaborative or Consultative Styles is that the data collection for clinician behaviors be jointly planned; that both parties be involved in some portions of the record-keeping; and that it is done systematically, not at the whim of the supervisor.

Rating Scales. Rating scales may be used in observation when behaviors to be observed are known ahead of time and there is a need for qualitative data. In such instruments, behaviors or events are listed and value judgments are made as to the quality of the behaviors—the degree to which the rater perceives that the behavior has been performed adequately or inadequately, appropriately or inappropriately. Degree is typically assessed using a Likert Scale. Rosenshine (1970) called rating scales "high-inference systems" because they call for inference and judgment on the part of the observer, as opposed to analysis systems, which he labeled "low inference" because of their relatively more objective nature. Many rating scales are of very poor quality, reflect the bias of those who constructed them, and have no validity or reliability.

Rating scales that have been developed to evaluate clinical competencies (e.g., W-PACC) are usually not appropriate for tallying behaviors in the clinical sessions, although they may sometimes be used in that way. If the descriptors are specific and are stated behaviorally, they might be modified for data collection, which would then feed into analysis and subsequent evaluation. Generally, however, rating forms used for evaluation are *not* useful for data collection because of the global nature of the items and the inherent judgmental factor that is built in. These types of instruments are, however, useful for making *summative* assessments about clinical performance over time, provided that ratings are based on data collected over time.

Verbatim Recording. Goldhammer (1969) dismissed all methods of data collection except verbatim transcripts, which contain everything done or spoken during a session. The transcripts are then examined in the analysis stage. Goldhammer's reasoning is sound—analysis systems or rating scales force behaviors into *a priori* categories, record supervisors' interpretations or perceptions, usually are not reliable or valid, and may miss important behaviors. Audio- or videotapes are unmanageable unless submitted to extensive analysis. Operationalizing Goldhammer's approach is more easily discussed than accomplished. Recording everything that happens during an observation, writing comments and questions in the margin, recording descriptions of nonverbal behaviors, and diagramming clinician and client positions requires practice and the skills of a stenographer. That is, one must be adept in taking notes, using symbols, abbreviations, diagrams and some type of shorthand, to complete verbatim transcripts. Realistically, most supervisors and supervisees need to prepare transcripts from videotapes.

Despite the drawbacks, Goldhammer's discussion of the need for *totality in recording* the activities observed is important. Verbatim recordings are particularly useful for obtaining baseline data with a new supervisee. They are also an excellent technique for making problem behaviors salient. For example, if a supervisee is having difficulty with accurate auditory discrimination of /r, ɝ/ and centering diphthongs, the supervisor can complete a verbatim transcript, employing narrow transcription. The power of seeing antecedent events; the

kind of stimuli that evoke correct, incorrect, and close approximations of the desired behavior; and the precise verbalizations and events used to consequate client responses enables a clinician to carefully analyze the clinical interactions and figure out what needs to be done differently to increase the client's success.

Selected Verbatim. An alternative to Goldhammer's method involves narrowing the scope and making a verbatim transcript only of certain events or categories of events selected during the planning stage by the supervisor and supervisee. Such recording may be done concurrently with the session or from a taped recording. Acheson and Gall (1980) list the advantages of selective verbatim recordings:

- The supervisee becomes sensitized to the verbal process in teaching.
- The supervisee does not have to respond to all aspects of the teaching–learning process, only those that have been selected.
- An objective, noninterpretive record of behavior that can be analyzed is constructed.
- It is a simple procedure.

These advantages may also be problems, according to Acheson and Gall. The supervisee, knowing what is to be recorded, may become self-conscious in using the behaviors or may use them more often during the observation period only. There is also the possibility of bias in the selection of behaviors and the way they are analyzed and interpreted, the possibility of selecting trivial behaviors, and the difficulty in keeping up with verbal behaviors.

Selective verbatim transcripts from tapes are a useful tool for self-analysis. Nothing reveals the inaccuracies, monotonies, ambiguities, and irregularities in a person's own verbosity as quickly as a written script. Although time-consuming, it is a potent tool for behavior change. For example, some clinicians have difficulty providing clear directions to their clients. Rather than a supervisor providing an evaluation after a session such as, "Your directions were too complex/confusing/

ambiguous," he or she could instruct the supervisee to complete a self-analysis. That is, the supervisee would be instructed to tape the session, then make verbatim transcriptions of each direction used during the session. These would be examined relative to how the client responded after each direction and the supervisee would identify those that caused confusion for the client. These would be rewritten to simplify and clarify the direction and discussed with the supervisor to refine if needed, and the supervisee would use the revised directions in the next session. The process would be repeated until the objective of clear directions is achieved.

Block (1982) developed an innovative method called the Pre-Conference Observation System (PCOS), which is a kind of selective verbatim method. It used a coding system for recording some client and clinician behaviors such as giving directions, models, responses, and verbal reinforcement. She also used a standard set of symbols, initials, abbreviations, and placements on a page to enable objective, systematic data collection to be completed. Supervisors may find it helpful to develop a similar technique, using their own personal shorthand. Following are some examples of Block's system:

Notation

+   clinician thought the response was good

–   clinician thought the response was bad

IM   Immediate model

DM   Delayed model

X   Model repeated

(+)   Supervisor evaluated response as correct*

Θ   Supervisor evaluated response as incorrect*

Clinician versus client talk can be distinguished by differential placement on the page. For example, clinician talk can always be started at the margin and client talk can always be indented.

Example
book – X – X +

Explanation
Clinician said *book*
Response was incorrect [–]
Clinician repeated model [X]
Second attempt was incorrect [–]
Clinician repeated model again [X]
Third response was correct [+]

Smith (1980a) provided some innovative techniques for collecting and recording data during observations. Her examples illustrated a combination of tallies, notations, and time sampling.

Interaction Analysis Systems

The most structured form of recording observations is the interaction analysis system, which has been used in education, counseling, and psychotherapy for years (Amidon & Flanders, 1967; Bales, 1950; Simon & Boyer, 1970a, 1970b, 1974). Systems are constructed so that interactions between events can be analyzed and patterns identified. They have been developed by taking the behaviors that occur in teaching or in clinical sessions and categorizing them into sets that are distinguishable from each other, relevant to the purpose of the observation, and mutually exclusive; that is, all behaviors with common characteristics are placed in a category. They enable users to examine the relationship between events and to correlate interactional patterns with outcomes.

The use of interaction analysis systems by supervisors or in self-study by the supervisee is based on the assumption that the supervisee will change behavior as a result of feedback. These systems are very useful but should not been seen as a panacea.

A few systems have been developed in speech-language pathology and audiology. They

*These symbols are used when SOR and SEE disagree.

may be used in supervision, research, and self-study to focus observations and structure data collection. Before discussing specific systems, the advantages and disadvantages of their use will be presented. (Several interaction analysis systems for use with the supervisory conference are available and will be discussed in Chapter 9. The advantages and disadvantages of the systems listed here also apply to those used for the conference.)

Advantages of Interaction Analysis Systems

There are many advantages in the use of interaction analysis systems. The quantity of behaviors generated in most observations is so great that it must be structured in some way that enables the observer to analyze the total. Some people may be able to do this without observation systems, but certainly they make such analysis quicker, easier, and relatively more reliable. The systems also help establish a baseline and a record of progress for included behaviors. Analysis systems are helpful for training individuals in the observation process—to sort individual behaviors out of the mass of new behaviors they may be encountering as they take on clinical or supervisory tasks (Golper et al., 1976). They help observers focus their attention. They allow comparisons between sessions and simplify both the recording of data and the feedback. They also provide the "grist" for the analysis component. When used by clinicians themselves, analysis systems help them become aware of components of clinical sessions as well as their own behaviors—this self-recognition and self-analysis is perhaps one of the best uses. They may contribute to clearer communication between supervisors and supervisees about clinical sessions. They are more objective in their classification and identification of behaviors because behaviors are operationalized and ground rules are usually provided for categorizing ambiguous behaviors. Certainly they reduce a large amount of the opinion, judgment, some of the inaccuracies, impressions, misinterpretations, and poor memory that may go into less structured observations.

Disadvantages of Interaction Analysis Systems

The disadvantages of interaction analysis systems may be found in their construction, their use, or their interpretation. The assumption that they are completely "objective" is a dangerous one. It is true that they do force a certain amount of objectivity onto the observer because the behaviors are preselected and defined. However, that very selection may reflect the bias of the authors or a specific theoretical approach. Additionally, the possibility of subjectivity in the form of interpretation, selection of one category over another, or perceptual errors is ever present.

Some interaction analysis systems focus on the clinical process but not on the content, giving incomplete information. Thus, a question may be checked as a question but nothing is known about the type of question or its appropriateness without additional analysis. Further, systems usually do not relate to the efficacy of treatment. What happened is identified and quantified, but its effectiveness is still open to the judgment of the observer. Additionally, most systems do not account for nonverbal behavior.

The volume of behavior included in the system may be so great that it is not only difficult to record all of it, even with the system, but it may also then be impossible to manipulate it to make it meaningful. At the same time, the types of behaviors are limited; therefore, many important behaviors may be missed.

Supervisors or clinicians may become too dependent on such systems, limiting their ability to examine the "large picture." Many systems are poorly constructed and have no established reliability or validity. But perhaps the greatest sin against analysis systems is when they are equated as evaluation systems, which they are not, nor were ever intended to be. Anderson (1988) reported that she often heard the *Content and Sequence Analysis System* devised by Boone and Prescott (1972) referred to as the "Boone evaluation form" or heard supervisors say, "I evaluated her on the Boone." This misconception and misuse is a distinct disadvantage.

Despite the negatives, interaction analysis systems are invaluable tools in the supervisory process when chosen well and used properly. The next section provides guidelines for choice and evaluation of the instruments.

Selection and Use

Certain guidelines must be followed in choosing and using interaction analysis systems. Individuals must know what data they wish to collect and select the system accordingly. In addition, users must be cognizant of the strengths and weaknesses of a particular system. Preparation and practice with a system is crucial for effective use. A valuable outline of criteria for developers and users of interaction analysis systems has been provided by Herbert and Attridge (1975), which includes three categories of criteria: identifying, validity, and practicality.

Identifying criteria are those that enable users to select the instrument that is correct for their purpose and application. These include such items as appropriateness of the title to the system's purpose, the rationale or theoretical support, the specificity of its uses, and the behaviors included.

Validity criteria include characteristics such as clarity, lack of ambiguity, and consistency with theory. Under this heading, Herbert and Attridge suggested questioning whether the items are exhaustive (i.e., include all behaviors of the kind being examined, even if it is labeled "other"), are representative of the dimensions of the behavior being studied (related to sampling and generalizability), and are mutually exclusive (i.e., behaviors can only be categorized into a single category). They also stated that in addition to procedures for use, ground rules should be provided to assist the coder in making individual decisions about borderline or unusual behaviors. Other aspects of validity include: the nature and degree of inference to be made from items, context, observer effect, reliability, and validity measures.

Practicality criteria include relevance of items, method of coding, qualifications and training for users, and provisions made for collection and recording of data.

Unfortunately, no known system meets all the standards of Herbert and Attridge. Nevertheless, users who are knowledgeable about the criteria will be able to identify the strengths and weaknesses of systems they use and make adjustments accordingly. Anyone wishing to use interaction analysis systems, especially for research, should become familiar with the Herbert and Attridge criteria.

ANALYSIS SYSTEMS IN SPEECH-LANGUAGE PATHOLOGY AND AUDIOLOGY

Although interaction analysis systems have not proliferated in our disciplines as they have in some others, there was a surge of interest in this methodology during the late 1960s and early 1970s, coming out of the behavioral paradigm originally described by B. F. Skinner (Johnson, 1971). Systems for use in studying the clinical process were developed by Boone and Prescott (1972), Brookshire, Nicholas, Krueger, and Redmond (1978), Conover (1979), Deidrich (1969, 1971a), Johnson (1970, 1971), and Schubert, Miner, and Till (1973). Other systems for studying behaviors in interviews have been developed (Farmer, 1980; Molyneaux & Lane, 1982; Shipley, 1997). Based on citations in the literature, the systems developed by Boone and Prescott (1972) and Schubert and colleagues (1973) are the most frequently used by speech-language pathologists and are two that have withstood the test of time. These systems will be discussed and examples presented. School clinicians providing classroom-based intervention may find useful systems in Simon and Boyer (1970a, 1970b, 1974).

Content and Sequence Analysis of Speech and Hearing Therapy (Boone-Prescott)

The Content and Sequence Analysis of Speech and Hearing Therapy (Boone, 1970; Boone & Prescott, 1972; Boone & Stech, 1970; Prescott, 1971), based on an operant model, provides a method of quantifying certain behaviors of clinicians and clients. Clinician behaviors include: (1) Explain, Describe; (2) Model, Instruction; (3) Good Evaluative; (4) Bad Evaluative; and (5) Neutral-Social. Client behaviors include: (6) Correct Response; (7) Incorrect Response; (8) Inappropriate/Social; (9) Good Self-Evaluative; (10) Bad Self-Evaluative. All behaviors are recorded on a matrix and a summary form is available for analysis of the data. The system and an example are found in Appendix 6B.

The publication of the system had a major impact on supervisors and clinicians. It was probably the first time that an instrument had so clearly "dissected" the clinical process. University supervisors found it useful in preparing students to observe and identify components of the clinical process, to quantify the behaviors included in the system, to keep records of changes in those behaviors, to identify patterns of interactions, and a multitude of other clinical activities.

The system meets many of the criteria delineated by Herbert and Attridge (1975), but not all. Users of the system, particularly for research, might wish to evaluate it more thoroughly on the basis of these criteria. It is useful for collecting data on client/clinician interactions, is easily learned, is practical, and quantifies the 10 behaviors contained in the system. Given the limited number of categories, it is important not to overuse it—keeping in mind that other behaviors are important in the therapeutic process. Furthermore, as previously stated, it is not intended as an evaluation tool. The data generated by the system are quantitative and, although inferences and assumptions can be made after data are analyzed, the system does not include qualitative ratings that are inherent in evaluation measures.

The Analysis of Behavior of Clinicians (ABC) System

The ABC (Schubert, 1978; Schubert et al., 1973) is identical in purpose to Boone and Prescott's system (1972)—to quantify behaviors in the clinical session so that supervisors and clinicians can more accurately recognize, recall, and analyze the behaviors and sequential patterns. The systems

differ in that the ABC is a time-based system. Behaviors are recorded at three-second intervals or when a behavior changes within a three-second interval, by writing down the number assigned to a particular behavior.

The ABC categories are derived from the categories of the original Flanders (1970) system, which was based on behaviors of teachers and children in the classroom. Clinician categories include: (1) Observing and Modifying Lesson Appropriately, (2) Instruction and Demonstration, (3) Auditory and/or Visual Stimulation, (4) Auditory and/or Visual Positive Reinforcement of Client's Correct Response, (5) Punishment, (6) Auditory and/or Visual Positive Reinforcement of Client's Incorrect Response, (7) Clinician Relating Irrelevant Information and/or Asking Irrelevant Questions, and (8) Using Authority or Demonstrating Disapproval. Client categories include: (9) Client Responds Correctly, (10) Client Responds Incorrectly, and (11) Client Relating Irrelevant Information and/or Asking Irrelevant Questions. Category 12 is silence. The system and an example are found in Appendix 6C.

In a comparison of the Boone-Prescott and ABC systems, Schubert and Glick (1974) found that the two systems obtain essentially the same information when therapy consists mainly of stimuli—response—reinforcement. However, in a long occurrence of one behavior, such as reading a story in a language lesson, the ABC naturally provides a clearer indication of the length of time spent on a particular behavior. They concluded that both systems provide useful, objective information about the clinical session.

The ABC should also be evaluated against the Herbert and Attridge (1975) criteria to determine its appropriateness for the situation in which it is to be used. The same statements can be made about the ABC that were made about the Boone-Prescott—behaviors are limited and the same opportunities for misuse exist.

Observing Nonverbal Behavior

The tendency to concentrate on verbal behavior makes it easy to forget the importance of nonverbal behavior, especially as it relates to affective components of interaction. Certainly interaction between people cannot be discussed without acknowledging the importance of nonverbal behavior in communicating meaning either through facial expressions, body positions, or gestures. Nonverbal behavior is assumed to be less consciously controlled than verbal behavior. Nonverbal behavior may support, contradict, substitute for, complement, accent, or relate and regulate verbal behavior. Where there are inconsistencies between the two, the listener is more likely to believe the nonverbal (Condon, 1977).

Unfortunately, popular literature in the past several years has encouraged an overemphasis on and overinterpretation of nonverbal behavior. Many of the "how to" books related to interpersonal interaction, communication, or success in life, careers, and social life have oversimplified the meaning of nonverbal communication. It is tempting to move ahead of complex scientific analysis and speculate about such behavior. "If we are at all serious about understanding our nonverbal expressiveness in interpersonal communication, we must be somewhat cautious. There is a great difference between reading and reading *into* the expressions of others" (Condon, 1977, p. 106).

This is a particularly important warning for the supervisor. It is difficult, if not impossible, for individuals to interpret most of the nonverbal cues directed at them. How much more difficult it is to interpret as an observer! Not everyone reacts in the same way to nonverbal cues. Much interpretation is dependent on the context as well as the observer's own perceptual processes, attitudes, beliefs, and expectations (Stewart & D'Angelo, 1975). Gender, cultural, and age factors may also account for differences in nonverbal behaviors, which lead to misunderstanding. Therefore, for the supervisor to interpret the meaning of the clinician's behavior to a client or its effect on the client, or vice versa, is folly.

Nevertheless, such behaviors are an important part of clinical interaction and, no doubt, are frequently recorded by supervisors, whether or not they can be interpreted accurately. Often they are obviously distracting; at other times the effect on the client can be observed in backing away from a clinician, facial expression, or other movement. Goldberg (1997) provided some basic information that gives clinicians and supervisors an introduction to the influence that nonverbal behaviors may have on the clinical process. Shipley (1997) addressed the influence of some nonverbal behaviors on interviewing and counseling in communicative disorders. Those interested in a more in-depth study of nonverbal behaviors may refer to counseling and interpersonal communication texts.

WHERE HAVE ALL THE SYSTEMS GONE?

Methodology for collecting data is a crucial variable in the supervisory chain of events, particularly in moving it toward the realm of the scientific. In actuality, the efforts to approach observation of the clinical process, and therefore its assessment, more scientifically through the development of interaction analysis systems seem to have had a brief history and limited attention in speech-language pathology and audiology. Most of the systems were never published; others have been abandoned by the developers for reasons such as loss of interest, complexity of the task, cessation of funding, or higher priority of other interests. Other disciplines, particularly education, have continued to examine the teaching–learning process through the development and use of interaction analysis systems (Evertson & Green, 1986).

Anderson (1988) raised several questions about the infrequent use of interaction analysis systems: Is this a reflection of the lack of concern in the profession about the clinical and supervisory processes resulting in a modicum of research on or with analysis systems? Does the minimal use of these systems reflect supervisors' lack of interest in using a structured form of data collection? Do the systems seem to involve too much work? Did the systems fail to tap important dimensions of the clinical process? Are they perceived not to be useful? Are researchers or supervisors any worse off for not having more validated ways of observing and recording those observations? Are they viewed only as another form of tallying, albeit more structured, providing more information, and slightly more objective?

Anderson believes that the possibilities of interaction analysis systems in our professions were never fully explored because so few were published and thus not well known to many supervisors. They have great utility for supervisors, particularly if used carefully with full knowledge of their limitations. They certainly provide a method for exploring and obtaining information about the important variables in the clinical process. Even though categories in the systems reflect the biases of developers, and users must make some subjective analyses of data, Anderson maintains this is no different than what occurs in the assessment process. That is, no matter how many tests are given, it is still necessary to subjectively integrate and interpret information.

Obviously, there is still much to be learned about the clinical process and the efficacy of various treatments. According to Kendall and Norton-Ford (1982), **treatment efficacy** is a term the encompasses effectiveness, efficiency, and effects. *Treatment effectiveness* evaluates the causal relationship between a particular treatment and documented changes in client behavior. *Treatment efficiency* compares two or more treatments to assess if one method is superior to another, or more cost effective than another (Olswang, 1990). *Treatment effects* studies examine which behaviors change in relationship to each other as an outcome of treatment (Olswang, 1990). These latter studies obviously necessitate a dependent variable that can measure relationships between certain clinician–client behaviors. It seems then that the time is ripe for the resurrection, refinement, and development of interaction analysis systems that can be used to examine the intricacies of the clinical process.

OTHER METHODS OF RECORDING OBSERVATIONS

Traditional approaches to clinical intervention and assessment techniques are being modified rapidly with the advent of new knowledge and technologies. Without question, the proliferation of the personal computer and access to the Internet and World Wide Web have influenced the clinical process for both clinicians and clients. One of ASHA's three focused initiatives for 2001 was related to the use of web-based and advanced technology. A major issue that professionals have had to deal with is the use of telepractices in the delivery of clinical services. Part of the ASHA initiative provided a plan for generating technical reports, position statements, and guidelines that consider reimbursement systems; provision of services to rural and underserved populations; and ethical, privacy, legal, licensing, and credentialing issues. Another part of the initiative addressed "the application of current and emerging technology to deliver services in a manner that will: reduce barriers to access and/or specialized expertise, be cost effective, enhance provider productivity and/or effectiveness, and create additional value/benefits for the health care provider and/or the consumer" (Bernthal, 2001, p. 23). Telepractices necessitate new strategies for collecting, recording, and analyzing data for both the clinical and supervisory processes.

Computer-based scoring for standardized tests is increasingly more available in speech-language assessment. It allows clinicians to input client data and raw scores and then view a variety of derived scores such as quotients, percentile ranks, and language/age equivalencies. This is an asset when scoring is complicated and thus time-consuming and subject to error. Computerized Phonological Analysis (CPA) and Computerized Language Sample Analysis (CSLA) takes clinician input and generates in-depth individual client profiles and normative comparisons that would be labor intensive to complete by hand. Advances in quantifying aspects of respiration, vocal intensity, fundamental frequency, resonance, and various aspects of vocal quality (e.g., jitter, shimmer, etc.) continue to improve with technological advances.

A number of types of software can be used for speech-language intervention:

- *Dedicated software*—commercial software designed to assist in the remediation of specific problem areas (e.g., vocabulary, phonological processes, grammatical structures etc.)

- *Educational software*—programs designed for use by teachers to assist in the instruction of reading, writing, and spelling that can be modified by clinicians to meet individual client needs
- *Entertainment software*—clinicians have traditionally used toys, books, and other materials to elicit target behaviors in therapy. Computer books and games can be used in a similar fashion
- *Productivity software*—word processing, e-mail, spreadsheets, calendar software, and so on, can facilitate the program management aspects of service delivery
- *Clinician-generated software*—technologically savvy clinicians can create tools for assessment and intervention using authoring tools such as HyperStudio, Toolbook, and HyperCard
- *Instrument-based biofeedback*—computer instrumentation provides immediate performance information on various aspects of speech production

ASHA's website (http://professional.asha.org) provides a wealth of information for ASHA members and consumers, including links to directories, support groups, newsletters, free therapy materials and software/shareware, and interactive forums. The most up-to-date information regarding technology resources is available at this site. Every aspect of speech-language pathologists' and audiologists' professional lives, as well as those of consumers, will change drastically in the next decades. What the future holds is uncertain but it will require a commitment to maintaining an awareness of impending improvements and changes, adjustment, flexibility, and innovation on the part of supervisors.

SUMMARY

Observation is a required task in the supervisory process and competence in observation requires skill in using a variety of data collection procedures. Verbatim or selected verbatim recordings, tallies of behaviors, and the use of interaction analysis systems are among the more objective data collection techniques, whereas rating scales and checklists are evaluative and subjective. To be effective, observations must be scientific in nature and observers must be actively involved in systematically collecting data. This scientific, active approach necessitates mutual planning and involvement in observing the clinical or supervisory process.

RESEARCH ISSUES AND QUESTIONS

Establishing the validity of these competencies is an unquestionable research need:

- Assisting the supervisee in learning a variety of data collection procedures
- Assisting the supervisee in selecting and executing data collection procedures
- Assisting the supervisee in accurately recording data

Certain quantitative issues provide additional areas of inquiry. For example, "How long does it typically take to train supervisees to use *X* procedure at an 80–85% interrater level of agreement? Establishing how accurately observers are able to record ongoing events in real time is another research need. The effectiveness and efficiency of training in light of observer (e.g., students, peers, supervisors, etc.) characteristics, the complexity of data being recorded, the speed of occurrence of the behaviors being recorded, and the extent to which simultaneous events are variables that impact real-time data collection need to be explored.

Identifying efficient methods or developing software to store data so they can be easily retrieved and manipulated is a challenge, particularly in light of the mandates for accountability at preservice and inservice levels. This need exists for both the clinical and supervisory processes. Ruder et al. (1996) described a computer-aided evaluation system that enabled comparison of the strengths and weaknesses of a particular clinician between and across supervisors. They also reported on the Behavioral Evaluation System and Taxonomy (B.E.S.T.) program for scoring clinical interaction data (Sharpe, Koperwas, & Wood, 1994) that supervisors used with laptop computers. Ruder et al. (1996) related that B.E.S.T. allows an observer to collect time-based and frequency-based data on any observable entity. It also allows for data collection: in real time, up to 102 different events, simultaneous recording of multiple events, and rapid transformation of data into usable tables and figures.

Needs assessments to generate new institutional or extramural funds, outcomes data for billing and contract/salary negotiations, and databases to generate supervisee formative and summative evaluations are only some of the many reasons to develop *efficient, easy-to-use* systems. Supervision data, comparable to NOMs for collecting data and analyzing clinical outcomes, is a critical need. This is a project that could be initiated across universities with leadership and financial assistance from ASHA's Special Interest Divisions 10 (Higher Education) and 11 (Administration and Supervision) and the Council of Academic Programs in Communication Sciences and Disorders.

Kansas Inventory of Self-Supervision (KISS)

SELF-ASSESSMENT: OVERUSE OF "OK"

Clinician _____   Date _____

When supervising beginning students in speech-language pathology, it becomes apparent that many tend to say "OK" an excessive number of times during the management session. Four main types of "OK" responses seem to be the ones overused. They are "OK" used as (1) a filler, (2) a positive reinforcer, (3) corrective feedback, and (4) tag question. The definitions are as follows:

> "OK" as a filler—This happens when the clinician says "OK" for no reason throughout the session. For example, "OK, now let's turn to the back page."

> "OK" as a positive reinforcer—This is used after the client has given a correct response. Used in this manner, it can often appear as if clinicians are really not committing themselves to the client's production.

> "OK" as corrective feedback—This often occurs when beginning clinicians are afraid to commit as to the correctness or incorrectness of a response. After an error, the clinician would say "OK" instead of giving a rich descriptive feedback.

> "OK" as a tag question—An example of this is, "Pull your tongue up and back, OK?" or, "Let's get out our speech books, OK?" The addition of "OK" makes a statement into a non-assertive request.

During a 20-minute session, count the number of times each of the following types of "OK" are spoken by the clinician.

TYPE	DATA
"OK" used a filler	
"OK" as a positive reinforcer	
"OK" as corrective feedback	
"OK" as a tag question	
Total number of "OK"s	

After listening to the tape, set a realistic goal for reducing the incidence of "OK." Audio- or video-tape sessions weekly until the goal is met.

SELF-ASSESSMENT: POSITIVE REINFORCEMENT

Clinician _____ Date _____

Positive reinforcement is a tool that is utilized daily by speech-language pathologists. This form assists the beginning clinician in categorizing the various types of positive reinforcement used, and in examining sequences of positive reinforcement. For example, the clinician might say, "Good talking," then smile at the client, then give him a token. Three types of positive reinforcement have been utilized and now can be categorized and counted. The clinician can analyze the type and amount of reinforcement being used, examine the amount of progress the client is making, and adjust the reinforcement sequences accordingly.

Utilizing the coding system below, tally the type of positive reinforcement given the client after a correct response in the blank matrix, placing only one code per box. (Note: For a young client who needs maximum reinforcement, one may chart type of positive reinforcement used after any responses.)

RESPONSE CODE
    C = correct response
    I = incorrect response

FEEDBACK CODE
    PV = positive verbal
  NVP = nonverbal positive (smiling, nodding, leaning)
    PT = positive touch
    T = token reinforcement
    E = edible reinforcement

Total number of responses (C + I) = _____

Percentage of correct responses $\dfrac{C}{C+I}$ = _____

Examine the matrix and circle the sequences of positive reinforcement used. For example, a correct response followed by a smile, positive touch, and a token would have a sequence code of C/NVP/PT/T. (Slashes indicate "followed by" in sequence counts). List the sequences and the number of times that sequence is used during the session.

SEQUENCE COUNTS

SEQUENCE	NUMBER OF EVENTS
C/PV	
C/NVP	
C/T	
C/E	
C/PV/NVP	
C/PV/NVP/PT/T	
Etc.	

SELF-ASSESSMENT: CORRECTIVE FEEDBACK

Clinician _____   Date _____

Corrective feedback is defined as the type of corrective measures the clinician will utilize after the client has made an incorrect response. Beginning clinicians have historically demonstrated difficulty in this area by (1) using ambiguous feedback resulting in confusion for the client as to whether the response was correct or incorrect and (2) using feedback lacking descriptive qualities such as modeling, phonetic placement, and motokinesthetic techniques. This critique form looks at types and sequences of corrective feedback used, then asks the clinician to review the percentage of correct responses to determine if the corrective feedback techniques utilized resulted in maximum gain by the client.

Utilizing the coding system below, tally the type of corrective feedback given the client after an incorrect or approximated response. Place the code for each event in one box of the matrix, working left to right.

RESPONSE CODE
  I = incorrect response
  A = approximated response
  C = correct response

FEEDBACK CODE
 NR = no response from clinician
 VN = verbal negative; e.g., "No, try again"
  M = model
 VC = visual clue
 PP = phonetic placement; e.g., "Put your tongue up and back"
 MC = motokinesthetic cue; i.e., giving tactile cues

Total number of responses (I + A + C) = _____

Percentage of correct responses $\dfrac{C}{I + A + C}$ = _____

Examine the matrix and circle the sequences of corrective feedback. In the space below, list the sequences and the number of times each sequence occurred in the session. The slash indicates "followed by" in sequence counts.

SEQUENCE COUNTS

SEQUENCE	NUMBER OF EVENTS
I/NR	
I/VN	
I/VN/PP/M	
I/MC/PP/M	

SELF-ASSESSMENT: GROUP MANAGEMENT ROTATION RATES

Clinician _____   Date _____

Group management is not the norm in most practicum sites for speech-language pathology. Therefore, when beginning students are faced with teaching two or more children at the same time, they often do not understand how to rotate from child to child quickly in order to keep all children as involved as possible and behavior problems at a minimum. With this self-assessment form, student clinicians can assess, in minutes and seconds, the amount of time spent with each child in a group management session. This not only gives information regarding how quickly the SLP rotates from child to child, but this count will also yield a total amount of time spent with each individual child so the clinician can note if more time is being spent with one client than the others.

Below, write out the session task for each child. This will help in the analysis because, for example, in articulation management, more time may appropriately be spent with a client at the level of concentration versus a client at the word level of remediation.

Task for Child A _____

Task for Child B _____

Task for Child C _____

Task for Child D _____

Using the matrix below, figure out in minutes and seconds the time spent with each child for "his turn" during the speech session. Compute the total amount of time spent with each child.

TURN

	1	2	3	4	5	6	7	8	9	10	11	12
Child A												
Child B												
Child C												
Child D												

Total time spent with Child A _____

Child B _____

Child C _____

Child D _____

$$\frac{\text{Total time with all children}}{\text{Total number of turns}} = \text{Mean length of each turn} = \underline{\hspace{3cm}}$$

SELF-ASSESSMENT: RESPONSE RATE

Clinician _____   Date _____

The response rate form was developed so the clinician can self-assess how many responses per minute are being elicited from the client. When a supervisor says that the pace of the session is too slow, the supervisee can count responses to see if this is an area that needs to be improved. The clinician can accumulate baseline data and attempt to improve the number of responses per minute until the supervisor and supervisee agree that the number of responses per session is appropriate.

To figure response rate, add together correct and incorrect responses and divide by the number of minutes of direct management. For example, if in an individual management session the client had 37 correct and 24 incorrect responses, add these scores together for a total of 61. Then divide by the time involved in direct drill (e.g., 20 minutes). The response rate for the session would be:

$$\frac{61 \text{ total responses}}{20 \text{ min. direct drill}} = 3.05 \text{ responses per minute}$$

An example of figuring group response rates would be:

Child A has 12 correct and 43 incorrect for a total of 55
Child B has 29 correct and 12 incorrect for a total of 41
Child C has 42 correct and 9 incorrect for a total of 51

Add these totals together to find a total number of responses for the session. In this example, the total equals 147. Next, divide total number of responses in the session by the time involved in direct drill, 23 minutes.

$$\frac{147 \text{ responses}}{23 \text{ min. direct drill}} = 6.4 \text{ responses per minute}$$

Client	Task	# Correct	# Incorrect	Minutes of Drill	Responses per Minute

Comments:

SELF-ASSESSMENT: CLINICIAN RESPONSE
TO CLIENT SOCIAL COMMENTS

Clinician _____

Task _____

Date _____

As you listen to the audio- or videotape, after each social comment from the client, note the category of the clinician's next remark by placing a checkmark in the appropriate space. Next, note the effect your behavior had on the child in the column marked "Consequence." Indicate the topic of the "Client Social" by paraphrasing the comment in a few words; i.e., "recess fight."

Client Social (Comment)	Clinician			Consequences
	Social	Bad Evaluation	Return to Task	
Example 1. "Mary hit Tom"—recess fight				Client returned
2.				
3.				
4.				
5.				
6.				
7.				
8.				
9.				

Comments regarding the data: _____

_____

_____

_____

_____

_____

_____

SELF-ASSESSMENT: CLINICIAN VS. CLIENT TALK—TIME

Clinician _____

Task _____

Date _____

For this self-analysis, you will need to have two stopwatches. As you listen to the audio- or video-tape, measure the clinician's talk-time with one stopwatch and the client's talk-time with the other.

Talk-time of the clinician _____

Talk-time of the client _____

Total talk-time for session _____

Percentage of the clinician talk-time _____

(Clinician talk-time / total talk = % clinician talk-time)

Comments regarding the data: _____

_____

_____

_____

_____

_____

_____

_____

Reprinted with permission from Mawdsley, B. (1985). Kansas inventory of self-supervision. Paper presented at the annual convention of the American Speech-Language-Hearing Association.

Boone and Prescott Interaction Analysis System

CATEGORY NUMBERS AND DEFINITIONS

1. **Explain/Describe**
    Clinician describes and explains the specific goals or procedures of the session.
2. **Model/Instruction**
    Clinician specifies client behavior by direct modeling or by specific request.
3. **Good Evaluation**
    Clinician evaluates client response and indicates a verbal or nonverbal approval.
4. **Bad Evaluation**
    Clinician evaluates client response as incorrect and gives verbal or nonverbal disapproval.
5. **Neutral/Social**
    Clinician engages in behavior that is not therapy-goal oriented.
6. **Correct Response**
    Client makes a response that is correct for clinician instruction or model.
7. **Incorrect Response**
    Client makes incorrect response to clinician instruction or model.
8. **Inappropriate/Social**
    Client makes response that is not appropriate for session goals.
9. **Good Self-Evaluative**
    Client indicates awareness of his own correct response.
10. **Bad Self-Evaluative**
    Client indicates awareness of his own incorrect response.

PROCEDURES FOR USING BOONE AND PRESCOTT 10-CATEGORY SYSTEM

1. The clinician records the middle 20 minutes of his or her therapy, using a videotape or audiotape recorder. Experience and investigation using these con-frontation devices have found that the first 5 minutes and the last 5 minutes of a half-hour therapy session are not particularly representative of the whole session. Our investigations (Boone & Goldberg, 1969) have also found that a 5-minute segment, selected either randomly or specifically because the clinician wishes to study a particular part of his therapy, will offer about as much information as scoring the total 20-minute segment. In any case, record approximately 20 minutes of therapy.

2. Select for playback and study about a 5-minute segment from the total 20-minute recording. This segment should be studied as soon after the session is completed as possible, particularly in self-confrontation. Whenever possible, playback should not be deferred more than one day from taping.

3. The clinician views or hears his or her total 5-minute segment first with no attempt to score what he or she sees or hears. He or she then plays back the 5-minute segment and scores the segment using a 10-category system analysis. An experienced scorer can do this with a minimum of stop-starting of the playback. Scoring a typical 5-minute segment takes a total of about 7–8 minutes.

4. The total number of events scored in the session and the particular sequences of events are then summarized on the speech and hearing therapy session scoring form. This permits the clinician to determine, for example, how many of the therapy events he or she did, how many the client did, and the client's percentage of correct responses. By computing a few ratios with his or her total number of events in particular categories, he or she can find such information as the ratio of good evaluative reinforcements, bad evaluative responses, and socialization within session. The average time for determining the summary data on the session scoring form is also about 7 or 8 minutes.

5. The total time required for tape playback, scoring, and summary tabulation should not exceed 20 minutes.

BOONE-PRESCOTT SCORING FORM

Therapist: _____   Client: _____   Date: _____

Scored By: _____

1.	Explain/Describe															
2.	Model/Instruction															
3.	Good Evaluation															
4.	Bad Evaluation															
5.	Neutral/Social															
6.	Correct Response															
7.	Incorrect Response															
8.	Inappropriate/Social															
9.	Good Self-Evaluative															
10.	Bad Self-Evaluative															

1.	Explain/Describe															
2.	Model/Instruction															
3.	Good Evaluation															
4.	Bad Evaluation															
5.	Neutral/Social															
6.	Correct Response															
7.	Incorrect Response															
8.	Inappropriate/Social															
9.	Good Self-Evaluative															
10.	Bad Self-Evaluative															

BOONE-PRESCOTT SESSION ANALYSIS SCORING FORM

Clinician: _____

Client: _____

Date: _____

Session Goal: _____

_____

Category	No. of Events	% of Total		Category	No. of Events	% of Total
1				6		
2				7		
3				8		
4				9		
5				10		

Clinician Total: _____

% of Session: _____

Client Total: _____

% of Session: _____

Total # Interactions: _____

Sequence Counts

Sequence	No. of Events
6/3 (6 followed by 3)	_____
7/4 (7 followed by 4)	_____
8/1, 2 (8 followed by 1 or 2)	_____

Ratio Scoring

Correct Response $\dfrac{6}{6+7}$ ____%

Incorrect Response $\dfrac{7}{6+7}$ ____%

Good Evaluation Ratio $\dfrac{6/3}{6}$ ____%

Bad Evaluation Ratio $\dfrac{7/4}{7}$ ____%

Inappropriate Response $\dfrac{8}{6+7+8}$ ____%

Direct Control $\dfrac{8/1,\,2}{8}$ ____%

Socialization $\dfrac{5+8}{\text{Total \#}}$ ____%

Reprinted with permission from Boone, D., & Prescott, T. (1972). Content and sequence analysis of speech and hearing therapy, *Asha, 14,* 58–62.

Analysis of Behavior of Clinicians (ABC) System

George Schubert, Ada Miner, and James Till

CATEGORIES AND DEFINITIONS

CATEGORY	DEFINITION
1. Observing and modifying lesson appropriately	Using response or action of the client to adjust goals and/or strategies
2. Instruction and demonstration	Process of giving instruction or demonstrating the procedures to be used
3. Auditory and/or visual stimulation	Questions, cues, and models intended to elicit a response.
4. Auditory and/or visual positive reinforcement of client's correct response	Process of giving any positive response to correct client response
5. Auditory and/or visual negative reinforcement of client's incorrect response	Process of giving any negative response to an incorrect client response
6. Auditory and/or visual positive reinforcement of client's incorrect response	Process of giving any positive response to an incorrect client response
7. Clinician relating irrelevant information and/or asking irrelevant question	Talking and/or responding in a manner unrelated to changing speech patterns
8. Using authority or demonstrating disapproval	Changing social behavior from unacceptable to acceptable behavior
9. Client responds correctly	Client responds appropriately, meets expected level
10. Client responds incorrectly	Client apparently tries to respond appropriately but response is below expected level
11. Client relating irrelevant information and/or asking irrelevant questions	Talking and/or responding in a manner unrelated to changing speech patterns
12. Silence	Absence of verbal and relevant motor behavior

Recording procedures. Raw data is collected by recording a number on the "Raw Data Collection Sheet" every 3 seconds. This number corresponds with the clinician–client interaction occurring at the time of the observation. Therefore, every 3 seconds, a number is placed on the raw data collection sheet.

The following basic steps are suggested for learning the recording procedures:

1. *Learn the categories* so you can identify a behavior by number. A cue word list may help you recall the behavior quickly. Make yourself a cue card using the suggested list or one of your own choosing.

   BEHAVIORAL CATEGORIES

   1. Modifies
   2. Instructs
   3. Stimulus
   4. P/R—Positive Reinforcer
   5. N/R—Negative Reinforcer
   6. R/Inc.— Reinforcement Incorrect
   7. Clinician Irrelevant
   8. Authority
   9. C/R—Correct Response
   10. I/R—Incorrect Response
   11. Irrelevant response
   12. Silence

It will also help if you remember that categories 1–8 are clinician behavior, categories 9–11 are client behavior, and 12 is silence.

2. *Learn the time unit!* Categories are identified and recorded at 3-second intervals. Form the habit of observing and then writing the number that identifies the behavior.
3. *Record the behavior* (write the numbers) in the squares shown on the raw data collection sheet.
4. *Analyze the data.* The data can be analyzed by completing either or both of the data analysis forms. The two forms are: Quick Analysis Form and the ABC Analysis Form.

RAW DATA COLLECTION SHEET—ABC FORM

Clinician _____

Client _____   Date _____

Session goal _____

ABC QUICK ANALYSIS FORM

Clinician _____   Date _____

Client _____   Time _____

Category	Number of Occurrences	% of Total
1. Modifies		
2. Instructs		
3. Stimulus		
4. P/R		
5. N/R		
6. R/Inc.		
7. Irrelevant		
8. Authority		
Subtotal—All Clinician Behaviors		
9. Correct Response		
10. Incorrect Response		
11. Irrelevant		
Subtotal—All Client Behaviors		
12. Silence		

CHAPTER SEVEN

ANALYZING THE SUPERVISORY PROCESS

Once data have been gathered—whether qualitative or quantitative—they have to be organized, or structured, in a manner that will permit the questions that they are intended to answer to be answered. You can easily be deceived if you attempt to answer questions merely by skimming through or eyeballing the data.

—Silverman (1998, p. 149)

Task 6.0—Assisting the supervisee in observing and analyzing assessment and treatment sessions, and Task 8.0—Interacting with the supervisee in planning, executing, and analyzing supervisory conferences, and the associated competencies that describe the ability to assist the supervisee in using self-analysis and previous evaluation in preparation of goals and objectives for professional growth (2.4), analyzing and interpreting data objectively (6.4), revising plans for client management based on data obtained (6.5), ongoing analysis of supervisory interactions (8.9), and analyzing, evaluating, and modifying one's own behavior (12.2) are integral parts of the fourth component of the supervisory process.

The Position Statement (ASHA, 1985b) makes it clear that analysis is a distinct component of the supervisory process and is separate from evaluation (Task 9), yet the literature indicates that it is often neglected or avoided. Supervisors proceed from observation to feedback and the feedback is typically an evaluation of what was observed or suggestions for future sessions (Culatta & Seltzer, 1976, 1977; Peaper & Mercaitis, 1987; Roberts & Smith, 1982; Schubert & Nelson, 1976; Smith & Anderson, 1982b; Tufts, 1984). Analysis should not be equated with evaluation; rather it should be the bridge between observation and evaluation. It is the time when the supervisor's "square box" is put on the shelf. It is also the time when the clinician/supervisee begins looking at her or his clinical activities with an objective eye.

Analysis is the process of making sense of the data that have been collected. As in research, analysis is driven by the questions formulated before data collection occurred—questions formulated from the goals/purposes of the project. It is the time when the behaviors of the clinician are related to the behaviors of the client and the behaviors of the supervisor are related to those of the supervisee (i.e., the search for relationships or a logical way to account for significant differences).

The focus of this chapter will be on Task 6. Task 8 will be addressed in Chapter 9. Readers are reminded that the basic principles of analysis are applicable to both clinical sessions and supervisory conference.

SCIENTIFIC ASPECTS OF ANALYSIS

In clinical endeavors, as in research, scientific procedures must be used for answering questions—not only the large, global questions, of which there are many, but also the day-by-day, session-by-session, conference-by-conference needs for information. After goals have been established and data collected, scientific principles are used to analyze the data. Then, conclusions can be drawn and inferences can be made. This scientific approach to supervision underscores the importance of analysis to the total process. In research, it would be ludicrous to formulate conclusions and make recommendations for the future immediately after collecting data. It is equally ludicrous to do so in the clinical or supervisory processes. Analysis counteracts the superior role of supervisors solely as *evaluators* or *overseers* and highlights their role as scientific co-investigator.

Ventry and Schiavetti (1980) stated, "We see the practitioner as an applied scientist or a clinical scientist who uses the clinic or school as a laboratory for the application of the scientific method toward the end of providing the best clinical services possible. The scientific method, we think, is at the heart of clinical enterprise" (p. 14). Schiavetti and Metz (1997) emphasized the need to eliminate the gap between clinician and researcher. They affirm that the search for knowledge depends on the use of a systematic method, commonly called the *scientific method*. "The scientific method includes the recognition of a problem that can be studied objectively, the collection of data through observation or experiment, and the drawing of conclusions based on the analysis of the data that have been gathered" (p. 8).

In a discussion of the "clinician-investigator," Silverman (1998) stressed that the most compelling reason for functioning as a clinical scientist is to comply with the ASHA Code of Ethics (2001a), which stipulates that individuals shall evaluate services rendered to determine effectiveness. This requires systematic evaluation of the impact of services rendered. Silverman (1998) described several benefits for the clinician who functions as researcher:

- It would "probably make one's job more stimulating, less routine, and would probably increase the possibilities for positive reinforcement" (p. 12).
- It would help satisfy an employer's requirements for *accountability* (Olswang, 1990).
- It would likely help an individual become a more effective clinician because it would enable a clinician to answer questions relevant to managing one's caseload, to compare the effectiveness of current approaches to new ones, to establish the reliability of nonstandardized diagnostic measures, and to provide documentation for the efficacy of new clinical services being offered, which in turn could improve funding.

With this approach, supervisors and supervisees are asking questions that are "answerable" and stating hypotheses that are "testable." Analyzing data for a research project may be more extensive or more formal than analyzing data from a clinical session or supervisory conference, but the process is the same. Relevant data have to be summarized, organized, and categorized in a manner that is meaningful to the users of the results.

Careful adherence to the scientific method in analysis will ensure a greater degree of supervisor objectivity. In addition, the organization and quantification of observable behaviors and events, inherent in a systematic approach, enhances accountability. This kind of approach forces supervisors and supervisees to test their hunches rather than use "gut instincts" exclusively when making judgments. The scientific approach does not automatically guarantee objectivity—supervisors and supervisees have to be vigilant in their quest for nonbiased practice. They must constantly be conscious of their own "square boxes" because it would be very easy to look for patterns or categories of behaviors and draw conclusions that support a hypothesis or bias.

IMPORTANCE OF ANALYSIS

It is at the point where supervisors and supervisees begin to use analysis techniques that their supervision style probably differs most from what has previously been called "traditional" supervision or an apprenticeship model of supervision. Developing analytical skills may well be the most important step in producing thoughtful, self-analytical professionals.

If supervisors are serious about what often seems to be platitudinous voicing of the goal of producing "self-supervising" clinicians, this is a crucial point in the development of that ability. If clinicians are to be clinically competent, independently functioning professionals, they must develop expertise in self-analysis. It is essential that clinicians be cognizant of their behaviors and the effect of those behaviors on their clients if they are to modify or strengthen those behaviors. The analysis process enables clinicians to extract from a mass of behaviors a design—a configuration—from which they can begin to see what is happening, to draw some inferences, to construct some hypotheses about what was effective and what was not, to test those hypotheses, and then to plan for the future on the basis of their findings.

Organizing raw data on both clinician and client so that they become coherent and usable sets up the supervisor and supervisee for a more meaningful and efficient conference. Also, when supervisors analyze clinician behavior, they are modeling an approach that is transferable to the clinician's analysis of client behavior. Later, as they study behaviors in the supervisory interaction, they will find the same techniques applicable. Such analysis shows supervisees a method for functioning within the supervisory process. They are learning how to use the scientific approach, observing that it applies to both the clini-

cal and supervisory processes and acquiring a valuable self-analysis technique.

Analysis—particularly joint analysis—should contribute in a major way to meeting the expectations of supervisees for fair and rational feedback and evaluation, because evaluation will be derived from objective data and supervisees will be involved in analyzing and evaluating their own behavior.

When analysis is done jointly, it offers supervisees some protection from the subjective judgments made by supervisors, emphasizing behavior rather than the person. As a result, there may be less defensiveness, which in turn enhances communication. Supervisees also participate in measuring progress toward their objectives. If well planned and executed, the analysis will enable supervisees to function as colleagues in the conference (Andersen, 1980).

Reconstructing or rehashing the clinical session during conferences is the antithesis of analysis. Note this statement from a tape of an actual conference:

> Well, one thing—he got out of his chair and then I couldn't get him to do anything. He was OK while he was sitting. So I was waiting for him to sit down. I said, "OK, I'll wait." He asked me something about my glasses and I answered him. I shouldn't have done that. Then he started talking about his mother's glasses. Finally, I asked him again to sit down. So he sat down but when I asked him to make his sound he just sat.

If this behavior had been what Cogan labeled a critical incident—that is, a one-time occurrence that affected the child's learning—it might have been appropriate to report this lengthy rehash of the client's behavior. In this particular conference, however, a similar monologue continued in excruciating detail for over half the conference, occupying nearly half as much time as the actual events. The supervisor followed it with, "Well, why don't you...next time." This exemplifies Culatta and Seltzer's (1976, 1977) findings. They found that 61% of all strategy statements were made by supervisors following provision of observation and information (i.e., reconstruction of the clinical session) by the supervisee. The pointlessness of the discussion in this example is underscored by the fact that the supervisor had observed the entire session and was aware of what had happened! Had the session been submitted to some type of organized data collection and analysis, the supervisor and supervisee could have quantified the data on the basis of certain patterns and interactions. The provision of a solution to the problem by the supervisor deprived the supervisee of the opportunity to problem-solve and draw inferences from the data.

If the analysis component is not taken seriously or, worse yet, not understood by supervisors who proceed directly to feedback, conferences will likely continue to consist of a mass of raw data or anecdotal reports used essentially to unnecessarily reconstruct the clinical session, evaluations communicated directly to the supervisee, or a collection of trivial items that have no importance in the learning process.

PURPOSES OF ANALYSIS IN SUPERVISION

The major purposes of analysis are rooted in the works of Cogan (1973), Goldhammer (1969), Goldhammer and colleagues (1980), and Acheson and Gall (1980), who were the first to verbalize the concept of analysis as an **essential** part of the supervisory process. One purpose is to distill the raw data to a point where it becomes coherent, manageable, and usable for the feedback component. Another is to organize the observational data in such a way that it can be used to draw conclusions and make rational judgments about what happened in the teaching–learning process. It then becomes the basis for further planning.

In discussing analysis of data collected on the behaviors of teachers and students in the classroom, Cogan (1973) listed the objectives of analysis:

1. Determining if objectives have been met
2. Identifying salient patterns in the teacher's behavior

3. Identifying unanticipated learning by the student
4. Identifying critical incidents in the interaction (teacher behaviors that occur once but that appear to significantly affect the learning that takes place or the relationship between teacher and student)
5. Organizing the data to determine what was learned
6. Determining if what was planned really was carried out
7. Developing a database for the rest of the supervision program

Cogan urged careful examination of interactions between the behaviors of students and teachers. In addition, he discussed the identification of process learning, which he identified as "learning how to learn." Goldhammer (1969) and Goldhammer and colleagues (1980) concentrated on the notion that all human behavior is patterned and stressed the point that it is the **cumulative** effects of those patterns that are important to the learning that occurs. Therefore, supervisors should concentrate on identifying *salient* patterns, not unusual or incidental variables. The aim of supervision, they said, is to strengthen, extinguish, or modify the salient behaviors.

METHODS OF ANALYSIS

Analysis may be performed by the supervisor, the supervisee, or cooperatively by the two (Cogan, 1973). Each fulfills a need at various times along the continuum of supervision. The new Standard V for the Certificate of Clinical Competence in speech-language pathology (effective 1/1/05) mandates a combination of formative and summative assessments of knowledge and skills. "Formative assessment is the ongoing measurement during educational preparation for the purpose of improving student learning. Summative assessment is the comprehensive examination of learning outcomes at the culmination of educational preparation" (ASHA, 2000a). Practicum experiences must encompass the breadth of the current scope of practice and be sufficient for competent entry-level practice. Formative assessment of clinical skills necessitates observations, analyses, and evaluations of an individual's clinical competencies by all supervisors of that student. Students must also have analytical abilities. Specifically, they must be able "to *analyze* (italics added), synthesize, and evaluate information about prevention, assessment, and intervention over the range of differences and disorders specified in Standard III-D."

Analysis by Supervisors

At the beginning of the supervisory experience, the supervisee's clinical repertoire may be a blank slate to the supervisor. If the supervisor is to determine the salient features of this repertoire, it will require a broad look at data and a dedicated effort to determine baseline. Supervisors must be cautious and avoid looking solely for patterns that fit their personal prejudices or pet assumptions. They must constantly strive to keep in mind that they are concerned about the *documented effect* of the behaviors. Initially, then, the task of the supervisor is to examine the data carefully, looking for patterns, critical incidents, behaviors related to session objectives or plans, the interactions between clinician and client, and the visible learning effects. This is *not a time for judgments*. Evaluation will come later after conclusions are drawn and inferences made. For supervisors who have been accustomed to providing direct evaluation, this will require a great amount of restraint at first.

At the Evaluation-Feedback Stage, little or no analysis is done; supervisors provide evaluations based on their perceptions and judgments. This is the prominent characteristic of the style used at this stage—judgmental statements from the supervisor's "square box." As supervisors move into the Transitional Stage, a collaborative style is apparent. Questions posed prior to and after the observation by supervisees and supervisors serve as the basis for quantifying and categorizing behaviors and interactions. For example, consider that data collected by the clinician during a session revealed 40% correct responses, 15% close approxima-

tions, and 45% incorrect responses. The supervisor's data revealed that correct responses and close approximations were intermittently followed by verbal praise; incorrect responses were consistently followed by "OK" and a subsequent model. Depending on client and clinician goals, a number of additional questions would be formulated to guide analysis. For example:

1. How many times did the clinician model, expand, instruct?
2. What clinician behaviors preceded correct responses, close approximations, incorrect responses?
3. What was the nature of the task(s) used to elicit responses?
4. What was the client's response rate (number of responses per minute)?
5. What was the content of the directions and instructions?
6. What client behaviors followed certain clinician behaviors?

Once additional analysis is completed, supervisors and supervisees can begin to draw some conclusions, make some inferences, and formulate hypotheses to be tested in future sessions.

Introducing Analysis to Supervisees

It is imperative that the supervisee be involved in analysis as soon as possible. Initially, supervisors will likely need to teach these skills. Clinicians are trained to observe client behavior but are rarely taught to extend this observation to their own behaviors. Teaching procedures will depend on the supervisee's level. Supervisees may be asked to read certain material about data collection and analysis (e.g., Brookshire, 1967; Mowrer, 1977). Practice using a particular method or system for coding clinical behaviors and interactions is essential (Boone & Prescott, 1972; Camarata & Rassi, 1991; Lougeay-Mottiger, Harris, & Stillman, 1987; Schubert, Miner, & Till, 1973). Supervisors may opt to demonstrate the analysis procedure after the observation by doing it alone at first and presenting the analyzed data as feedback during the conference. At some point, supervisees must be involved. The supervisor may present data recorded during an observation to the clinician prior to the conference so that the clinician can do the analysis and bring the information to the conference. A supervisor may choose to perform the analysis *with* the supervisee, again modeling the behaviors that contribute to the analysis. Gillam, Stike-Roussos, and Anderson (1990) demonstrated that joint analysis effected positive changes in supervisees' clinical behaviors. Supervisors may use, or suggest that the supervisee use, interaction analysis systems and their summary forms to learn how to identify categories and patterns of clinical behavior (Brasseur & Jimenez, 1994; Francis, 1993). In a study of two supervisees with 200+ clock hours, who prior to the study had not self-analyzed, Camarata (1992) concluded that "there was something inherent in observing and analyzing their own work that allows for more productive evaluation and change" (p. 48).

The literature reveals that an initial client-centered focus is typical of *beginning* clinicians and that they must develop adequate clinical skills and a certain level of comfort in interactions with their clients before they will be able to be involved in data collection and analysis (Brasseur & Jimenez, 1994; Dowling, 2001; Francis, 1993). Beginning clinicians are focused on planning appropriate activities for therapy sessions, finding adequate materials, writing progress notes, and just making it through a session. This is likely to be the case for any supervisee in a new assignment who has learned neither how to self-analyze nor the importance of analyzing prior to evaluating one's behaviors. They are not ready to be active participants in the supervisory process. In addition, there may need to be some sort of contingency for completing assigned analyses (Dowling, Sbaschnig, & Williams, 1991) or a period of time when commitments are written (Shapiro & Anderson, 1988). The supervisor may need to be direct and establish professional development goals for the novice supervisee (Dowling, 2001; Lubinsky & Hildebrand, 1996). Yet it appears that there must be some method for facilitating ownership and a commitment to change

before novice supervisees will care about setting goals and collecting and analyzing data (Brasseur & Jimenez, 1994, 1996). The supervisor also must provide timely feedback for the supervisee about their performance in self-analysis (Freeman, 1982; Maloney, 1994).

Beginning supervisees need to learn that there is a core of categories of clinical behaviors that are important to most clinical interactions—recording and charting client behaviors, determining types and schedules of reinforcement, giving instructions, establishing types of cues and feedback to provide to clients, staying on task, and other behaviors appropriate to the specific client. Goldberg (1997) described two types of foundation skills—technical and process—that "should be learned by new clinicians, preferably before they begin therapy" (p. 93). The technical skills are divided into four categories containing 47 techniques and behaviors. In discussing fundamental process skills, Goldberg (1997) noted that trust is essential to a therapeutic relationship and described 11 categories of skills containing 58 techniques and behaviors that will contribute to the development of trust. In addition, Goldberg described higher-level technical and process skills that are needed to demonstrate clinical competence. These skills certainly could provide a focus for clinicians beyond the Evaluation-Feedback stage on the continuum. Hegde and Davis (1995) provided a number of methods that are vital to effective therapy in speech-language pathology and could operationalize important categories for supervisees. Whatever framework is selected, the supervisor and supervisee will need to establish the supervisee's baseline relative to selected categories. Mawdsley's (1985b) self-assessment instrument, KISS (discussed in Chapter 6) is a useful tool for beginning clinicians because of its simplicity. It is helpful for learning to assign behaviors to certain categories. Goldberg (1997) also provides a number of checklists that could be helpful in establishing baseline and tracking change over time. From here, the analysis proceeds to a less-structured search for other patterns that affect the clinical interaction.

If interaction analysis systems such as the Boone and Prescott system (1972) or ABC (Schubert, Miner, & Till, 1973) have been used, the summary forms that accompany them facilitate analysis. If other systems are used that do not have summary forms, they can easily be constructed. As previously noted, interaction analysis systems do not cover all possible categories, interactions, or behaviors, so supervisors must identify categories for other data they have collected.

Whatever strategy is selected to initiate the supervisee in analysis, the supervisor's objective should always be increased responsibility on the part of the supervisee for self-analysis. If supervisees are involved initially with their supervisors and then gradually assume responsibility for themselves, they will develop skills with which they can continue to be self-analytical even when they are working alone or with no supervision. Supervisors who do all the analysis for supervisees inhibit and prevent their learning. Similarly, the supervisor who uses the analyzed data to develop all the conclusions and inferences and— even worse—to evaluate and provide the strategies, is abrogating the responsibilities of supervision. As they move along the continuum, the balance of supervisor/supervisee responsibility for analysis should progress toward increased supervisee participation.

Organizing the Data for Feedback

Once data have been collected by either supervisor or supervisee, they are then categorized. Interactions are analyzed to determine the amount of client learning that has occurred, the clinical competencies apparent in the interactions, and so on. Client and clinician behaviors to be strengthened, extinguished, or modified are identified. Decisions are made about achievement of objectives.

Goldhammer and colleagues (1980) discussed at length the principles of organizing the data to determine patterns related to learning. Although they stressed the importance of being able to demonstrate consequences of behavior in the data and the ability to support the patterns on the basis of theory, they also said that patterns may be selected simply because one has hunches about them. The latter principle is discouraged because it is less persuasive, most likely wrong, and implies that "hunching one's way through supervisory practice" (p. 88) is acceptable.

Cogan (1973) suggested first analyzing the data on the behavior and learning of the student (client) and relating both to the objectives to determine if they have been met; then, analyzing the teacher's (clinician's) behaviors and forming hypotheses about the relationships between the behaviors and the learning. He also stressed the importance of dealing with interaction, not isolated parts. Some patterns will be more obvious than others, some will be more important than others, and some will reflect biases and inaccurate perceptions.

Cogan (1973) suggested that **critical incidents** should receive a high priority in the analysis because the one-time occurrence that has a profound impact on an individual's learning affects outcomes. Cogan's examples with regard to teaching involve aggressive teacher behaviors, behaviors related to discipline, and incidences that have positive consequences—where students gain insights that have lasting effects. Certain skills for managing clients affect the clinical interaction and may constitute a critical incident. On the positive side, the clinician's ability to capitalize on spontaneous learning—for example, the sudden insight of the client or the unexpected accomplishment of a task—might be a critical incident that, once identified, the supervisor and supervisee may want to convert to a strategy.

The supervisor may very well have seen important patterns of behavior emerge during the observation and recorded them. If not, analysis is where the search begins. Data are perused, categories of behavior are quantified, and consequences of certain behaviors are identified (i.e., when the clinician did X, the client did Y). Some questions to be asked in analyzing data were listed previously (p. 194). Additional areas of interest in analysis might include clarity of instructions/directions, task difficulty, pacing, clinician talk-time, turn-taking in group therapy, number/ variety/creativity of activities, client response rate, client self-evaluations, and so on. Gradually, the detective work will yield results and the data will fall into place. Out of this quantification and categorization, both the supervisor and supervisee begin to draw some conclusions, make some inferences, and state some hypotheses to be tested. As treatment efficacy and clinical effectiveness studies reveal, there is no single variable/ strategy/technique or simple cause–effect solution that results in a perfect session. When session goals are or are not achieved, it is important to examine *all* the plausible reasons for success or failure.

Consider the following scenario. Session data reveal that 60% of the client's responses were incorrect. Incorrect responses increased as the session progressed. Two patterns are immediately obvious in the clinician's behavior: (1) he or she positively reinforced 35% of the incorrect responses and (2) direction giving and modeling for all productions (accurate and inaccurate) followed the same pattern throughout the session. Twenty percent of the time, the client had observable nonverbal reactions (facial grimaces, head shaking, or sighing) to his own incorrect productions. The clinician did not respond to these reactions but presented the task again in the same way. The nature of individual tasks and task difficulty obviously need to be analyzed. Consequences for correct responses and frequency with which they were applied are among the other variables that should be examined. Additional questions might emerge as the data are analyzed.

What follows such a session will depend on the dyad's place on the continuum. In the Direct-Active Style at the Evaluation-Feedback stage, feedback will be delivered by the supervisor in writing or during the conference and consist of value judgments or strategies the supervisee is directed to use in the next session.

In the Collaborative Style, there are a variety of ways to use the collected data. During the early part of the Transitional Stage, the supervisor will complete the analysis by categorizing and quantifying the behaviors, quantifying types of interactions, comparing clinician behaviors with client responses, summarizing client nonverbal reactions, and other methods. Data and the analysis are presented to the supervisee in the conference. As an alternative, the analysis might be done jointly to demonstrate the process. A bit further along the continuum, the supervisor will give the analyzed data, and later the raw data, to the clinician for study prior to the conference. At whatever point it seems appropriate, the clinician will begin recording data from tapes in preparation for the later stage of self-analysis.

In the beginning stages of analysis, the clinician may be assisted by using a technique that has a built-in method for analysis (e.g., KISS, Boone-Prescott, and ABC) or by certain questions that provide a focus and some structure. For example, "What evidence is there that your objectives were met or not met?" or, "Can you see anything in your models and directions that related to the client's responses?" The supervisor may want to have supervisees examine data with a wide-angle approach or in terms of long-range objectives.

Finally, as clinicians progress along the continuum, they assume more responsibility for data collection and self-analysis. Supervisors and supervisees analyze data separately. The analyses are brought to the conference where they become the basis for the conference agenda.

One may ask, "Why take the time to do all this when it is so much easier to tell them and get on to other matters?" First, self-analysis is essential to the competencies listed at the beginning of this chapter. Second, learners must be actively involved in their own learning. Third, although teaching self-analysis skills may take more time than giving direct evaluations or feedback, over time there will be "pay-offs" in terms of the supervisee's increasing independence and ability to analyze and problem-solve. Fourth, time should not be the prime consideration. It is assumed that if supervisors and supervisees are assigned to each other for a learning experience that *some* time is spent together. The question then becomes one of the *quality* of that time. Fifth, teaching these skills contributes to accountability in supervision. Analyzed data can be compared across sessions and clinician growth can be accurately documented, not "guestimated." More accurate hypotheses can be made about methodologies and their results. Sixth, a skill is being taught in the analysis stage that clinicians must have if they are to continue to grow and be self-sufficient, competent clinicians. Further, this skill is absolutely essential when clinicians become supervisors themselves.

DETERMINING THE CONTENT OF THE SUPERVISORY CONFERENCE

One purpose of analysis is to determine the content of the conference. Analysis that really reduces the data and places a priority on items to be discussed in the conference leads to an efficient, organized, and focused conference. It is the prelude to the conference. Here is another place where components overlap—analysis and planning flowing together.

The content of the conference will be discussed in the next chapter but the possibilities for topics are almost limitless. In addition to general topics, which may vary by situation, the infinite amount of behavior observed in most clinical sessions makes it reasonable to think that not everything observed or identified through analysis can be dealt with in the conference, although it often seems that participants in conferences try to do just that. The premise here is that conferences or other forms of feedback must be *planned*. Anderson (1988) in the first edition of this text stated that her observations of many hours of tapes of conferences made it obvious that conferences frequently are unplanned, unfocused, and disorganized and contain an unbelievable amount of trivia. Analysis does not ensure the elimination of trivia—trivia are trivia, even when quantified. But analysis does make it easier to establish higher priorities for the discussion of some events or issues than others.

Three criteria for selecting items for the conference from all the patterns were provided by Goldhammer and colleagues (1980).

- *Saliency.* The frequency with which behaviors are found in the data, their significance, their relationship to theory, their relationship to other patterns or to commonalties among teachers (clinicians), and the relationship to what the supervisee sees as important or has requested to discuss.
- *Accessibility of patterns for treatment.* The patterns related to emotionally charged issues that may be too threatening for the supervisee.
- *Fewness.* Because time in conferences is limited and supervisees may only be able to assimilate a certain amount of input, patterns of behavior can be selected or rejected on the basis of certain criteria. These criteria include easy and clear identification of patterns in the data, the subsuming of some patterns under others, the similarity or difference to other patterns, the emotional content of the patterns, the amount of time needed to cover the patterns adequately, and the orderly transition from one issue to another. In other words, each pattern of behavior does not stand alone. It is related to others.

There are other important decisions to be made during the analysis that directly influence the content and organization of the conference. The foundation for an organized, problem-solving, meaningful conference is built during the analysis. Questions that must be asked are:

Are there data on clinician strengths as well as weaknesses?

Are there appropriate data to measure the accomplishment of objectives?

Have clinicians participated in the analysis to an extent that will enable them to have meaningful input into structuring the conference?

How much should they be expected to participate in the analysis?

Are there enough data for an analysis? How much data are enough?

Although there is some indication that three to five minutes of observation and data collection are sufficient to represent the entire session (Boone & Prescott, 1972; Schubert & Laird, 1975), these findings came from the use of specific interaction analysis systems with limited numbers of behaviors. The same kind of information does not exist for other kinds of clinical analysis. The answer to this final question may depend on what clinical skills are being addressed.

Is the information from the analysis to be considered as infallible? Will there be times when it is inconclusive? Will there be crisis times—or even noncrisis times—when the analyzed data will need to be discarded in favor of some more urgent issues? Is it possible to miss some important issues through the effort to be analytical?

Supervisors need to be sensitive to the fact that overutilization of analyzed data can lead to a conference that is too structured.

There are many factors that need to be considered in planning the agenda for the conference. The use of the analyzed data is only one facet, but it is an important one in promoting a scientific approach to supervision and in helping supervisees become aware of their own behavior and their own needs.

EVALUATION

"What about evaluation?" the reader is probably asking at this point. Is it eliminated entirely? Is it legitimate for supervisors to provide a direct evaluation? Certainly; in fact, it is the responsibility of supervisors to evaluate *at appropriate times.* It is unrealistic and unprofessional to assume that evaluation should never happen; it is not the intent of the writers to imply that. As stated previously, standards for CCC in speech-language pathology (effective 1/1/05) mandate formative assessments. Thus, periodic evaluation must be built into each practicum experience. It is also a part of the clinical fellowship and likely a part of employment in any setting. Additionally, studies about what supervisees want and expect indicate a desire for critique, identification of weaknesses, and guidance about specific techniques. Thus, expectations may not be met unless supervisees (1) receive some evaluation or (2) understand the reasons why the supervisor is encouraging self-evaluation and not providing it all themselves.

When the supervisor goes directly from the observation to evaluation, it should be done rationally, however. Clinicians who are at the Evaluation-Feedback stage and are unable to participate in joint- or self-analysis can be assumed to need some direction, which must come through evaluation and direct feedback. If certain behaviors have been identified as needing specific attention and it has been agreed that the supervisor will provide a rating of these occurrences of the behavior, this type of feedback is essential. Sometimes the use of direct evaluation is a more efficient procedure and certain features of the situation make it reasonable to employ direct evaluation: the seriousness of the impact of the behavior on the client may demand immediate evaluative feedback; the behavior may be too trivial or too obvious to justify any lengthy analysis procedure; the behavior may be one that is being dealt with on an ongoing basis and the clinician may need only a reminder; or the significance of the issue may be too complex for the clinician at the moment either intellectually or emotionally. Supervisors must use their best judgment here as to when to provide direct evaluation as related to teaching or when to involve the supervisee in self-analysis or self-evaluation. The important point of the decision should be, "What will the supervisee learn and how will she or he learn it best?"

The topic of feedback will be dealt with in greater depth in the next chapter on Integrating. The broader topic of formal, organizationally based evaluation is another issue, and is included in Chapter 10, Accountability. Formative evaluations should be scheduled periodically during a practicum and should include data collected and analyzed to substantiate ratings. An evaluation tool that could be used in completing formative evaluations is found in Appendix 7A.

SUMMARY

The Analysis component of the supervisory process, like the Observation component, is a point where the scientific approach is essential. It is a time when the supervisor and supervisee utilize the recorded data to hypothesize about what has happened and to plan subsequent events. Analysis is not synonymous with evaluation, but it is a necessary step that leads to objective, disciplined judgments by the supervisor and to independence through self-analysis and self-evaluation by the supervisee.

RESEARCH ISSUES AND QUESTIONS

As stated in Chapter 3, the purpose of the research sections at the end of some of the chapters in this text is not to provide an exhaustive review of the studies that have been completed to date. Rather, it is an attempt to highlight some of what we currently know from research and to suggest some directions for future research. Our hope is that it will stimulate interest and collaboration among supervisors and supervisees in universities, schools, and medical settings and lead to publications of new investigations that demonstrate the effectiveness of clinical supervision.

Some research has been completed that has examined the impact of joint analysis and self-analysis of therapy on supervisee's clinical behaviors. Results reveal that clinicians can develop an awareness of their abilities through the analysis of their own audio- or videotape recordings (Boone &

Stech, 1970; Schubert & Gudmundson, 1976). Studies of inexperienced student clinicians have demonstrated that they are able to learn to systematically score audio- or videotapes of their sessions after a few hours of training (Brasseur & Jimenez, 1994; Camarata, 1992; Camarata & Rassi, 1991; Francis, 1993; Lougeay-Mottiger, Harris, & Stillman, 1987) but the impact of training on clinical performance has varied. In the Camarata (Camarata & Rossi, 1991; Camarata, 1992) investigations, clinicians who scored videos of their own treatment sessions improved the accuracy of targeted clinical behaviors whereas about half of the students in the Brasseur and Jimenez (1994) study, but none of the clinicians in Francis' study, increased their target behaviors. Some of the variables that may account for the differences in findings include:

- The length of time in which self-analyses were completed (whole term vs. part of the semester)
- The complexity of the analysis (two or three behaviors vs. an interaction analysis system)
- Feedback on or evaluation of the completed analysis
- Consequences for completing the assigned analysis and completing it on time

Camarata (1992) questioned whether the positive effects could be achieved if supervisees were to score a portion of the therapy session rather than the entire session. In a follow-up study of the same subjects (1994), Brasseur and Jimenez (1996) concluded that some didactic training in the supervisory process might have been an important prerequisite to self-analysis. At minimum, supervisors probably need to share their philosophy of supervision as well as their expectations and goals for the supervisory process with supervisees if supervisee attitudes and behaviors are to change. Each of these discussion points would make interesting questions for future research. Further, all of the bulleted variables could be systematically manipulated in future studies with supervisees who have different levels of experience and who are at different stages of their careers (e.g., students, clinical fellows, SLPs in medical and school settings, etc.).

Another aspect of self-analysis that is important is that of commitment. Shapiro and Anderson (1989) found that clinicians demonstrated greater completion of commitments when written commitments were introduced early in the supervisory relationship and gradually faded. Written commitments proved more effective for beginning clinicians than for experienced clinicians. Experienced clinicians completed commitments when no written agreement was required and seemed to benefit from less structured, collegial interactions. Maloney (1994) investigated the influence of clinician journal writing on interpersonal communications skills and the affective nature of the relationship with clients. Lubinsky and Hildebrand (1996) examined the impact of journal writing in facilitating the attainment of personal goals in practicum. With these latter two studies, some of the same variables that were noted previously (target behaviors or skills, time, feedback, contingencies for completion) seemed

to influence the results, and thus would be interesting to explore in future investigations.

Gillam, Strike-Roussos, and Anderson (1990) demonstrated the functional relationship between joint analysis of session data and desired changes in clinicians' therapy behaviors. This experimental study introduced yet another variable to consider. Specifically, it may be important to ease clinicians into the process of self-analysis by **jointly** developing observation and data analysis strategies. It would be interesting to compare clinicians who engage in joint analysis with those who independently complete self-analyses.

The competencies listed at the beginning of this chapter also provide important areas for research. Supervisors and supervisees could use Casey's instrument (Appendix 4G) to calculate discrepancy scores and devise plans to minimize the gap. The effectiveness of the techniques contained in plans could be scientifically explored to address the validity of the competencies across different work settings and levels of supervisee experience and expertise.

Formative Evaluation Tool

This instrument has been developed as a tool for clinical educators to monitor the ongoing clinical development of individual student clinicians. Complete skill ratings at least two times during a practicum experience (midterm and final) on this sheet. Color code the time segments (e.g., green ink for midterm and red ink for final).

Student clinician _____

Semester _____

Previous experience/clock hours accrued prior to current semester _____

Supervisor _____

Practicum site _____

Number of clients _____   Ages of clients _____

Types of problems. Circle all that apply:

A   Articulation

F   Fluency

VR   Voice and resonance, including respiration and phonation

L   Receptive and expressive language (phonology, morphology, syntax, semantics, and prag-
          matics). **Indicate modality: sp**eaking listening, **r**eading, **w**riting, **m**anual

H   Hearing, including the impact on speech and language

SW   Swallowing (oral, pharyngeal, esophageal, and related functions)

COG Cognitive aspects of communication (attention, memory, sequencing, problem solving,
          executive functioning)

SOC Social aspects of communication (including challenging behavior, ineffective social
          skills, lack of communication opportunities)

Communication Modalities. Circle all that apply:

Oral   Manual   Augmentative and alternative communication techniques   Assistive technologies

Clinical Skills Evaluation

	1	2–3–4	5–6–7	8–9–10	NA
Conducts screening and prevention procedures					
Collects case history information					
Integrates case history information with information from clients, family, caregivers, teachers, relevant others, and other professionals					
Selects and administers appropriate evaluation procedures (e.g., behavioral observations, standardized and nonstandardized tests and instrumental procedures)					
Adapts evaluation procedures to meet client needs					
Interprets, integrates, and synthesizes all information to develop DX and make appropriate recommendations for TX					
Completes administrative and reporting functions necessary to support evaluation					
Refers clients for appropriate services					
INTERVENTION					
Develops appropriate TX plans with measurable and achievable goals that meet clients' needs					
Collaborates with clients and relevant others in planning TX					
Implements TX plans. Involves clients and relevant others in the TX process					
Selects or develops and uses appropriate materials and instrumentation for prevention and intervention					
Measures and evaluates clients' performance and progress					
Modifies TX plans, strategies, materials, or instrumentation as appropriate to meet the needs of clients					
Completes administrative and reporting functions necessary to support intervention					
Identifies and refers clients for services as appropriate					

	1	2–3–4	5–6–7	8–9–10	NA
INTERACTION AND PERSONAL QUALITIES					
Communicates effectively, recognizing the needs, values, preferred mode of communication, and cultural/linguistic background of the client, family, caregivers, and relevant others					
Collaborates with other professionals in case management					
Provides counseling regarding communication and swallowing disorders to clients, family, caregivers, and relevant others					
Adheres to ASHA Code of Ethics and behaves professionally					

Ratings

Users should refer to Figures 3 (quantitative) and 4 (qualitative) in the W-PACC for matching clinician behaviors to numerical values.

1   Specific directions from the supervisor does *not* alter unsatisfactory performance

2–3–4   Needs specific directions and/or demonstrations from the supervisor to perform effectively

5–6–7   Needs general directions from supervisor to perform effectively

8–9–10   Consistently demonstrates the ability to effectively function at high levels of independence. Makes changes when appropriate.

NA   Does not apply

Supervisor's Signature _____ Date _____

Clinician's Signature _____ Date _____

Please return this to the university clinic director.

CHAPTER EIGHT

INTEGRATING THE COMPONENTS

It is a matter of some curiosity that, with a few exceptions (Mosher and Purpel, 1972; Goldhammer, 1969), a reader of supervisory texts is rarely confronted by what really seems to happen in the course of the inevitable meetings that take place between the parties to the supervisory process.
—Blumberg, (1980, p. 1)

At some point, everything that happens in the supervisory process—the preparation, the observation, the analysis—must be integrated through some form of communication between supervisor and supervisee. This typically occurs during a conference. Communication about the tasks and associated competencies for effective supervision (ASHA, 1985b) usually occurs during the conference as well. Traditionally, the conference was viewed as a time when the supervisor provided feedback to the supervisee about the observation. This feedback was perceived to be something of a one-way street—from supervisor to supervisee. This is characteristic of the Direct-Active Style. For the Collaborative or Consultative Styles, Anderson (1988) stated that the broader term of *integrating* seems more appropriate than *feedback* in describing the interaction that takes place when supervisor and supervisee meet. Although feedback will be one aspect of the integration component, it is here where the components of Understanding, Planning, Observing, and Analyzing will merge. Since those components have been discussed previously, the content of this chapter is related to the communication that takes place about them and

their results and suggests a richer synthesis of ideas than the old concept of supervisor-to-supervisee feedback. The integration component includes other activities such as planning, problem solving, analyzing, and many other topics necessary to maintain a profitable relationship. The conference itself will not only include feedback about the clinical session but also discussion of procedural topics such as administrative issues or report writing, the supervisory process, professional issues, personal concerns, and general information relevant to the development of all participants. Task 8—Interacting with the supervisee in planning, executing, and analyzing supervisory conferences—and its nine competencies (ASHA, 1985b) are focused on the conference. The competencies describe the supervisor's ability to assist and involve the supervisee in: determining when a conference should be scheduled (8.1), planning a supervisory conference agenda (8.2), jointly establishing a conference agenda (8.3), joint discussion of previously identified clinical or supervisory data or issues (8.4), making commitments for changes in clinical behavior (8.8), and ongoing analysis of supervisory interactions (8.9). They also describe the

205

supervisor's ability to interact with the supervisee in a manner that facilitates the supervisee's self-exploration and problem solving (8.5), adjust conference content based on supervisee's level of training and experience (8.6), and encourage and maintain supervisee motivation for continuing self-growth (8.7).

In examining the other tasks and competencies (Appendix 3A), it becomes apparent that many of the competencies are an integral part of the self-exploring and problem-solving necessary for growth. Consider these, for example:

3.3   Ability to assist the supervisee in providing rationale for assessment procedures

4.2   Ability to facilitate an integration of research findings in client management.

4.3   Ability to assist the supervisee in providing rationale for treatment procedures

These particular competencies are necessary for problem-solving and evidence-based practice.

Some additional competencies that require self-exploration and problem solving include:

4.8   Ability to assist the supervisee in integrating documented client and clinician change to evaluate progress and specify future recommendations

6.5   Ability to assist the supervisee in revising plans for client management based on data obtained

7.3   Ability to assist the supervisee in organizing records to facilitate easy retrieval of information concerning clinical and supervisory interactions

9.2   Ability to assist the supervisee in the description and measurement of his or her progress and achievement

SCHEDULED CONFERENCES

Competency 8.1 focuses on scheduling conferences. For some time, conferences have been the most commonly used structure for communicating feedback in professions where there is applied training—education, social work, counseling psychotherapy, and certainly speech-language pathology. *Regularity* is a critical factor. Geoffrey (1973) reported that 96% of the 111 facilities responding to her survey conducted regularly scheduled conferences. Of the 501 supervisors studied by Schubert and Aitchison (1975), 98% reported the use of posttherapy conferences. The importance of regular conferences continues to be emphasized (Brasseur, 1989; Dowling, 2001; McCrea, 1994; Strike-Roussos, 1988) and is a basic expectation of supervisees (Dowling & Wittkopp, 1982; Larson, 1982; Tihen, 1984). Dowling (2001) emphasized that the "catch me when you can" method is ineffective—it "will negatively affect the establishment of trust, the quality of the interpersonal relationship, and the effectiveness of the conference" (p. 128). Dowling suggested that weekly conferences be scheduled for students in training. Clinical Fellows and professional staff may not need, nor may they want, weekly conferences, but there needs to be some regularity and a definite schedule (e.g., monthly) if the conferences are to be productive and facilitate professional growth.

COMMUNICATION IN THE CONFERENCE

The implementation of the continuum of supervision is dependent on the communication skills of both supervisor and supervisee. The ability to be clear, specific, and concrete is essential to sharing feedback, perceptions, expectations, planning, discussion of data, and to determining the effectiveness of the supervisory interaction. Further, the supervisor's ability to encourage supervisee participation in self-exploration and problem solving during the conference is essential to movement along the continuum. Supervisors need to monitor their talk-time to prevent dominating the conference. At times supervisees will need to plan some of their verbal behavior to achieve clear, concise discourse.

Clarity in Communication

Nothing is more powerful and frequently distressing to speakers than to see their verbal behaviors written in script. Even some of the most proficient language users are horrified by their excessive and irrelevant fillers (*OK, you know, um, er, uh*), redundancies, fragmented sentences, and incorrect syntax or grammar. Consider the following excerpt from a supervisee in an actual conference:

> Um, I think that—I guess that some or a lot of— well, you know—I think a lot of the words we've worked on—not, you know—I think it's near the, it's the same type of sound that we've been working on—you know—the voiceless—well, it's not a stop plosive, you know—um the other sounds we um—you know—worked on were stop plosives but the poorer articulation was— you know—would be /s/ you know—pretty much the same, I think.

This was in response to a supervisor question asking how to proceed with the client. This type of utterance may be the result of several conditions—the supervisee's natural lack of facility with the language, anxiety, lack of preparation, poorly stated objectives, and other reasons.

Supervisors are not immune to such cluttered and imprecise verbalizations, as any number of conference transcripts reveal. Individually, they produce confusion and sometimes frustration for the listener. Multiplied for an entire conference or a whole semester, they are inefficient, time wasting, and nonproductive.

Listening to an audiotape or viewing a videotape of a conference early on in the supervisory relationship will likely reveal many types of behaviors that are obvious targets for objectives for supervisors and supervisees. The basis of such scattered, unclear communication may be in the planning and analysis components. If the agenda is planned carefully and the plan followed (8.2, 8.3, 8.4), there may be less rambling. If that planning is combined with skill in analysis, the data can be presented clearly and concisely.

One role of supervisors is to improve the communication behavior of their supervisees and themselves (10.2). Not only can improvement in verbal and nonverbal skills increase the efficiency and effectiveness of the conference, it should carry over to the clinical process. The supervisee who cannot clarify issues in the conference probably cannot give clear, precise directions to clients either, and may fill clinical sessions with unnecessary verbiage.

Strategies for this task must be carefully planned. Supervisees may perceive their verbal style as a personal characteristic that no one has a right to change. That may be true with regard to an individual's private life; when it becomes an issue in terms of professional interactions, it is another story. Anderson (1988) reported on a student in a supervision practicum who demonstrated a voice and manner of speaking that was coy, passive, and flirtatious, and that conveyed an attitude of dependence and immaturity. In actuality, the student was a highly intelligent, mature, capable professional. The behaviors were easily identified by Anderson and the student and objectives were set for modifying them. The student was highly motivated and made significant changes. In her final conference, she shared, "My friends tell me I don't sound like a little girl anymore."

Some of the techniques for collecting and analyzing data in the clinical process are applicable to the supervisory process. For example, one method for decreasing the verbosity of a supervisor or supervisee is to complete verbatim transcripts of a portion of a conference tape. The individual who is redundant *ad nauseum* can then rewrite the transcribed text in a clear, concise style. This individual soon becomes conscious of the behavior in subsequent conversations and better able to change it.

From the counseling literature (Carkhuff & Truax, 1964), four facilitative dimensions in interpersonal interactions have been identified. McCrea (1980) adapted them for use in analyzing supervisors' behavior in speech-language pathology and audiology (Appendix 9C). One of these dimensions is *concreteness,* and it is relevant to the issue of clarity discussed here. Concreteness means being specific, and the scale used for its measurement ranges from the lowest Level 1—supervisor statement that is extremely vague, causes confusion, and greatly detracts from the flow of the discussion—to the highest Level 7—supervisor statements must be specific with an example and a rationale. Roberts and Smith (1982) indicated that supervisors do not give rationales and justification for their statements, and McCrea (1980) found that concreteness in supervisor behavior in the conferences she studied occurred below the minimally facilitative level of functioning needed for self-exploration. Because examples and rationales clarify topics being discussed, the findings of these studies suggest that supervisors need to examine their own conferences. Further, supervisors are expected to model professional conduct (Task 12) and what better way to induct supervisees into evidence-based practice than to provide rationales that are grounded in research.

SKILLS FOR FACILITATING COMMUNICATION IN THE CONFERENCE

Any of a multitude of books on counseling, the helping relationship, and interviewing contain descriptions of skills that facilitate communication (Brammer, 1985; Condon, 1977; Goldberg, 1997; Hackney & Nye, 1973; Knapp, 1972; Luterman, 1984; Molyneaux & Lane, 1982; Shipley, 1997; Tannen, 1990, 1994). Such information may be familiar to many supervisors, having been part of their basic training as clinicians. Today, however, basic communication theory and methods for effective interpersonal communication may or may not be part of the curricular offerings in training programs. Thus, it may be necessary to provide some didactic training for supervisees or to upgrade skills through reading, self-study, and continuing education.

Listening Skills

Effective listening is essential in counseling, therapy, and in conversations with friends. Kagan (1970) noted that people, in general, are not particularly good listeners. "We really don't listen to each other. I tell you about how much I hurt and you're just waiting for me to finish so you can tell me how much you hurt" (Kagan, 1970, p. 95). Pickering and McCready (1990) stated that the skill of listening is related to intent—deciding if you really want to hear what someone has to say—if that person is valuable enough to listen to.

The literature on expectations reveals that supervisees want to be listened to and have supervisors pay attention to them and take them seriously. In addition, if supervisors want supervisees to be active in conferences, they must not only listen but also must offer encouragers to talk. Encouragers are signals to continue talking and include behaviors such as saying "fine," I see," "good," "yes," "mmm," or "uh-huh" (Shipley, 1997). Verbally and nonverbally attending to and acknowledging the supervisee, and restating or paraphrasing the speaker's basic message are important basic skills (Pickering & McCready, 1990). Eye contact, positive head nods, appropriate facial expression, forward body leans, and, at times, touching are ways to convey that you are listening and function as minimal prompts to a speaker to continue. One of the categories in Blumberg's (1980) interaction analysis system is "Accepts or Uses Teacher's Ideas," and is defined as statements that clarify, build on, or develop ideas or suggestions by teachers. This is an activity extremely important to both the Collaborative and Consultative Styles. It should be apparent that listening is more than just hearing what the supervisee has said. It is responding to the input, rephrasing it to test understanding, clarifying it, restating it to better interpret intent, focusing the discussion, and checking the accuracy of listener perceptions. The flip side of active listening is apparent in a "Yes, but…" response. It's difficult to think of anything that squelches communication quicker than a "Yes, but…."

Barbara (1958) maintained that there are at least four essential factors in effective listening: concentration, active participation, comprehension, and objectivity. Concentration requires mental alertness and clearing the environment of distractions. Active participation requires openness, flexibility, and the use of some of the attending behaviors listed in the previous paragraph. Comprehension necessitates attending to the content, intent, and feelings being conveyed in a message. Objectivity requires that listeners not allow their personal feelings or attitudes to interfere with the message or their regard for the speaker.

Listening is not a one-way street in which supervisors must assume all responsibility. Supervisors can help supervisees become aware of their own listening patterns. A brief look at a videotape of a conference will reveal quickly what is happening between participants. If the supervisee is not using good listening skills in the conference, she or he may not be using them in the clinical session either. Establishing active listening skills as a supervisory objective and working on it as part of the supervisory process should facilitate generalization to the clinical process.

Carl Rogers (1980), in a retrospective discussion of the development of his theories about dealing with people, related that in his early years as a therapist he discovered that simply listening to clients was important in being helpful. "So, when I was in doubt as to what I should do in some active way, I listened. It seemed surprising to me that such a passive kind of interaction could be so useful" (p. 137).

Questioning Skills

The ability to ask questions may be the most important skill in the supervisor's repertoire—questions that generate thinking by the supervisee, questions that do not already contain the answer desired by the supervisor, and questions that have a purpose and are carefully thought out before they are uttered. In fact, it is possible that the type of questions asked by supervisors may, in many instances, be the determining factor in whether supervisees move along the continuum. Their impact may be either positive or negative.

Carin and Sund (1971), Cunningham (1971), and Davies (1981) suggested that learning in the classroom is determined largely through questioning techniques. Carin and Sund (1971) amplified this further when they said,

> Involved in any deep communication between persons is the ability to ask appropriate questions and to listen. This is the genius of communication. To listen and question at just the right place and degree delineates the truly brilliant instructor from the average. An insightful question appropriately delivered may stimulate the individual to reach a new level of mental mediation. We learn to think only by thinking. We become creative only by having opportunities to be creative. A properly phrased question often is the necessary "input" needed to ignite student's thinking and creative process. (p. 2)

The use of questions in the classroom has received extensive coverage in education literature. Questioning is the most frequently used utterance of teachers, but questions are least commonly used to stimulate thinking. Rather, teachers use questions in giving directions, managing the classroom, initiating activities, and in other learning situations. Critical thinking, however, seems not to be stimulated by teachers through questioning (Cunningham, 1971). Is this true of supervisors?

Questioning has many purposes—to obtain feedback or responses, to get data, to encourage thinking, to promote problem solving, to evaluate the student's preparation or participation in planned activities, to determine strengths and weaknesses, to review or summarize, to help the student recall, understand, synthesize, or apply, and to focus (Carin & Sund, 1971; Cunningham, 1971: Davies, 1981; Whiteside, 1981). Pederson and Ivey (1993) maintain that "questions have a great deal to do with power" (p. 131). Questions can provide a means to control a conversation.

There is an assumption that high levels of questioning behavior raise the cognitive level of students, forcing them to reflect, refocus, clarify, expand, and be more creative in their thinking, although the research is somewhat contradictory. Nevertheless, many systems for classifying and studying questions have been proposed and they are worthy of attention in the self-study of verbal behaviors in the conference. Sanders (1966) used seven categories: memory, translation, interpretation, application, analysis, synthesis, and evaluation. Lowery (1970) suggested three categories: broad, narrow, and miscellaneous, with broad questions subcategorized into open ended and valuing, narrow into direct information and focusing. Probably the most useful category system for questioning is presented by Cunningham (1971). He divided questions into narrow and broad categories, which he then broke down further. The narrow category includes cognitive memory questions (recall, identify/observe, yes or no, define, name, designate) and convergent questions (explain, state relationships, compare and contrast). The broad category includes divergent questions (predict, hypothesize, infer, reconstruct) and evaluative questions (judge, value, defend, justified choice). It is easy to see the increasing complexity of these classifications of questions. Recognizing the importance of these levels of questioning in encouraging thinking and problem solving by supervisees is an important part of any supervisor's approach to supervision.

Questioning in Speech-Language Pathology and Audiology

Interest in questioning by speech-language pathologists increased with the profession's involvement with the language-disordered child and the emphasis on the study of children's questions and answers (Ervin-Tripp, 1970; James & Seebach, 1982; Leach, 1972; Tyack & Ingram, 1977). Interest in discourse analysis focused attention on questions in relation to language development (Gallagher & Prutting, 1983). Although questioning has always been a tool of the clinician and, thus, a concern of supervisors, there is no indication of it having been a major topic of study as related to clinician behavior.

Questioning in the Supervisory Conference

Questioning in the supervisory conference was an important issue to Blumberg and Cusick (1970) in the development of their interaction analysis system for studying the supervisory process, as evidenced by their inclusion for both participants of items related to requesting information, opinions, and suggestions. Their analysis of conferences revealed certain information related to questioning—supervisors did less asking for ideas and suggestions than telling, and less asking of opinions than giving of opinions. In fact, asking for suggestions was the least-used supervisory behavior, and supervisees never asked "Why?" when given advice. Thus, they said, teachers are not involved in problem solving about conditions they face in their classrooms. The interaction is *not* collaborative. Additionally, teachers reacted most negatively to supervisors asking for information, assuming that they were being "trapped." Blumberg and Cusick did not analyze the type of questions being asked but, if they had, they might have found a clue to the hostility engendered by such question asking.

Blumberg and Cusick also reported that conferences rated High Direct, High Indirect and those rated Low Direct, High Indirect were perceived as more productive than the High Direct, Low Indirect and the Low Direct, Low Indirect. Recall from Chapter 2 that High Direct, High Indirect includes telling, suggesting, giving information, and criticizing, as well as reflecting and *asking* for information and suggestions. The Low Direct, High Indirect contains less telling and more reflecting and asking. It is not known, of course, from Blumberg and Cusick's data if the conferences *were* more effective, only that teachers perceived them in that way. Thus, although there was a preference in terms of productivity or effectiveness for both kinds of behavior, there was a stronger emphasis on the asking and reflecting behaviors.

Smith and Anderson (1982b) also found questioning behaviors of supervisors and supervisees to be related to the perceived effectiveness components (direct and indirect supervisory behaviors) of the conference. Smith (1979), in another study, provided an extensive description of questions used in 45 supervisory conferences in speech-language pathology and audiology. Questions were usually cognitive and dealt with objectives or methods and materials. They asked primarily for factual information such as, "What did Mary do when you asked her…" and, "What are John's objectives?" (p. 11). Thus, they would fall in Cunningham's (1971) narrow category, and probably in the cognitive-memory subcategories. Smith found that supervisors asked 81% of the questions. The only difference in type of questions was that supervisees asked more opinion questions than supervisors. It did appear that supervisors varied their types of questions on the basis of such supervisee variables as experience and grade point average. Smith concluded that supervisors are dominating the questioning process and, by asking for the type of factual information indicated in her study, they are depriving supervisees of a vital opportunity for problem solving. She reflected,

> If, as clinical supervisors, we intend to relinquish power and authority and utilize the clinical supervision model while training supervisees to problem-solve, self-analyze, and self-direct their own behavior, we must critically analyze and change, if necessary, our use of questions during conference interactions. (p. 9)

Sbaschnig, Dowling, and Williams (1992) analyzed 45 conferences for 15 supervisor–supervisee pairs from two universities and found that supervisors talked more than six times as much as supervisees. Further, they asked twice as many questions as did supervisees. The supervisors had a direct, unchanging style. These results are consistent with those of Smith (1978, 1979).

The way in which questions are posed will determine not only the answer but also the type of thought that must go into the answer. This is readily apparent by examining Cunningham's (1971) classification. For example:

NARROW/COGNITIVE MEMORY QUESTIONS
Recall: How many responses did you elicit with *X* activity?

Identify/observe: What kinds of disfluencies are apparent when he talks with his dad?

Yes or no: Did the stickers work as a reinforcer?

Define: What do you mean when you say he is hyperactive?

Name: What is the term for a slushy /s/ and other sibilants that is characterized by airflow over the sides of the tongue?

Designate: Who brought tapes to the last conference?

NARROW/CONVERGENT QUESTIONS
Explain: What happened when you used toys instead of pictures to elicit your targets?

State relationships: What is the impact of doing therapy with Mrs. Jones at 10:00 a.m. versus 4:00 p.m.?

Compare and contrast: Which of the three strategies resulted in the most correct responses?

BROAD/DIVERGENT QUESTIONS
Predict: What would happen if…?

Hypothesize: How could you determine if *X* is really causing the change in his behavior?

Infer: Given these varied research findings, what techniques seem to be the most plausible for your aphasia group?

Reconstruct: Given these facts about adult learning styles, what things might you have done differently with the parent support group last Tuesday?

BROAD/EVALUATIVE QUESTIONS
Judge: What theories and research suggest that full inclusion is the best service delivery mode for these students? Which strategies will likely effect the greatest amount of generalization?

Value: Why might you be inclined to do that?

Defend: Why do you think that is so?

Justified choice: Despite the fact that all of the treatment goals have not been achieved, why do you think he is ready to be dismissed from therapy?

Strike-Roussos (1988) trained supervisors to use broad questions and subsequently examined the cognitive level of supervisor questions and supervisee responses (1995). Her results suggested that without specific education, supervisors tend to use predominantly narrow questions, and that the frequency of higher-level questions increases in conjunction with education. "More interestingly, the effectiveness of the higher-level questions in facilitating higher-level thinking by supervisees also improves after supervisors participate in an educational program focused on question asking" (p. 17).

Some questions have an effect opposite of that intended. Consider, for example, the clinician who utters to her 4-year-old client, "Can you say____?" That question probably evokes other familiar "yes or no" questions that have been observed in treatment sessions where clinicians are attempting to encourage a client to talk. One of the first lessons the inexperienced clinician may learn is to avoid such questions; yet it is easy to do, even with experience, unless there is constant monitoring and planning of new behaviors. The same can be said of supervisor utterances. "Do you think it would be better if he wrote it out?" is deceptive. It may appear to request an opinion, but to the supervisee it is a directive and requires an automatic "yes" answer.

In addition to "yes or no" questions, Cunningham (1971) listed several other problem questions. The ambiguous question does not include enough criteria to enable the respondent to define a good answer. "What about the session?" may appear to be a broad question to the supervisor, but the supervisee may feel that he or she must play a guessing game to find out what the supervisor wants to hear.

Another type of problem question is the "spoon-feeding" question, sometimes called leading or rhetorical, where the answer is embedded in the question. This type of question ranges from simple to complex. From transcripts of tapes of conferences, the following stand out as spoon-feeding: "That's more appropriate, isn't it?" "That was mostly nonverbal, wasn't it?"

Confusing questions, according to Cunningham (1971), include too many factors for the answerer to consider at one time. Consider this example from a tape of a conference: "What would you say—how high a success rate? Have you noticed, like, if he is succeeding at 60 or 70% of the time, is he usually OK versus 20% of the time if he's getting one out of five right? Does that make a big change in behavior for you, in your situation or not? Or have you been able to determine any of that? What do you think?" The obvious answer is, "I think this is a very confusing question," but most supervisees would not have the courage to answer that way. This supervisee responded, "What do you mean? In the group?"

Shipley (1997) cautioned against the use of "why" questions "because they put many respondents on the defensive" (p. 59). He suggested that "could" questions are a better alternative. For example, "Could you explain that a little?" as opposed to "Why do you think that is a good thing to try?" Whiteside (1981) reported on "tugging questions" such as, "Well, come on, you know that" or, "What did you do? Come on now, you can tell me about that. What did you do?" These are perhaps more commonly used by clinicians in attempts to get a response from an unresponsive client. Molyneaux and Lane (1982) included in their categories of interview questions a similar type that they labeled "bombardment"—one that contains three or more questions of any type.

The kinds of questions posed not only influence the kinds of responses evoked, but also the kinds of thinking the respondent must use to answer the question. Furthermore, they can impact the relationship of those involved in the relationship.

The Answers

The importance of listening has been stressed. Acceptance of answers to questions and the responses to them are important in future participation and problem solving. Responses to incorrect or inaccurate answers require diplomacy involving response, redirecting, helping the respondent move closer to a better answer, and not blocking communication by responding negatively (Carin & Sund, 1971). In supervisory conferences there are often answers that are neither right nor wrong and appropriate responses will encourage further discussion.

Responses are important, but frequently silence is just as important. Silence may mean resistance or simply mean that the responder is engaged in exploring the issue (Brammer, 1985). Wait time between questions and answers has been a popular area for study in education. Carin and Sund (1971) reported on a study that found that a teacher's wait time was one second. When the wait time was extended, it resulted in longer student responses, less "I don't know" answers, more whole sentences, increased speculative thinking, more questions from children, revised teacher expectations of children, and a wider variety of questions asked by the teacher. Supervisors, too, need to learn to tolerate silence. Some people need more time to get their thoughts together than others, and the wait may result in a better answer.

INTERPERSONAL ASPECTS OF THE CONFERENCE

It was stated earlier that the interpersonal aspects of the supervisory process would not be treated extensively in this book—that addressing that topic requires a book of its own. There are volumes of material on interpersonal communication, helping relationships, and the helper skills needed to facilitate change in the helpee. Readers are implored to make themselves familiar with some of this literature. Among the many sources from the counseling and communication literature are Anderson and Guerrero (1998), Brammer (1985), Danish and Kagan (1971), Deetz and Stevenson (1986), Duck (1997), Faiver, Eisengart, and Colonna (2000), Feltham (2000), George and Cristiani (1981), Luft (1969), and Young (2001). Regardless of the coverage, it must be clear to readers that the approach presented here is based on assumption of attitudes of respect, empathic understanding, facilitative genuineness, concreteness of expression, unconditionality of regard, congruence, and self-exploration—all the interpersonal qualities proposed by Rogers (1957, 1961), Carkhuff

(1969a, 1969b), Carkhuff and Berenson (1967), and the many others who followed them.

Although Pickering (1986) stated that the profession of speech-language pathology has *not* been exemplary in "probing aspects of interpersonal communications in its helping, clinical relationship" (p. 16), it is encouraging that there has been some focus in recent years on the interpersonal communication aspects of the supervisory process. The research of Pickering (1979, 1984) and McCrea (1980) were discussed earlier. In addition, Pickering has continued to explore this area (1987a, 1987b), as have many others, including Caracciolo (1977), Caracciolo and colleagues (1978a, 1978b), Crago (1987), Hagler, Casey, and DesRochers (1989), Klevans, Volz, and colleagues (1981), Volz (1976), Volz, Klevans, Norton, & Putens (1978), and McCready and colleagues (1987, 1996). Ghitter (1987) explored the relationship between the interpersonal skills of supervisors and the impact on supervisees' clinical effectiveness in 88 dyads. Her results affirmed what has been demonstrated in studies by Caracciolo and colleagues (1978a) and other studies in helping professions: when supervisees *perceive* high levels of unconditional positive regard, genuineness, empathic understanding, and concreteness, their clinical behaviors change in positive directions. Perceptions of those core behaviors facilitate high levels of clinical effectiveness.

The supervisory relationship may be one of the most intense interpersonal experiences in which a person can engage. The emotional dimensions of this vital relationship may influence both participants in ways that have not even begun to be identified. Mosher and Purpel (1972), in discussing the personal development of prospective teachers during student teaching, asserted that not only does learning to teach require the student to change what she or he does, it also requires "that he change what he is" (p. 115). They stressed the need to assist the student in his or her process of changing from a *person* to a *professional person* and offered suggestions for a supervisor to deal with this critical period in a student's life. In examining actual behaviors, not merely perceptions, Pickering (1984) and McCrea (1980) found only minimal evidence of facilitative interpersonal interaction between supervisor and supervisee in speech-language pathology. Is this the state of the art today? Hagler, Casey, and DesRochers (1989) found that providing supervisors with data about their facilitative behaviors from analyses of conferences, along with some suggestions for change, was not sufficient to induce a change in supervisors' behaviors.

Decades ago, Ward and Webster (1965a, 1965b) expressed their concern about personal needs of students in their growth and development as clinicians. Pickering (1977) stressed the importance for supervisors to have an understanding of four concepts of human relationships—authenticity, dialogue, risk taking, and conflict. In a later report of her research, Pickering (1984) contended that neither students nor supervisors appear to know "how to analyze the interpersonal dimensions of therapeutic relationships" (p. 194).

Much of the counseling literature reflects the need of counselors to help counselees express themselves about their feelings, their concerns, and their anxieties. Although supervisors are not counselors and a line must be drawn between the two roles, supervisors will find times when they need to reflect the supervisees' words and focus on their feelings. There are situations when dealing with feelings is essential.

Despite the data that suggest that supervisors have traditionally focused on teaching and instruction to the neglect of attending to supervisees' interpersonal needs, there are signs that the profession is turning its attention to this area of study. If it is as important as it seems to be, then every supervisor in her or his role as facilitator of the supervisory process should become familiar with the literature and assist supervisees in learning about it. More than that, however, they need to study their own interpersonal interaction to determine its possible impact on the supervisory process.

PLANNING FOR THE CONFERENCE

Competencies 8.2, 8.3, and 8.4 substantiate the importance of planning. Planning the interaction between supervisor and supervisee is a primary aspect of the clinical supervision model. Cogan (1973) and Goldhammer and colleagues (1980) discussed strategies for planning the conference and emphasized the importance of planning for maximizing the teaching–learning process in supervision. This planning comes out of the analysis of the clinical and supervisory processes, when decisions are made about what to do with the collected data and priorities are set for conference discussion. Goldhammer and colleagues discussed such issues as doing a full or partial analysis of the data; the order in which such issues will be presented; dealing with strengths or weaknesses; the balance between the past (analysis of previous data), the future (planning), and the present (discussion of the supervisory process); how to record what is happening in the conference; reviewing the contract, if there is one, for possible modification; and how and when to end the conference. They suggested that although there may be appropriate times for an open conference, it is easy to "squander an open conference on superficialities or on peripheral or irrelevant issues" (p. 136). The link between analyzed data and planning the conference has also been discussed in the previous chapter.

Although most studies of conferences have centered on what has already happened, Peaper (1984) conducted one of the first studies that focused on planning for the conference. Graduate students were divided into two groups. One group planned agendas for their conferences after listing potential topics for discussion under three categories—client-centered, clinician-centered, and supervisor-centered issues. Students in the other group did not participate in such a listing. Students in Peaper's study valued the conference, as opposed to the subjects of Culatta and colleagues (1975), who did not feel a need for regularly scheduled conferences. The group that preplanned agendas for their conferences felt that they set the tone of the conference—not a surprising fact, but an important consideration for the supervisor who wishes to have supervisees feel more "ownership" for the experience.

Experimental studies by McFarlane and Hagler (1992a, 1992b) and Jans, Hagler, and McFarlane (1994) have demonstrated the positive effects of supervisee-prepared agendas. These investigations substantiated that students were more actively involved in conferences for which they prepared agendas. Students initiated more and were less reflexive in conferences they planned. Sbaschnig, Dowling, and Williams (1992) examined conference outcomes when supervisors planned agendas, when the agendas were jointly planned, and when supervisees planned them. Their dependent measures were talk-time and question usage and the results revealed that supervisors talked more and dominated the conferences regardless of who planned the agenda. However, how the agendas were used in conferences was unknown. McFarlane and Hagler (1992a) suggested that supervisees may not accept ownership even when they planned the agenda. The ownership issue may be related to supervisee experience and should be investigated. Specifically, as students gain experience in their dual roles as clinicians and supervisees, they may be better able to assume responsibility for agenda planning and to be more active in conferences. Establishing goals for the supervisory process, to decrease supervisor control and increase supervisee participation, and monitoring progress in goal attainment also should be examined more closely. Obviously, goals should be directed toward the supervisee's movement along the continuum.

The agenda will identify conference content but how feedback will be provided also needs to be planned. Such planning should include decision making about purpose, type, content, amount, timing, and rationale as well as evaluation of the appropriateness of the feedback. Feedback should usually result from the analysis of data collected during the observation. Kurpius and his colleagues are among the many experts who have clarified the purposes and established criteria for giving helpful feedback.

When given to another person, feedback has three primary purposes (Kurpius, 1976):

- To identify discrepancies between what the recipient assumes and what actually exists— that is, the difference between perceptions and reality

- To support or reinforce desired behaviors
- To modify behavior so content and actions are congruent with the intended message.

A supervisor should delineate these purposes for supervisees, and should also state the criteria for giving feedback. Criteria include (Kurpius & Christie, 1978):

1. Be descriptive rather than evaluative.
2. Be specific in describing behaviors.
3. Consider the appropriateness (i.e., based on recipient rather than self needs).
4. Determine the usefulness of feedback—to be useful, the recipient must be able to act on it.
5. Assess who desires the feedback—solicited is the most helpful.
6. Attempt to determine receiver readiness— feedback must be well timed (i.e., timely feedback is provided close to the time when the event occurred and to a recipient who is psychologically ready to receive it).
7. Seek clarification—check to see if the recipient understood. Encourage questions, ask the recipient to restate in his or her own words, and so on.
8. Check the accuracy of feedback prior to giving it. It should be objective—for example, derived from data collected during observation or based on standards (ASHA, APA) or clearly identified competencies.

Further, it is important to control the amount of information the user receives—too much will be overwhelming.

Feedback is *not* solely evaluative, just the end product of the supervisory process, or exclusively provided by the supervisor. It is, instead, an exchange of ideas that occurs throughout the entire interaction, emanating in a variety of ways from all the participants in all directions. It may come during or immediately after an observation, or it may be delayed. It may be verbal or written. Optimally, it is based on data collected during the observation but at times it may consist of judgmental or evaluative statements. Whatever its form, it serves both as closure to preceding events and transition to further planning. The conference is the typical vehicle for this interchange (Cogan, 1973). Supervisors and supervisees will be both recipients and providers of feedback for each other, their peers, and themselves. Dowling (2001) emphasized the importance of reciprocity and stated that, "Reciprocity is achieved by encouraging the supervisee to question, ask for clarification, compare analyses of data, and to provide feedback to the supervisor regarding the helpfulness of the information" (p. 85).

Readers are reminded that the integration component includes but is not restricted only to feedback. Given that feedback has not been thoroughly addressed in the previous chapters, some expanded discussion seems prudent.

FEEDBACK

Many of the expectations of supervisees about supervision are related to feedback behaviors of both supervisors and supervisees. In fact, feedback may constitute a major portion of what many supervisees think of as "supervision." A document generated more than a quarter of a century ago illustrates the point that feedback is a basic expectation, that it involves clinical teaching as well as evaluation, and that participants in the supervisory process are involved in both giving and receiving feedback.

This classic document, the "Bill of Rights" for supervisors and supervisees (Gerstman, 1977), includes a **supervisee** category entitled *Right to Expect Supervisor to Provide Means and Method of Feedback,* and contains feedback-focused items such as systematic monitoring, ongoing mutual feedback, opportunity to express self, formal and informal conference time, honest appraisal of job performance, oral and written evaluations, the possibility of appealing decisions, and the opportunity to say "No." The **supervisor** section contains a category entitled *Right to Offer and Get Mutual Feedback.* Items include the right to make justified criticisms, expect staff to expect and accept criticism, judge and criticize effects of services, honestly criticize and suggest other ways of operating, get

feedback from supervisees about supervision received, expect supervisees to say, "You're a lousy supervisor" or even a good one, and determine some of the ground rules of how often they will be observed. The group of supervisors who developed the Bill of Rights obviously took a broad look at the many aspects of feedback.

Studies on expectations reviewed in Chapter 4 revealed a variety of views about what supervisees and supervisors want and need with regard to feedback. Supervisees frequently expressed a desire for direct feedback about their work—a critique. This issue must be clarified in operationalizing the continuum. Supervisees must learn the appropriate balance between direct feedback from the supervisor and self-analysis. Unless this is clarified, it may be a source of frustration and dissatisfaction for the supervisee in conferences. Anderson (1988) offered an anecdote to illustrate. In the early days of the doctoral program with concentration in supervision at Indiana University, a Ph.D. student and an insightful, advanced clinician were paired in supervision practicum and had established an excellent collaborative relationship. The supervisor trainee was observed to be supportive, encouraged problem solving, and stimulated creative thinking. The clinician was self-analytical, creative in planning, self-evaluative, and participated productively in conferences. A supervisory dyad created in heaven! Yet, about two-thirds of the way into the semester, as the two walked down the hall after a conference, the student said, "Well, when are you going to start criticizing me?" The implications in terms of expectations, unexplored and unmet, need not be belabored. The experience, Anderson said, provided a valuable lesson for her, the trainee, and the clinician. Expectations must be identified and discussed, and ways to meet the ones deemed important and appropriate must be incorporated into the planning.

Providing Feedback

Feedback may be provided in a variety of situations using many different methods. Although the scheduled conference seems to be the most frequently used setting for the exchange of feedback, there are other procedures. These include written feedback, spontaneous verbal interaction, and feedback during sessions. These procedures are primarily *one-way delivery of feedback*—supervisor to supervisee—and thus are almost always direct evaluations or suggestions.

Written Feedback. Many supervisors use checklists, rating scales, evaluation forms, or messages written during the observation period that are given to the supervisee after the *clinical* session (Geoffrey, 1973); but the type of feedback provided and received about the *supervisory* process has received minimal attention in the literature. The conference rating scale developed by Smith (1978; Smith & Anderson, 1982a), modified by Brasseur (1980a), and contained in Appendix 4F has been used to examine direct and indirect supervisory styles (Brasseur & Anderson, 1983; McFarlane & Hagler, 1992b; Smith & Anderson, 1982b). Supervisors and supervisees may use this scale to obtain feedback about conferences and to compare perceptions.

Kennedy (1981) studied the effects of two types of preconference written feedback—subjective statements and verbatim transcripts of events—on verbal behaviors of supervisors in conferences. Both supervisor and supervisees showed differences in conference behaviors, depending on which form of feedback had been provided. Weller's (1971) *Multidimensional Observational System for the Analysis of Interactions in Clinical Supervision* (MOSAICS) was the dependent measure and the verbatim condition yielded more supervisor Explanation, Opinion, and talk about supervision than the subjective condition. Supervisees in the subjective condition used more Justification of Opinions than those in the verbatim condition. Despite some limitations, this study addressed an important issue: Does type of feedback make a difference?

Peaper and Mercaitis (1987) and Rocchio and Iacarino (1990) studied written feedback and found it to be highly evaluative. Jans and colleagues (1994) examined the effects of supervisors' written session comments on their verbal feedback during conferences. They compared supervisors who provided written feedback to those who withheld it and found no differences in verbal conference content between the two groups. Supervisors in both conditions tended to provide facts, explanations, and suggestions rather than evaluations and opinions. Both supervisors and supervisees engaged in limited evaluative discussion. Jans and colleagues suggested that supervisor experience and the tools used to analyze feedback and verbalizations might account for differences in the evaluative behavior of supervisors. Education and training would also likely be a factor—that is, training supervisors to refrain from immediate evaluation and training supervisees to analyze their own behavior.

The content of the written message is of great importance in encouraging the collaborative approach to supervision. If the written message handed to the supervisee after the observation is observational data collected by the supervisor, it should be useful to the supervisees in the analysis that precedes the conference. Certain types of questions from the supervisor may also enhance self-analysis by the supervisee. If the written feedback is a direct evaluation, however, the opportunity or motivation for supervisee self-analysis and self-evaluation may be lost and the tone of the conference preset. If the written message is used without further verbal interaction, it may be misunderstood. The intent of the message may be clearer and the opportunity for misunderstanding reduced if the purpose and content have been discussed during joint planning.

Report writing is one area in which written feedback is always provided to supervisees. Task 10 and its associated competencies (ASHA, 1985b) focus on reporting and editing. It is not uncommon to hear supervisees say that a report was returned with so much red ink that it appeared to have "bled to death." On the other hand, supervisors report that helping supervisees develop *good* report writing skills is one of their toughest challenges but one that can yield significant benefits. If a student can write coherently about behavior, they most likely understand it and their work with their client.

In an investigation of feedback on written reports, Gunter (1985) examined the degree of consistency between supervisors' judgments of the most important constituents of a report and their evaluations of an actual report. The components considered of highest value were related to content as opposed to style. Analysis of comments on an actual report, however, were inconsistent with this because they revealed more comments on style than on content. It is obviously easier to provide written feedback on style than content and Gunter pointed out the great need for a method to ensure that feedback on both are provided. She also reported that supervisors' comments on the report were not consistent, indicating that important components of feedback may be left out. She urged some means of consistency, such as a checklist for supervisors to use in reacting to reports.

Ruder et al. (1996) developed several evaluation forms designed to improve the "consistency from one supervisor's expectations to the next" (p. 107). Among their forms is one used to evaluate the written work of student clinicians, specifically semester treatment plans and end-of-semester reports. Twenty-four items are scored on a 5-point rating scale (5 = very good, 4.5 = good, 4.0 = satisfactory, 3.5 = less than satisfactory, 3.0 = poor, below 2.5 = unsatisfactory). The items are related to content, style, and general professional behavior. Sample **content** items include:

- Background information is accurate and complete—only pertinent history included
- Diagnostic data are displayed in a table or figure
- Tests results are accurately scored
- Protocols are completed and attached to report
- Goals and objectives are appropriate for age, disorder, and severity level
- Clinical impressions thoroughly integrate information from other sections

Sample **style** items include:

- Spelling and punctuation
- Morphology and syntax (grammar use)
- Report is free of unnecessary words, repetitions, and meanderings
- Information reported in terms that are appropriate for the recipient

Sample **professional** items include:

- Met deadline for report
- Report is in correct format
- Exercised caution in making statements outside professions

As noted in Chapter 6, Ruder et al. (1996) developed a computer-assisted program for supervision in their university clinic. The program creates a spreadsheet for individual students and enables individual supervisors to enter data and for all staff to share ratings. The spreadsheet analysis allows for a comparison of strengths and weaknesses of a particular clinician across and between supervisors. This type of approach and the written feedback inherent in it would make it easy to monitor an individual's acquisition of clinical competencies and thus be very helpful in providing the kind of formative assessments mandated by the new ASHA Standards (ASHA, 2000a).

Spontaneous or Unscheduled Verbal Interaction. Supervisors and supervisees have many opportunities for verbal interaction between the time of the observation and the conference. Regardless of setting, they meet in halls, the lunchroom, or the classroom; they may be working together on other tasks; or they may interact in a variety of other ways. The opportunities and temptations to discuss fragments of the observed clinical session in such interactions may be great.

One must ask what purpose is to be served by such spontaneous interactions. If a very specific goal has been set for the supervisor to rate certain interactions during the session, feedback may be given to the supervisee immediately. If immediate reinforcement is the goal, then this type of feedback is appropriate. Supervisors should resist the temptation to respond automatically with a stereotypic positive or negative statement without considering its purpose or effect. Further, a brief interchange may not do justice to the complexities of a clinical session. There likely has been no time for analysis by either party. A quickly delivered message may be misinterpreted. As with the written message, the probability is high that this type of interchange will take the form of an "instant evaluation" or directive for the future, which removes the need for self-analysis or self-evaluation by the supervisee. On the other hand, if a session has been a devastating failure, the supervisee may be greatly in need of an understanding word that will sustain her or him until the scheduled conference. Social rules usually encourage some kind of verbal exchange when two people meet—no one wants to be met with a stony stare after a session. Whatever is said, the tone of the subsequent discussion may be influenced by the supervisor's words.

The remarks made by supervisors between observation and conference may be more important than they realize, especially in terms of the Collaborative Style. Such spontaneous remarks may take any of several forms, but certainly deserve some thought—and their goals and purpose should be an important part of planning the supervisory interaction. If the activities that make up the observation and analysis components as well as the type of feedback have been planned previously, there will be less uncertainty about what to expect in the conference and probably less need for spontaneous verbal interaction.

Direct Feedback During Clinical Sessions.   This form of feedback includes such behaviors as communication through the "bug-in-the-ear" referred to in Chapter 6, slipping notes to the clinician that suggest changes in activities, interruption of the session to make suggestions or to demonstrate, and other forms of attracting the attention of the clinician in an attempt to alter the direction of the session.

Interruption of the Session.   No data are available on the topic of interruption of the session by the supervisor. Countless discussions with supervisees indicate, however, that there are mixed reactions to this technique, depending on the supervisee's maturity, the supervisor's manner, the relationship between the two, the purpose and nature of the intervention, the amount of planning that preceded it, and the clinic/organization culture. Demonstrating for and participating with the

supervisee is a distinct supervisory task, but jointly determining when it is appropriate is the first competency for Task 5 (ASHA, 1985b).

Some clinicians report that they consider "swooping into the clinical session" without warning and taking over the work with the client to be the most reprehensible behavior supervisors can exhibit. There is a general feeling that when supervisors enter unexpectedly and begin to interact directly with clients or to make suggestions in the presence of clients, it threatens the professional status of the clinician, damages credibility, and is demeaning. Other clinicians indicate that they welcome suggestions or demonstration. In fact, when present or former students are asked what was missing from their preparation, they often express a wish to have had more demonstrations from their supervisors. They do, however, consistently prefer to have some warning that it is going to happen or to have requested it.

In keeping with the theme of collaboration presented here, such unannounced or unplanned intervention would be especially inappropriate. Sensitivity to the supervisee's feelings and advanced planning would deter feelings of resentment and threat that might occur. The optimal way to deal with the issue of intervention and demonstration is to include it in planning activities, both long range and specific instances, so the supervisor's presence can be explained to the client. For example, the supervisee may indicate in the conference that she or he wishes a demonstration of a particular procedure. Or the supervisor may be concerned about the supervisee's evaluation and reinforcement of client responses and may wish to join the supervisee to assist in discriminating responses. If planned, the supervisee can easily explain the supervisor's forthcoming visit and be prepared for the interruption. Without further study, it seems safe to surmise that unplanned interruption may reinforce the supervisee's subordinate role and increase supervisee dependence.

Anderson (1988) stated that the only justification for *unplanned* interruptions would be if the client's welfare was in serious jeopardy. This is a particularly cogent issue in settings where clients are paying fees. The client's right to high-quality service must be considered; at the same time, supervisors must be sure that their judgments about negative features of a session are accurate and not merely from their own "square boxes." In other words, the techniques may be different from those the supervisor would use. The issue at stake here is the learning that is taking place.

A special situation is presented in the case assessment sessions, especially if it is a one-visit evaluation where there will be no other opportunity to obtain reliable data. Incorrect test administration may warrant interruption. However, adequate planning and preparation may prevent such problems, or at least alleviate potential defensiveness.

When there is no observation room, a totally different situation is created. In some settings, supervisors may have to sit in the room where the session is being conducted. Intervention in such cases might be planned in such a way that the supervisee could request the supervisor to join in the session or to demonstrate a specific activity without infringing on the supervisee's relationship with a client. In some situations, supervisors and supervisees may work cooperatively as a team on a fairly regular basis, thus giving the supervisor a natural opportunity to demonstrate. Sensitivity and planning are obviously important when supervisor and supervisee share the same space.

Rassi (1978) described a supervisory procedure in audiology assessment in which the supervisor demonstrates for the student, explains rationale between questions of the patient, and then has the student perform the tasks while the supervisor remains in the room. The supervisor then listens in an adjacent room and "if deemed necessary and/or appropriate, supervisor may intervene to assist student or give him suggestions" (p. 46). Rassi stressed the dangers of dependence on the supervisor and said, "Beware of transforming the student into robot" (p. 47). Rassi (2001) discussed some fundamental differences in supervision of student or staff clinicians in audiology as compared to their counterparts in speech-language pathology, suggesting a more apprenticeship approach. The nature of clinical tasks involved in the practice of audiology, the number and variety of clients served, the physical environment dictated by the equipment used in clinical audiology, time constraints, and the probability that students may not be present for a particular client's return visit necessitates a more directive supervisory style (explaining, telling, modeling).

Live Supervision

The term *live supervision,* referred to briefly in the discussion of observation, has developed in the training of professionals in marriage and family counseling (Goodman, 1985) and has potential applicability for speech-language pathology and audiology. Whiffen and Byng-Hall (1982) traced the evolution of family therapy supervision from case discussions, audiotapes, role playing, exploring the therapist's own family, videotapes, and methods that only allow a retrospective view of therapy. As supervisors in that discipline have tried to have more immediate contact with the trainee, they have developed various techniques—consultation behind a screen with a supervisor at prearranged time, a telephone in the therapy room, the earphone or "bug-in-the-ear," and finally, supervisors joining trainees in the room with the family. This model of training may also be applied to individual therapy (Goodman, 1985).

In the live supervision approach, the supervisor assumes the role of *co-therapist.* Kaslow (1977) noted that there are many advantages to this model, where "the student can be exposed to intensive learning by direct observation and participation with the supervisor. Such experiences can be exhilarating and highly productive" (p. 224). This type of supervision also has its disadvantages, according to Kaslow—the possible assertiveness of the supervisor, the modeling that may take place, and the repression of the supervisee's spontaneity. It is hoped that, for supervisees, "the supervisor will help them maintain their individualities, find their own styles, trust their hunches, and gradually feel free to move in more rapidly, so that ultimately the teams will be well balanced" (p. 225).

Does this approach have application in our professions? Discussions with supervisors have revealed instances where a comparable approach is used, but Rassi's approach to audiology supervision is the only detailed account in the literature (Rassi, 1978, 1987, 2001; Rassi & McElroy, 1992). Anderson (1988) reported that she frequently encountered this approach in off-campus settings. Certainly, it deserves investigation. Although at first glance it may appear to be the antithesis of the model advocated in this text, this approach may be suited to interactions at either end of the continuum. At the very early stages, there may be a need for modeling, demonstrating, immediate intervention, or reinforcement of beginning clinicians to help them develop some foundation skills. This methodology may also be viable with the marginal student. At the Consultative end of the continuum, it may be the ideal way for peers to work together in solving certain problems. Gillam (1999) advocated an apprenticeship model in which faculty function as master clinicians and clinical researchers who teach students a research approach to the clinical process through demonstration, mediated learning experiences, and coaching. Determining when an apprenticeship model is most efficient and what effect it has on the potential development of collaborative and consultative styles provide interesting matter for efficacy research.

Supervision by Earphone.   A form of live supervision that has received some attention in the literature is that of the bug-in-the-ear technique. This method uses electronic equipment such as an FM transmitter and receiver, allowing the supervisor to communicate directly with the clinician in such a manner that the client is not privy to the conversation. Called the most intrusive device in use in supervision, both cognitively and emotionally, by Loewenstein and Reder (1982), it has been used for many years in social work and psychotherapy (Kadushin, 1976).

The speech-language pathology literature contains a few references to the bug-in-the-ear procedure. Brooks and Hannah (1966) reported it as a supervisory tool, but warned that the supervi-

sor must avoid dominating the instruction and "causing the student to become a voice-operated automaton." They also indicated that it is sometimes difficult for the supervisor "to hold himself in check in this regard" (p. 386) and cited dependency of students as one of the dangers of such a system. A similar procedure was described by Starkweather (1974) for use in behavior modification training of clinicians, but he warned, "The whole procedure rests on the assumption that the supervisor's judgment is perfect, which is obviously unrealistic" (p. 610) and followed that with the cogent statement that the same problem exists in traditional training, but that the degree of independence of the student in traditional training "may enable the excellent student to overcome some of the shortcomings of his mentor" (p. 610). Hagler and Holdgrafer (1987) and Wilson, Welch, and Welling (1996) suggested that the technique has the advantage of enabling supervisors to provide immediate feedback to clinicians in an unobtrusive manner. Hagler and Holdgrafer (1987) used it to attempt to modify the amount of clinician talk-time as they obtained language samples. Results demonstrated that directives to "talk more/less" had the desired effect on the amount of talking done by student clinicians. In a comparable study, Hagler (1986) found that supervisors were able to reduce their verbal behavior during conferences as a result of verbal directives to "try to talk less" delivered at two-minute intervals.

Other Structures for Feedback

Microteaching and video confrontation methodologies, described in Chapter 6, involve the provision of feedback, often from peers and usually immediate. In some settings, case presentations and discussion provide opportunities for feedback, which are typically client centered. The case presentation, or staffing, rather than the conference, has been the classical means of supervising in psychiatric education. With this method, the trainee evaluates a case, presents it to the supervisor and peer group, or conducts an interview before a group. The trainee's performance is then discussed and critiqued by the supervisor and group (Kagan & Werner, 1977). This format has been used in speech-language pathology, but has not been formally studied. Group conferences are a commonly used opportunity for sharing feedback and will be given more detailed attention later. Demonstration therapy provides another method for providing feedback. Wagner, McCrea, and Spigarelli (1992) studied advantages and disadvantages of using e-mail to conference. They noted that it is an effective means for providing feedback about specific issues such as scheduling, lesson planning, or sharing information from observations but suggested that it not be used as a replacement to traditional face-to-face conferences.

CONFERENCES

Competency 8.9 stipulates that supervisors must involve supervisees in the analysis of supervisory interactions, competency 8.5 stipulates that interactions should facilitate the supervisee's self-exploration and problem solving, and competency 8.6 states that conference content should be based on the supervisee's level of training and experience. To achieve these competencies, and to encourage and motivate supervisee development (8.7), it seems imperative that supervisors understand the nature of conferences and what has been learned through research.

Anderson's thinking and study about conferences was initially influenced by a large body of descriptive literature in education. Work by Cogan (1973), Blumberg and associates (Blumberg, 1974, 1980; Blumberg & Amidon, 1965; Blumberg & Cusick, 1970; Blumberg & Weber, 1968), Dussault (1970), Goldhammer and associates (Goldhammer, 1969, Goldhammer et al., 1980), Weller (1969) and others provided a foundation for most of the dissertation studies Anderson directed for more than a decade at Indiana University. Although addressed more extensively in the first edition of this text, salient findings from some of the key studies have been discussed in earlier chapters. A brief summary of a few key findings from selected studies follows; it provides a frame-work for the conference studies in speech-language pathology.

Education

The pioneering work of Blumberg and his associates addressed the nature of the human relationships between supervisor and teacher, the place where Blumberg believed most of the problems in supervision arose. The main point of interaction in these relationships is the conference and therefore Blumberg turned his attention to analyzing conferences.

Blumberg and Cusick (1970) developed an interaction analysis system and used it to analyze 50 conferences. The results provided the first published view of what was actually occurring in conferences and the first use of the terms *direct* and *indirect* to describe supervisor behaviors. In their analysis, Blumberg and Cusick found that supervisors talked slightly less than teachers (45% for supervisors, 53% for teachers, and 2% silence). What was more interesting than the amount of time, however, was the type of verbal interaction. Supervisors were about 33% more direct than indirect (i.e., they were giving information, telling or suggesting to teachers what they should do, giving opinions, criticizing). They gave information five times more than they asked for it. Supervisor talk was heavily weighted toward telling, as compared to asking, in both problem solving and task-oriented discussions. They spent about seven times as much time telling supervisees what to do as they did in asking teachers for their ideas or suggestions. Supervisors asked opinions of teachers about one and one-half times more often than they gave opinions, and this was interpreted by teachers as an attempt to "box them into a corner" (Blumberg, 1974, p. 109). Teachers asked very few questions.

Further discussion of results included the interpretation that supervisors did not deal directly with teachers' negative feelings in a way that helped teachers. Interaction was mainly instruction from supervisors. Teachers did not perceive supervision as helpful—probably the reason they asked so few questions.

During the time supervisors engaged in accepting and clarifying teachers' ideas, 90% of the time was spent in giving short responses such as "I see" or "Uh huh." Very little time was spent in clarifying the supervisees' remarks. When teachers did exhibit negative socioemotional behaviors, the responses from the supervisor were not "therapeutic" but tended to be hostile and defensive. In trying to create a positive atmosphere, supervisors often used brief praising such as "good" or "I like that."

In another discussion of the 1970 study, Blumberg (1974) proposed that the behavior of supervisors was antithetical to the accumulated knowledge about helping relationships. The supervisors studied did not maintain a collaborative, problem-centered relationship with teachers. This is particularly significant because they were talking about employed professionals—not inexperienced students.

Although their analysis system focuses only on behavior, not content, Blumberg and Cusick (1970) discussed their impressions and stated that supervisors tended not to deal directly with teachers' complaints; that when supervisors gave advice and information, teachers did not question or ask for a rationale; and that the bulk of discussion revolved around "maintenance procedures" such as schedules, movement of children in the room, and so forth. Further, supervisors backed away from dealing with teachers' defensiveness and the researchers perceived the whole process as a rather stereotyped, role-playing process. Very little behavior was related to action or problem solving, resulting in conferences in which the interaction was not related to critical problems in the classroom, nor was it collaborative.

Other studies of the content of conferences in education at that time reported similar data (Heidelbach, 1967; Lindsey, 1969; Link, 1971; Michalak, 1969; Pittinger, 1972). Weller (1969), whose interaction analysis system will be discussed in the next chapter, found in a study of conferences that over 93% of the conference was spent in analysis of instruction. Items related to this analysis were evenly divided between methods and materials (37.3%) and instruction and interactions (35.9%), while objectives and content received only 20% of the time. Over two-thirds of the conference content was cognitive rather than affective or social-disciplinary.

These early descriptive studies of teacher education conferences formed an important foundation for the study of conferences in our professions. Substantial evidence indicates that conferences in speech-language pathology and audiology are very similar to those described in education.

Speech-Language Pathology

Several descriptive studies of conferences are available in the speech-language pathology (SLP) literature. It seems reasonable to assume that the process information derived from these investigations may be generalizable to audiology and SLP assessment conferences. Content will obviously differ.

Hatten's (1966) pioneer work reported descriptive data concerning the temporal, topical content, and social–emotional characteristics of 40 mid-semester supervisory conferences in a university clinic. Supervisors talked approximately 60% of the time. In the 35% of the time supervisees spoke, their responses were brief, most frequently "Uh huh" or other kinds of agreement. Mean length of conference was approximately 16 minutes and the range of topics discussed was from 4 to 10, with a mean of 6.5. The number of topic changes within a conference, including returns to a previous topic, ranged from 5 to 49, with a mean of 24. Topics, in the order of the time spent on each, were: therapy techniques (41.97%), client's qualities (21.86%), therapist's qualities (13.87%), motivation (7.54%), clerical (4.21%), social (2.86%), parents (2.74%), interpersonal (2.58%) theory (1.7%), and equipment (.64%). Thus, the first three topics accounted for almost 78% of the conference time. Only one category (client's qualities) was present in all conferences. Hatten suggested that percentages might change depending on the time in the semester the conference was held.

Underwood (1973) used Blumberg and Cusick's (1970) interaction analysis system to investigate SLP conferences and reported results similar to those of Blumberg and Cusick. However, she found that SLP conferences with students were longer than those with teachers—a 24-minute average versus 13 minutes in education. The least-used supervisory behavior was "supervisor asks for suggestions," as in Blumberg and Cusick's study. Least-used supervisee behavior was "negative social emotional behavior."

Another view of SLP conferences comes from a study of 10 supervisor–clinician pairs over a 12-week period (Culatta & Seltzer, 1976). As a group, the trend was for supervisees to provide raw data about the sessions; supervisors then used the data to suggest strategies for the next session. Sixty-one percent of all strategies came from supervisors, who asked about 70% of the questions (although the types were not indicated). There were no conferences in which clinicians made more statements than supervisors. Culatta and Seltzer noted the absence of evaluation statements by supervisors or self-evaluation by supervisees. Only 9% of all responses were evaluative; two-thirds provided by supervisors. In addition, even though supervisors thought they changed their behaviors during the 12-week term, there was virtually *no change* in the relative proportion of responses of supervisors and clinicians, talk-time, and the categories of response. In a follow-up study (Culatta & Seltzer, 1977), the same proportions occurred across conferences and confirmed the fact that supervisors did not change, even on self-selected behaviors.

Similar data were provided by Schubert and Nelson (1976), who used Underwood's interaction analysis system (modified from Blumberg & Cusick, 1970) to analyze nine conferences. Behavior used most frequently was clinician positive social, including responses such as "mmhm" and "OK" (21.4%). Next most frequent was supervisors providing opinions/suggestions (20.6%), followed by providing factual behavior. Supervisor talk consistently accounted for a larger part of conferences (65%) than supervisee talk. No supervisor criticism or negative social behavior from clinicians was found.

Irwin (1975, 1976) studied conferences that were conducted after microtherapy sessions and also found that the direct style (instruction, modeling, negative reinforcement) was used significantly more than the indirect style (asking questions, positive reinforcement). Supervisees responded to supervisors, rather than initiating.

Similar behavior was cited by Roberts and Smith (1982), who described behavior of 15 supervisor–supervisee pairs in 45 conferences over a six-week period from data obtained in Smith's (1978) extensive dissertation study. Using Weller's (1971) MOSAICS as the dependent measure, they found that supervisors assumed the initiatory role by structuring and soliciting responses and by contributing more pedagogical moves (uninterrupted verbal utterances). Supervisees assumed a predominantly reflexive role—participating less and, when they did, they responded and reacted to supervisor moves. Supervisors set the content and interaction patterns and directed the dialogue, thereby affecting and controlling the conference. Supervisors talked less about previous behavior and more about what should be done in future sessions. As in the Culatta and Seltzer study, supervisees appeared to present data about the session; supervisors prescribed what supervisees should do and gave opinions and suggestions for future sessions. Supervisors provided more facts, experiences, and observations than evaluative statements, again in agreement with Culatta and Seltzer. Both supervisor and supervisee used simplistic rather than complex statements, meaning there was little explanation, justification, or rationalization of statements from either party. Behavior did not change over time.

Tufts (1984) developed a content analysis system to quantify the topical content of supervisory conferences and found results similar to the other studies. About half the time in conferences was spent on two categories—clinical procedures (techniques, materials, client management) and lesson analysis (discussion of what the client did). When the category Client Information (general comments about the client not related specifically to the observed lesson) was added, approximately 70% of the time was accounted for. Less emphasis was placed on client information and planning for future sessions. Tufts looked for differences in content based on supervisee experience and found no major differences between three experience levels, except in lesson planning. Supervisees with the most experience spent much more time planning and assumed more responsibility for planning than those with less experience.

Shapiro's (1985b) study of commitments made in conferences revealed that 47% of the total commitments made were in the areas of planning, analysis, and evaluation of the clinical process, with particular focus on the client. Second most frequent commitments (39%) addressed implementation of treatment or assessment techniques for the client. Only 8% of commitments included planning, analysis, or evaluation of supervisee behavior. Findings reinforce that conferences focus on client and the clinical process.

Two studies have focused entirely on the interpersonal aspects of the conference. McCrea (1980) adapted scales developed by Gazda (1974) for measuring the supervisor facilitative behaviors of Empathic Understanding, Respect, Facilitative Genuineness, and Concreteness as well as the ability of the supervisee to self-explore, all concepts from Rogerian theory (Carkhuff, 1967, 1969a, 1969b; Carkhuff & Berenson, 1967; Carkhuff & Truax, 1964; Rogers, 1951, 1957, 1961, 1962). After modification of the scales, she analyzed 28 conferences. Respect, Facilitative Genuineness, and Concreteness were demonstrated only at minimal levels and Empathic Understanding and Supervisee Self-Exploration were not identified often enough to be included in statistical analyses. Two limitations of this study were that conference audiotapes were used, thereby eliminating the nonverbal behavior through which much affect is carried, and that behaviors were identified by trained raters and did not reflect *perceptions* of supervisees. Despite this, it appears clear that the emphasis in these conferences, too, was not on clinician affect or behavior, but on such cognitive content as client problems, discussion of activities, planning strategies, and procedural matters.

Pickering (1979) used a descriptive, naturalistic approach to examine interpersonal communication in 40 samples each of therapy sessions and supervisory conferences. Although her qualitative

methodology was different from other studies of conferences, her results were not. Supervisors' communication in conferences was predominantly instructional, giving suggestions, advice, opinions, directives, and questions. Supervisors seemed to have an individual style that they maintained. Emphasis was on resolving issues regarding clients, not supervisees; content was cognitive and analytical. Supervisors shared few feelings; they were sympathetic, supportive, and reinforcing when supervisees expressed feeling and concerns, but did not aid supervisees in expanding those feelings or expressing their own. Supervisors frequently failed to attend to supervisees' expressions of feeling associated with therapy, often asking a cognitive question to turn conversation back to solution of client problems. The supervisors and supervisees rarely discussed the supervisory relationship or their feelings about each other. At the same time, supervisors were keeping journals in which they indicated the importance of the students' feelings in the therapeutic relationship with the client. Supervisees, too, focused on cognitive issues and shared feelings more frequently than supervisors, but they were frequently vague and reflected past feelings rather than current (probably because the discussion was the typical recounting of the clinical session).

Group Conferences.   Although one-to-one conferences seem to be the traditional method in speech-language pathology and audiology, group or team conferences seem to be used frequently. Supervisors may be motivated to use groups because their workloads prevent individual scheduling or they may have strong beliefs in the value of group interaction in the learning process.

Among the advantages of group supervision are: economy in terms of time and effort in dealing with common issues, sharing experiences and problem solving, emotional support, safety in numbers creating a comfortable learning environment, and peer influence (Kadushin, 1976). A supportive environment for change, and one in which supervisees do not feel their anxieties or problems are unique, should enhance professional self-esteem. In addition, supervisees are exposed to a wider variety of cases so the context for learning is expanded. Supervisees are able to learn directly and vicariously. Problem solving skills should be enhanced as supervisees explore various solutions to dilemmas and learn that several approaches may be effectively implemented to solve a particular problem. Participation in a group can also enhance an individual's interpersonal communication abilities as they practice active listening, questioning, and giving and receiving feedback, and learn how to manage resistance to change. Supervisees will be more active in the supervisory process because all members must assume equal responsibility for group functioning and share the responsibilities in accomplishing the tasks involved in supervision. This should foster supervisee independence/decrease dependence on the supervisor and facilitate the development of a personal, individual clinical style. Risks to effective and efficient group functioning involve issues of cohesiveness, trust, and ensuring that all members share the work and have comparable responsibilities. Obvious disadvantages of group conferences are that some individual needs will not be met and that supervisees do not receive the amount of attention that occurs in one-to-one interactions.

Dowling (1979) has been the main proponent of group methodology in our professions with her work and research on the *Teaching Clinic.* Developed for teacher training, the Teaching Clinic is a specifically structured peer-group form of supervision. As described by Dowling (2001), the Teaching Clinic consists of six sequential phases: (1) review of the previous teaching clinic, (2) planning, (3) observation, (4) data analysis and critique preparation, (5) problem-solving and strategy development, and (6) clinic review. The group consists of a demonstration clinician who contributes a videotape of a clinical session, and a clinic leader who serves as facilitator. Other participants are a group monitor, who observes the process to see if roles are being fulfilled and ground rules followed, and peers of the demonstration clinician.

Basic operation of the Teaching Clinic is as follows.

1. The previous clinic is reviewed to maintain continuity. The demonstration clinician discusses the results of implementing the suggestions made in the previous clinic. Any problems from the previous clinic are discussed. Ground rules are reiterated.
2. During the planning session, the demonstration clinician presents his or her therapy objectives and plans, and requests certain data she or he would like to have collected. The leader then discusses data collection tasks to be carried out by peers.
3. The team members, including the demonstration clinician, view about ten minutes of the tape.
4. The demonstration clinician leaves the room to analyze data independently and the leader and peers analyze their data, problem-solve, and determine how to provide feedback in the most supportive manner.
5. The demonstration clinician returns, presents his or her self-analysis, which is followed by group feedback, problem solving, and the generation of strategies for the next clinical session.
6. In the review, the monitor assesses the effectiveness of the group interactions.

A comprehensive description of the Teaching Clinic is available in Chapter 10 of Dowling's most recent text (2001).

A number of studies has been completed to analyze the efficiency and effectiveness of the Teaching Clinic. Dowling and Shank (1981) compared it to conventional supervision and found the two yielded similar outcomes. In a subsequent analysis (Dowling, 1983a) using a more sensitive dependent measure (MOSAICS), there were some differences in that the Teaching Clinic contained more direct behaviors. Johnson and Fey (1983) compared individual conferences and the Teaching Clinic and found no differences with regard to student attitudes about therapy or perceived clinical effectiveness. In a 1987 investigation, Dowling found that teaching clinics were clearly viewed more positively than typical conferences and were *perceived* by the 46 graduate students in her study to be more indirect than typical conferences. McCrea (1994) described using an adaptation of the Teaching Clinic as part of the curriculum for a Master's degree thesis option in supervision. This provided opportunities for students to apply what they learned in a three-credit-hour course the previous semester to their own supervisory practice. McCrea reported that students increased their self-awareness and abilities to self-analyze the supervisory process as a result of their experience. Dowling and colleagues (1992) described some adaptations and unique uses of the Teaching Clinic. Descriptive data and anecdotal information supported the use of the Teaching Clinic as a primary or augmentative procedure. It was useful in (1) increasing satisfaction with the supervisory process; (2) identifying parameters of effective therapy; (3) teaching self-analysis, problem solving, and strategy development skills; and (4) analyzing and enhancing the quality of supervision. Given her expertise and years of studying this approach, and consulting with others who have experimented with the Teaching Clinic, Dowling (2001) recommends that it be used "as a supplement to traditional supervision rather than a substitute" (p. 321).

McFarlane and Hagler (1992a) compared the traditional approach to peer groups in which 47 undergraduates with less than 16 clock hours served as subjects. The hypothesis that student clinicians would be more initiatory in conferences with a peer than with a supervisor was not substantiated. Overall, peer supervisors initiated significantly less than supervisors in conferences. Supervisees remained passive regardless of the type of supervision they experienced. The results "suggested a need to re-think past explanations of supervisors' apparent inability to alter their largely direct-evaluative behavior" (p. 80). An important variable seems to be the level of supervisee experience; supervisees at the Evaluation-Feedback end of the continuum need a Direct-Active style and are not yet ready to assume a leadership role in conferences.

Bowline, Bunce, Polmanteer, and Wegner (1996) described an innovative approach to clinical teaching developed at the University of Kansas out of frustration with the traditional method of supervision and the need to teach students to be effective team leaders and members. Clinical faculty manage a team in an area of individual expertise (e.g., AAC, adult neurogenics, child language, etc.). Students are assigned to a team and each graduate clinician provides between 5 to 10 hours of therapy per week. Teams meet weekly for a two-hour period; students rotate the facilitator and recorder roles. Students set their own agenda and run the meetings; supervisors may add items to an agenda. In addition, undergraduates in a pre-practicum course rotate through three different teams in four-week blocks of time. They write observation reports, note teams skills, and track the team process. The major benefits of this team approach are "that it is more efficient in terms of clinical operations and instruction, provides broader and more self-directed learning experiences for students, and better teaching by faculty" because they can focus on individual interests and experiences (Wegner, 1999, p. 104).

Farmer (1987a) addressed the advantages and disadvantages of dyadic versus group approaches to conferences. Among the advantages of groups are that they are more time efficient; they expand exposure to a variety of ideas, methods, and materials; information can be disseminated quickly to all supervisees; the possibility of lack of information, misinformation, or misunderstanding is decreased; networks are developed; and supervisee dependence on the supervisor is less likely to develop. He cautions that groups may be too confusing for marginal supervisees, they may create interpersonal competition, and they are less useful for appraisal/evaluation than the traditional conference. Farmer (1994) also distinguished between group and team supervision, maintaining that "a team has a task focus with a strong relationship orientation to support the efforts to complete the task" (p. 141).

Supervisors who wish to use group conferences should be sensitive to the needs of supervisees. Many students prefer to have the opportunity for some individual contact with the supervisor along with group interaction. Certain aspects of the Collaborative Style lend themselves to a group methodology. For example, much of the introductory aspects of the first component, Understanding, could be done in a group, not only to save time, but also to allow supervisees to share insights and experiences. Teaching supervisees data collection and analysis techniques, as well as demonstrating certain clinical techniques, are other tasks that could be easily managed in groups.

For the Consultative Style, groups may be especially appropriate. Self-supervising clinicians have much to share with each other and such conferences could be an effective means of promoting professional growth, whatever the setting.

An important issue in implementing group supervision is how well prepared supervisors are in group dynamics and group processes. There is an analogy to be found in group therapy. Most supervisors have observed so-called group therapy, which was simply a few minutes of individual therapy for each client who happened to be sitting in the group. Among the reasons for this are the fact that the group has been defined on the basis of scheduling convenience rather than on common goals or problems or the ability to work together, and their needs are so varied that even the most skillful group leader would have difficulty managing the group. Another reason is the lack of preparation, experience, or insight about group processes, which results in ineffective use of group time. Clinicians become supervisors and their lack of skill in group management generalizes to the supervisory process. Although group supervision is thought to be valuable, effectiveness is contingent on the skills of the leader. As many experts (Bowline et al., 1996; Dowling, 2001; Farmer, 1994) have noted and as any instructor who has tried to implement problem-based learning or other forms of group teaching can substantiate, supervisees need some orientation to group work. Complaints about group members who don't carry their weight or conflicts between individuals are not uncommon. Techniques to ensure trust, openness, cohesiveness, and goal accomplishment have to be planned. Any supervisor who wishes to use a group approach would be wise to investigate the vast resources on group processes in the counseling (therapeutic groups), business (task groups) or communication literature. Understanding how to form groups (e.g., homogeneity, optimal size, and so on), identifying how groups and individuals within groups will be evaluated, clarifying group goals, developing mutual understanding of each person's roles, clarifying members' right and responsibilities, establishing ground rules (e.g., regarding confidentiality, attendance, honesty) are among the many concerns that need to be considered. Understanding group dynamics will not only be an asset in supervision, but also in all other professional domains in which we find ourselves to be part of a working group.

Varying Perceptions of Conferences

There is evidence that supervisees and supervisors perceive the activities within conferences differently. This fact, coupled with the data that indicate the supervisory process is not discussed, increases the opportunity for misunderstanding and frustration (Brasseur & Jimenez, 1996; Culatta et al., 1975; Dowling, 2001; McCrea, 1980; Pickering, 1984; Roberts & Smith, 1982; Shapiro, 1985a, 1985b; Tufts, 1984).

Culatta and colleagues (1975) found that supervisees and supervisors frequently reported "completely contradictory interpretations of the same event" (p. 152). The discrepancies relative to lesson planning were reported in the Planning chapter. Other areas where discrepancies existed are relevant. For example, supervisors said they believed it was important to have supervisees review client's case history and confer with the supervisor before client contact. Seventy percent of the supervisees, however, reported that supervisors did not attend these conferences, resulting in disappointment and confusion on the part of supervisees. Supervisors felt positively about viewing videotapes; supervisees did not. There were differing views about the value of various types of reports and of the supervisory conference. Most important, the areas of difference were never discussed during conferences. Similar results have been reported by others (Anderson & Milisen, 1965; Russell, 1976).

Such differences in perceptions are illustrated by the following situation. An off-campus supervisor says to the university supervisor, "I wish the student would use more of her own ideas and not just do what I do," while the supervisee says, "I feel that I have to do therapy the way she does it. That is what she wants." And, as in the study by Culatta and colleagues (1975), they seldom discuss these differences except with the university supervisor. In fact, this may become a major function of the university of the off-campus practicum—bridging the "communication gap."

In an extensive study of the conference, Smith (1978) and Smith and Anderson (1982b) found that supervisors, supervisees, and trained raters each perceived different effectiveness variables in conference content. Such differences of perception are not surprising. What is significant is the lack of discussion about the differences. It might be assumed that such differences between expectations and reality would be clarified at some time, as an integral part of Understanding, but such does not seem to be the case. Relevant to this fact is the recommendation

> that supervisors and supervisees should keep their self-perceptions of the conference at a conscious level, investigating them at frequent intervals to determine if perceptions are similar. A lack of information regarding the convergence or divergence of perceptions of those involved in conference interactions, if allowed to exist over time, may greatly diminish the effectiveness of the conference. (Smith & Anderson, 1982a, p. 258)

The mass of descriptive data on the conference and the consistency of the finding that supervisor behavior does not change over time or according to the supervisee's experience raises some interesting issues. There are, admittedly, weaknesses in some of the studies. Change has been measured over a relatively short period of time, possibly not sufficient to expect change. The questions asked, the settings in which research was conducted, instruments used to measure change, and the preciseness of methodology vary across studies. It must be assumed that the outcomes do not typify every conference, yet the striking similarities enhance collective credibility. The knowledge that supervisors' perceptions of their own behavior and its change are inaccurate does not give comfort to the supervisor who says, "But my

conferences are not like that. I use different styles and behaviors to meet the needs of individuals." Although this may be true, no one can say it with certainty until they have engaged in some type of objective study of their conferences.

WHAT'S A SUPERVISOR TO DO?

What do all these studies and all this discussion tell the supervisor about the provision of feedback or conferences? Except for general knowledge about learning, motivation, communication, interpersonal interaction, leadership, and other relevant topics, there is not enough specific information to support the merits of any method of feedback or any particular type of conference. Anderson (1988) maintained that this allows freedom to speculate— **professional growth, including specific behavior change in supervisees, will or will not take place mainly as a result of the interaction in the conference.** It is the theme of this book that the conference, although only one of several types of interaction between supervisor and supervisee, is probably the most important. This belief comes not only from the fact that it appears to be the most commonly used occasion for communication, but also because of the sheer dynamic of this interpersonal "happening"—this event that can be so important to its participants. Further, there is an assumption that it is through the intensive study of the conference that the positives and negatives of the supervisory process will begin to unravel.

What *is* known about the conference from research is that it is consistent with the Direct-Active Style appropriate to the Evaluation-Feedback Stage, not with the Collaborative Style nor with the Consultative Style. If the continuum and the styles appropriate to its different point are accepted, conference behavior can be measured against that standard.

Conferences Using the Collaborative Style

Some of the characteristics of the Collaborative Style appropriate to the Transitional Stage are listed here. This is not an all-inclusive list, nor are items listed in order of importance. Any single conference must not necessarily include all the items. Content will be determined by individual needs, place on the continuum within the Transitional Stage, supervisory objectives, and other factors.

- The conference will include some evidence that it has been planned—there will be some type of agenda.
- There will be evidence that both long-range and short-range goals have been set for all participants: client, clinician, supervisee, and supervisor.
- There will be evidence of data collection on both client and clinician by both supervisor and supervisee.
- The data will be presented in an organized manner that gives some evidence of planning data collection. For example, it will be obvious that data are related to goals. It will be obvious that planning took place to determine what data would be collected, how, by whom, and how they will be presented.
- There will be emphasis on analysis of data related to the relationship between client and clinician behavior, not a single focus on the client. Inferences will be drawn about the relationship between client and clinician.
- Analysis will be related to goals and objectives.
- There will be data collection, analysis, and discussion of goals and objectives for supervisee and supervisor; that is, the supervisory process will be studied to determine if appropriate learning is taking place.
- There will be a combination of direct and indirect supervisor behaviors. The balance will be determined by continuum placement.
- Topics other than data from sessions will include procedural or administrative issues, academic topics, research relevant to practice, personal or affective concerns, professional issues, unexpected events, and other pertinent issues.
- Although the emphasis will be on analysis, particularly self-analysis by the supervisee, leading to self-evaluation, there is a time and

place for varying degrees of evaluative feedback and information given by the supervisor.
- The supervisor will assume responsibility for structuring joint problem solving through open, thought-provoking questions, appropriate responses to the supervisee, types of objectives set, and other techniques. In turn, the supervisee will accept responsibility for participating in problem solving.
- Part of the learning process will be the expansion of verbal statements by supervisor and supervisee—explanations, justifications, rationale for opinions and suggestions, and questioning each other for such expansions if they do not occur. Research demonstrates that, traditionally, utterances are simple and short rather than the type that lead to in-depth discussion and information exchange. To optimize learning and generalization, more discussion of options, justifications, and explanations of suggestions by supervisors should be apparent in conference dialogue.
- The interpersonal interaction in the conference will be supportive and facilitative, with both participants being sensitive to the needs and feelings of the other.
- Supervisor and supervisee will periodically review their own objectives for the supervisory process, compare their perceptions of whether objectives are being met, and make appropriate adjustments.

The Consultative Style

The Consultative Style, appropriate to the Self-Supervision Stage, is not as clear-cut as the other two styles. It may include behaviors from each of the other styles, but the supervisor and supervisee will maintain a different type of relationship. Referred to commonly in the literature in other helping professions, consultation is not so frequently discussed in speech-language pathology and audiology.

According to Hart (1982), consultation in counseling is "an informal educational experience usually used in place of supervision" (p. 12). Kurpius and Robinson (1978) called the consultant a "collaborator who forms egalitarian relationships with the consultee to bring about change. In this collegial relationship, there is a joint diagnosis with emphasis on consultees finding their own solution to their problems" (p. 322). The consultant serves as a catalyst for problem solving. Kurpius and colleagues (1977) said that consultation is a frequently employed approach to supervision and it "implies shared problem definition, problem solving, and evaluation…there is a suggestion in the literature that consultation becomes a more dominant mode of supervision as the trainee becomes increasingly able and professional in his performance" (p. 288).

The Consultative Style of supervision is a style that results from the need to solve a problem. It has a voluntary and possibly an intermittent or temporary aspect not found in the other styles. The supervisee identifies the need. The supervisor's role is not only to help the supervisee solve the immediate existing problem, but also to develop problem-solving abilities so that future problems may be anticipated and managed. A democratic, collegial relationship is essential to this style. Developing this type of relationship requires that the supervisor exhibit nonjudgmental and nonevaluative behaviors (Kurpius, 1978), in addition to behaviors that convey openness, supportiveness, interdependence, equal power, and professional respect. The supervisor is responsible for building the relationship and for using skills to facilitate the problem-solving process. Supervisees have the knowledge and expertise in their area of work, as well as the necessary abilities and resources to solve their problem, although some of these may need to be developed. Supervisees are responsible for acknowledging ownership of the problem and for learning new skills and behaviors to solve their problem. The nature of the situation and the presenting problem may require the supervisor to perform different roles and use various skills and approaches during the process. The *process of problem solving* must always remain the primary focus even though at times during the relationship there may be attention to content and the supervisor provides information, shares knowledge, gives rationales or assumes other content-related roles. The emphasis on problem solving, fundamental to this style, will enable supervisees to function more effectively in the future.

A brief description of the components of the "clinical problem-solving" process seems appropriate here. The supervisor facilitates this process while the supervisee functions as the actual agent of change. First, the presenting problem needs to be clearly defined. Next, information must be gathered. This may involve doing library research, administering tests or other assessment protocols, interviewing, and so on. As data are being collected, they are analyzed, weighted, and used to generate multiple hypotheses about the precise nature of the problem. The problem is clarified, refined, and translated into a goal statement. The next step involves formulating optimal interventions or solutions to solve the problem or achieve the goal. It is important to brainstorm a variety of alternatives (Kurpius & Robinson, 1978), and creativity is important. During brainstorming, criticism is withheld, free-wheeling is encouraged, quantity is desired, and combination and improvement of ideas are sought. The forces that support and impede change should be examined. An action plan is then devised, which will enable the hypotheses that were generated to be tested and evaluated. When the plan is implemented, both the process and the product should be evaluated. It is essential to include evidence-based practice into the action plan strategies and criteria for evaluating the effectiveness of the results. The process is a dynamic, cyclic, reiterative process in which observation, analysis, synthesis, deduction, induction, hypothesis generation, hypothesis testing, strategy design, and implementation are interrelated (Barrows & Pickell, 1991).

This Consultative Style may seem minimally different from the Collaborative Style. Actually, the difference is a matter of degree. Consultation is an expansion of the Collaborative Style to meet the needs of supervisees who have truly reached the point where they are capable of self-supervision, are able to analyze their clinical work, and can identify their own needs. The time when an individual reaches this stage varies. If reached during the educational program, the supervisor may become a monitor, may help supervisees expand their clinical activities and assume new challenges, or may assist them in spending more time in the analysis of the supervisory process. If reached during off-campus practica or the Clinical Fellowship (CF), consultants may need to adjust their expectations and behaviors to truly operate as a consultant; that is, to assist supervisees in using their knowledge and skills to solve problems. In the service delivery setting, where supervisor and supervisee are both fully qualified professionals, the interactions will vary even more. Conference content will be determined not only by the nature of the problem to be solved but also by the frequency with which the supervisor is able to interact with the supervisee in the work setting. Despite professional standards, not every professional in the work force has the ability to be self-supervising in every situation. A person may reach the Self-Supervision Stage in one area of clinical expertise but not in others. And herein lie the hazards in the use of the Consultative style in any setting—the possible inaccurate perception of supervisees of their own ability, either positive or negative, or the inability of the supervisor to accurately determine the true nature of the supervisee's skills. This is why the suggestions in the Planning chapter for determining placement on the continuum are important.

You'll know you've achieved a Consultative Style when:

- You say "we" and mean it
- You feel you've learned from your supervisee and can tell him or her so
- You're not afraid to say, "You're right—I was wrong"
- The supervisee solves a problem with little or no input from you
- You accept the supervisee's input as important as your own
- You are able to work jointly on the supervisee's performance evaluations

Flower (1984) summed it up when he stated, "Good consultation resembles any other professional service; it is valuable only if offered in a way that is useful to the recipient"(p. 12). Consultation, he said, will be helpful only when it is sensitive to the recipients' needs and is "relevant, practical, and applicable" (p. 13).

SUMMARY

This last component, Integrating, is also the beginning. It is the place where everything that has happened in the other components comes together and the future is determined. Understanding, Planning, Observing, and Analyzing feed into this component.

Because the other components have been discussed individually, this chapter focuses on the communication that takes place between supervisor and supervisee. The conference is discussed at some length because this is the usual place where communication between supervisor and supervisee occurs.

This chapter includes extensive discussion about feedback, which is defined as interaction between all participants about all components of the process, not as just the traditional reporting on observation. This component, then, becomes the culmination of all the effort and time that have gone into the supervisory process.

RESEARCH ISSUES AND QUESTIONS

As a beginning in the process of validating the competencies associated with Task 8, several studies have examined the impact of supervisee input into conference *agendas* (Jans, Hagler, & McFarlane, 1994; McFarlane & Hagler, 1992a, 1992b; Peaper, 1984; Sbaschnig, Dowling, &Williams, 1992) and a couple have investigated the effects of written and verbal *commitments* (Gillam, Strike, & Anderson, 1987; Shapiro, 1985b). The effect of involving supervisees in preparing conference agendas on their active involvement in conferences is mixed. Written commitments appear to facilitate follow through with beginning clinicians whereas verbal commitments are sufficient in promoting action for more advanced clinicians. It is evident that more research is needed to identify the competencies that enhance the effectiveness of the supervisory process at various stages on the continuum

Only the surface has been scratched in investigating the effect that communication skills have on supervisees' decision making, problem solving, and critical-thinking abilities. For example,

Strike-Roussos (1995) demonstrated that supervisors can be trained to use convergent and broad questions and these higher-level questions facilitate higher-level thinking in supervisees. The limited sample size in her study makes replication essential. A number of other studies have examined supervisors' interpersonal skills. Caracciolo and colleagues (1978b) and Ghitter (1987) have demonstrated that it is important for supervisees to perceive high levels of unconditional positive regard, genuineness, empathic understanding, and concreteness being offered by supervisors but McCrea (1980) and Pickering (1979) have shown that in actuality, these behaviors occur in conferences only minimally, if at all. Hagler, Casey, and DesRochers (1989) found that providing data to supervisors about the amount of these behaviors in their conferences and written suggestions for change was not sufficient to induce change. They suggested that subsequent studies should attempt to train specific facilitative behaviors, including opportunities to role play or practice. Active listening, on the part of both supervisees and supervisors, is another communication behavior that needs to be examined. What is the extent of active listening in individual and group conferences—and what impact does it have on problem solving and decision making? Other behaviors, such as supervisor self-disclosure, have been identified as important facilitators for supervisee change (Pickering & McCready, 1990), but their frequency of occurrence and influence on supervisee behaviors has not been investigated. Those interested in the interpersonal aspect of the process will be able to generate many more important questions that need to be answered.

In looking at the composite characteristics of conventional speech-language pathology conferences described in Chapter 2, we need to find out if things have changed in the last couple of decades. For example, past research indicated that very little explanation and justification, and few rationales, are offered for ideas and strategies by either supervisors or supervisees (Hatten, 1966; Roberts & Smith, 1982; Smith and Anderson, 1982b). If evidence-based practice is to be the norm, as mandated in the new certification standards (ASHA 2000a), rationales for practice should be abundant in conferences. Culatta and Seltzer (1976) noted the absence of supervisor evaluations and supervisee self-evaluations, and this was evident in a number of other studies (Jans, Hagler, McFarlane, McCrea, et al., 1994; Roberts & Smith, 1982; Schubert & Nelson, 1976; Tufts, 1984). Other studies have reported that *written* feedback from supervisors is highly evaluative (Peaper & Mercaitis, 1987; Rocchio & Iacarino, 1990). Future research is needed to identify strategies that effectively elicit supervisee self-evaluations and to find out how these strategies affect clinical behaviors.

Although Dowling has conducted numerous studies on the Teaching Clinic (1981, 1983a, 1983b, 1992, 2001), the advantages and disadvantages of other group models need to be established through careful study. It seems that groups and teams are appropriate for specific kinds of tasks at the Evaluation-Feedback Stage (e.g., orienting supervisees to the supervisory process, teaching data collection strategies, and so on) and, as supervisees progress through the transitional stage, peers may be able to assume more leadership in conferences. Training in the supervisory process and in group dynamics are apparent prerequisites to effective functioning in group conferences, but this remains to be demonstrated. Because of the exposure to clients being served by peers, groups would also appear to be conducive to providing numerous opportunities "to critically evaluate and incorporate research relevant to professional practice," as stipulated in the new standards (ASHA 2000a). Comparing and contrasting the knowledge acquired in group versus individual conferences with regard to this would be interesting.

Lastly, readers will notice that many references to support practices in Chapters 4 through 8 are dated. This suggests a compelling need to rejuvenate the research that was being done in the 1970s and try to regain the momentum and productivity that was apparent in the 1980s. Research initiatives are important for advancing the science and the art of the supervisory process.

CHAPTER NINE

PREPARATION FOR THE SUPERVISORY PROCESS

Supervision, as a field of study, is filled with myths, unclear
definitions and distinctions, and untrained supervisors who
operate with good intentions as their main resource.
—Hart (1982, p. 5)

Preparation for supervisors? Unnecessary in the opinion of some, crucially needed in the opinion of others. Speech-language pathologists and audiologists are expected to have extensive preparation to become professionals. Psychologists, social workers, teachers, doctors, counselors—all the helping professions—have varying amounts of education to prepare them for their professional roles. Much of the preparation of such professionals—the applied aspect of it—is provided by supervisors. Yet it has been generally assumed in most of those disciplines—certainly in speech-language pathology and audiology—that preparation of those supervisors who provide a critical part of the education of practitioners is not necessary. In many disciplines, the apprenticeship model has been the prevalent model for transferring skills from one professional generation to another, "learning by doing," or copying a master practitioner (Kurpius et al., 1977).

The Position Statement (ASHA, 1985b) legitimizes supervision as a distinct area of expertise and practice and stipulates that special preparation

is needed to enable individuals to function competently as supervisors. Preparation may be in the form of preservice or in-service curricular offerings, continuing education at professional meetings, practicum at universities, self-study, or research. Until the Position Statement was adopted, many speech-language pathologists and audiologists assumed that CCC automatically enabled a professional to be an effective, competent supervisor. Education, on the other hand, had for many years recognized the need for preparation and special certification for supervisors. However, a review of relevant literature revealed that the focus had not been on the interaction between supervisor and supervisee; rather it had been on more general topics (Blumberg, 1980). Data are hard to come by on the number of supervisors in various related disciplines such as counseling and social work who are working with or without special preparation. While perusal of curricular offerings in programs accredited by ASHA's Council on Academic Accreditation (CAA) reveals that many programs have courses in clinical supervision on their books, it is unclear how often the courses are offered, what kind of enrollments these courses have, and the precise content of the offerings. A number of early surveys in our disciplines revealed that supervisors felt the need for training in supervision (Anderson, 1972, 1973a; Schubert & Aitchison, 1975; Stace & Drexler, 1969), and, interestingly, supervisors who have been exposed to some kinds of special preparation begin to see the process as a more complex phenomenon—they seem to begin "to know what they don't know."

Yet the notion that *anyone* can supervise still seems to be alive and well—particularly among non-supervisors. People state, "Our supervisors have been supervising for years and we're doing okay," "We can't afford to add another course to the curriculum," or "We have no data to prove that training makes supervisors any more effective." Even the new standards (ASHA, 2000a) continue to focus on the amount of observation, not the quality of the experience or the competence of those providing the supervision. The cost of increasing education requirements or adding faculty to teach supervision courses is a serious concern in the days of reduced budgets, but perhaps it is a matter of establishing priorities. Culatta and colleagues (1975) treated the issue of cost in relation to time spent in supervision in a statement that is relevant to the cost of preparation for supervisors.

> The implicit suggestion is that we re-examine our educational priorities to redetermine how critical a factor adequate supervision is in the training of new professionals. Although the knowledgeable administrator will quickly point out the cost of clinical supervision, with its necessarily low student-faculty ratio, one can scarcely venture a guess as to how many poorly trained students, economically produced, equal one expensively well-trained professional successfully meeting the needs of her or his clients. (Culatta, Colucci, & Wiggins, 1975, p. 155)

Similarly, efficiency and effectiveness of well-prepared supervisors may eventually balance out additional costs accrued in their education and produce better clinicians in the bargain. O'Neil (1985) emphasized the importance of supervision, stating that given the number of clock hours of supervised practicum required for the master's degree, "clinical supervision and the qualifications of the supervisors should be of major importance" (p. 23). Hardick and Oyer (1987) said:

> Increasing attention has been directed toward the preparation of trained clinical supervisors and the identification of desirable characteristics of supervisors and the supervisory process. Research in supervision and the teaching of this content are legitimate components of the educational process…. The expanding literature on the subject also makes it feasible for university clinics to offer in-service training for staff supervisors, including faculty members who participate in supervision. The administration of a university speech and hearing clinic should provide encouragement and support for staff participation in workshops, courses, or less formal activities designed to improve the supervisory process and individual skills. (p. 49)

Interestingly, when licensure boards in states such as California mandate minimal training in supervision for those who will supervise aides and assistants, it would seem that at least comparable mandates would exist for supervisors of students and professionals. Indeed, some states have special certification requirements for program supervisors in schools. And some states or university programs require at least a course in supervision for field supervisors of all school internships, including speech-language pathology. In the first draft of the 1985 ASHA Position Statement (ASHA, 1982), a recommendation for *minimum* qualifications for supervisors included that, in addition to the Master's degree and CCC in the area supervised, supervisors should have at least two years of professional experience (after the CFY) and some coursework in supervision. Coursework was to consist of six semester credit hours or nine continuing education units applicable to the supervisory process, of which at least one half must be specific to the supervisory process in speech-language pathology or audiology, *and* a practicum in supervision in which at least 50 clock hours of supervision would be supervised. In light of the trend in doctoral programs across disciplines to prepare candidates not only as researchers but also as instructors, it seems like an opportune time to revisit the 1982 recommendation to assist professionals in acquiring the skills necessary for effective supervision.

PREPARATION IN SPEECH-LANGUAGE PATHOLOGY AND AUDIOLOGY

Although there had been a limited amount of preparation in the 1960s, it was not until the 1970s that the profession saw the real beginning of formal education programs in the supervisory process. A survey done by the ASHA Committee on Supervision revealed that such educational offerings were sparse (ASHA, 1978a). Of the 279 programs responding to the survey, 41.5% reported some form of preparation in the supervisory process. When analyzed, the data revealed that less than half of those offered a course and/or practicum; 25% included content in other courses and about the same number offered an independent study. It is time for an updated survey. Perhaps the Council of Academic Programs in Communication Sciences and Disorders (CAPCSD) or SID 11—Administration and Supervision will undertake this task.

Impetus for preparation, besides self-motivation, may come from several sources. Some individuals may take courses or workshops to obtain continuing education units (CEUs). Some states have special certification requirements for program supervisors in schools that include coursework in the supervisory process as it pertains to speech-language pathology and audiology. A few states or universities require at least one course in supervision for school supervisors of all student-teaching experiences. And, some employers are beginning to look for preparation, rather than experience alone, as part of the credentials of people they wish to hire as supervisors.

Content of Supervisory Preparation

It is important that supervisors remain current in the disorder areas in which they are supervising.

For supervisors in educational programs who are also instructors in the disorder areas, the study of the disorder areas is a given. For full-time supervisors in university programs, it is essential that they be knowledgeable about what is being taught in the academic coursework in the program. For supervisors outside an educational program, such as off-campus, CFY, or service delivery settings, the need to maintain current information is just as essential.

Content will vary depending on the orientation of the program and the instructor's philosophy. This book presents Anderson's (1988) approach, which was based on the clinical supervision model (Cogan, 1973; Goldhammer, 1969; Goldhammer et al., 1980) and influenced by situational leadership theory (Hersey & Blanchard, 1982). Anderson (1988) stated, "It has never been assumed that this is the only way to supervise" (p. 229) and she acknowledged the merit of other approaches. What *is* assumed to be absolutely essential is that those who supervise or those who teach others about the supervisory process have some model, some theoretical base, some solid foundation on which they can build their procedures, form hypothesis, and develop their plans. Too much supervision, and presumably the teaching of it, is not rationally and logically planned on such a foundation. Thus, it likely to be fragmented, inconsistent, and lacking in direction and focus, with no rationale and justification.

There are certain types of information and certain skills related to the supervisory process that supervisors must attain. The question about the content of such preparation is not what it *should* be, but what can be *selected* from the vast array of knowledge important to the supervisor. The tasks and competencies (ASHA, 1985b) provide a focus for training.

MODELS FOR PREPARATION IN THE SUPERVISORY PROCESS

There are many ways in which preparation in the supervisory process can be implemented. The models that will be discussed here range from inclusion of information in early clinical management courses to preparation at the doctoral level.

At each level there are different purposes and different procedures.

Inclusion in Clinical Management Courses

Training programs typically offer a course on clinical methods/clinical management procedures prior to or in conjunction with practica. It is highly recommended, as discussed in Chapter 4, that basic information about the supervisory process be included in such a course. A basic introduction to the supervisory process at this point makes it easier for individual supervisor/supervisee dyads to begin a discussion of their own individual interaction. The purpose at this level is to assist supervisees in learning what to expect of supervision, their rights and responsibilities, and how to maximize the benefits of their clinical training.

McCrea (1985), in describing a component on supervision in an undergraduate clinical management class, listed the objectives as (1) to encourage undergraduate students to view the clinical and supervisory processes as complementary and interactive, (2) to introduce undergraduate students to the participants and their primary roles and responsibilities within both processes, and (3) to introduce undergraduate students to problem-solving strategies to enhance both processes. McCrea then made the points that each part of the clinical process has its counterpart in the supervisory process and that they can be taught in such a way that the complementary and interactive nature of the two processes is emphasized. For example, evaluation and goal setting for the client have their counterparts in goal setting for the clinician's development, as do observation, data collection, and data analysis. Because time may be limited in such courses for inclusion of the topic, the instructor must be knowledgeable about the process and able to distill the information into meaningful concepts appropriate to the students' level. Such content should extend beyond the undergraduate level. Even advanced graduate students will profit from opportunities to discuss their changing roles as supervisees. McCrea (1985) suggested such procedures as lecture, problem solving, and in-class discussion, as well as "hands on experiences…through the presentation of actual samples of supervisory problems, experiences with observation tools, and viewing and analysis of videotaped samples of supervisory conference behavior" (p. 3).

Some programs pair inexperienced clinicians with more advanced clinicians, easing the inexperienced clinicians into the clinical process by having them first observe then gradually assume some responsibility for therapy. This is an excellent opportunity for the supervisor to present some basic supervisory concepts to the advanced clinician, and to provide them with opportunities to "try-on" the supervisory role with the assistance of the supervisor. They will be able to learn something about the dynamics of the process at an early stage in their careers.

Basic Course in Supervision

Coursework in supervision is provided for master's- or doctoral-level students in some colleges and universities. It is also often taken by professionals in the field who are supervising or preparing to do so. The wisdom of providing a course in supervision as part of the Master's degree curriculum is seen in the fact that, historically, the major portion of the supervision is done by professionals who hold Master's degrees, most of them without preparation or even much clinical experience (Anderson, 1972, 1973a, 1973b; Schubert & Aitchison, 1975; Stace & Drexler, 1969). Additionally, it is reasonable to assume that students and professionals who have the opportunity to take a course in supervision become better supervisees. Knowledge of the process seems to give them more confidence about their own participation and what they can expect to gain from supervision.

The wisdom of such a course for doctoral-level students is similar. Most of them intend to obtain positions in academe where their responsibilities are apt to include supervision of students preparing to become clinicians, or they may become supervisors in other settings. Further, if they have CCC, they may be engaged in supervision as doctoral students at the time they are taking the courses.

Such a course should include at least the following topics: relevant information on supervision from related disciplines; preparation for the role of supervisor; professional/political issues in supervision in speech-language pathology and audiology; the planning, observation, and analysis role of the supervisor relative to the clinical process; the planning, observation, and analysis of the supervisory process; supervisory techniques; interpersonal aspects of the supervisory process; variations in supervision across sites; accountability and evaluation in the supervisory process; preparing supervisees for the process; and research in supervision. Assignments should include extensive reading from the speech-language pathology literature as well as some from other disciplines, viewing of videotapes of conferences, a self-study of students' interactions in taped conferences (as supervisor or supervisee), a research proposal or review of literature on a specific topic, or other assignments that meet individual needs and interests. The course should be oriented so that it could be taken by both speech-language pathologists and audiologists.

Such courses and their content were discussed by Anderson, Rassi, Laccinole, Casey, Brasseur, McCrea, Ulrich, Ganz, and Hunt-Thompson at an ASHA convention short course moderated by Smith (1985). Rassi described an introductory course for advanced students in the audiology graduate program who aspire to supervisory positions or have an interest in supervision and to on- and off-campus supervisors. Rassi noted that the course provided an opportunity for potential supervisors to study the process as they experienced it. Content included an examination of supervision research, methodology and theory in communication sciences and disorders, clinical decision making, competency-based instruction, supervisory competencies, leadership and supervisory styles, data collection, conference analysis, interpersonal relationships, observation, attribution and judgment, and evaluation and self-evaluation. Activities included participation in laboratory experiences or practicum that is monitored by a regular staff supervisor, listening to conference tapes, keeping a journal, and roleplaying.

Coursework described by Casey (1985) had content and requirements similar to Rassi's, but fo-

cused more on ASHA's (1985b) tasks and competencies. It included a practicum experience, conference analysis, and the use of self-assessment instruments related to the ASHA competencies. Casey reported that the material in the course not only prepares people to supervise, but also enhances the student's performance as a supervisee. Dowling (1993, 1994) has repeatedly demonstrated the benefits that completing a course in supervision has for graduate students. Harris and colleagues (1992), in a training project conducted in North Carolina, noted that the graduate students who completed a course in supervision appeared to be more self-analytical and to function within the framework of Anderson's model better than those who did not take it.

Practicum Experiences in Supervision

Each of the courses described has included a very important laboratory or practicum component. Just as clinicians need practice in gaining clinical skills, supervisors also need opportunities to try out the skills they are learning about. The ASHA competency list provides a guide for such practice.

The practicum experience as part of a doctoral-level preparation program has been described by Anderson (1981) as probably the most significant component of the program. "This experience is a necessary step in gaining insight about the supervisory process, in the modification of the supervisory behavior of trainees, and in defining the questions that lead to research in the supervisory process" (Anderson, 1981, p. 80).

Procedures for the doctoral-level practicum in supervision as conducted by Anderson was dependent on need. Some doctoral students had experience in supervision—all had clinical experience and CCC. They were assigned a certain number of student clinicians to supervisee. The doctoral student planned, observed, and analyzed the clinical work and held conferences with the students. Similarly, their work was planned, observed, analyzed, and discussed in conference with the faculty directing the supervision practicum. Extensive use of audio- and videotape and interaction analysis systems provided conference content.

Practicum or laboratory experience for the master's-level students must be handled differently because they do not have CCC and, therefore, cannot be independently responsible for supervising student clinicians. Thus, they will need to be assigned to a clinical supervisor and involved in the supervisory process at whatever level is appropriate. At the beginning of the experience, the clinical supervisor, the master's-level student, and the student clinician who is to be supervised discuss the purpose of the experience, set objectives, and develop a plan for the semester. This plan includes the master's-level student's role in observation, data collection, and analysis of the clinical sessions. It also includes procedures for observation, data collection, and analysis of conferences between the supervisor and the student clinician or the master's-level student and the supervisor. The plan will specify procedures to be used—use of certain observation systems or other data collection methods, journal writing, observation of others, methods of analysis and reporting in the conference, and other suitable activities. Portfolios would certainly provide a useful procedure for measuring growth. Depending on the dynamics of the situation, the student may participate to some degree in the conference when appropriate. If this is done, the student will have opportunity for self-analysis of his or her interaction in a conference situation. The student will also have weekly conferences with the supervisor to discuss his or her progress toward the objectives that were set.

Master's-Level Preparation

McCrea (1994) developed a two-part Master's degree option that included a three-credit-hour seminar and a modified practicum experience. The seminar fully developed the dynamics of each component of Anderson's model. For example, addressing the Integration phase strategies for structuring supervisory conferences are discussed as are the concepts of immediacy, relational communication, and conflict resolution, and the importance of both verbal and nonverbal communication behaviors. Students learn a variety of strategies to observe, analyze, and evaluate both the clinical and

supervisory processes. The second component involves a modification of the Teaching Clinic (Dowling, 2001; Michalak, 1969) to allow students to apply what they learned in the seminar in the development of their supervisory skills. In using the Teaching Clinic for guided practice in supervision, each demonstration supervisee contributes a segment of a videotaped supervisory conference and states what data he or she wants to be collected to determine if objectives were met. The demonstration supervisee also indicates what data collection tools are to be used. The peer observers then view the video, gather and analyze the data, problem solve the interaction, and decide how to provide feedback in the most supportive manner. The demonstration supervisee may remain in the room during this phase or not, at his or her discretion. Once the analysis phase is complete, the demonstration supervisee presents his or her own self-analysis followed by the group feedback, problem solving, and generation of strategies for the next conference. This cycle repeats itself for as many student supervisees and weeks as there are available.

In a case study, Dowling and Biskynis (1993) examined the impact of a course in supervision and a subsequent practicum on the behavior of a graduate student. Pre- and post-measures of conferencing ability were obtained using a simulation experience to assess course outcomes. After studying Cogan's clinical (1973) and Anderson's (1988) continuum models of supervision and discussions with the instructor, the student established three goals and contracted to change these in her final conference at the end of the semester. In the subsequent term, the student enrolled in a practicum. She was assigned to supervise a first-semester clinician, teaming with the instructor who was certified. Over the course of the semester, the trainee assumed increasing responsibility for the student clinician although the instructor jointly observed all treatment sessions. The instructor met regularly with the trainee and also observed supervisory conferences. They also completed joint analyses of conferences. Academic training resulted in changes in the trainee's supervisor talk-time. Those behaviors for which grade contingencies were established consistently improved. During the practicum, behaviors that were targeted changed as well.

The practicum portions of each of these models highlight the importance of providing opportunities to apply concepts learned in a course and to practice skills that are discussed. As stated previously, developing new behaviors requires practice, analysis of performance, and feedback. These models also provide workable models of how supervision practicum can be arranged for master's students who obviously don't have the CCC required for autonomous supervisory practice.

Preparation for Off-Campus Supervisors

Supervisors of off-campus practicum are very influential in the development of clinical skills by students. If preparation can make a difference in the effectiveness of supervisors, as is assumed, it should be extended to off-campus sites.

Many programs provide educational offerings for their off-campus supervisors in the form of regular credit course or in-service offerings. One of the roles of the university supervisor of off-campus practicum may also be seen as assisting site supervisors to develop their supervisory skills.

In the short course presented at ASHA, a program for this purpose, funded by the U.S. Department of Education, was described (Brasseur, 1985). The target population was clinicians who were working in the schools and supervising students from the university and persons who wanted to supervise students in the future. Some graduate students also opted to enroll in the beginning course for two reasons: (1) it would help them be more participative, analytical supervisees and (2) there is a high probability that they will become supervisors at some time during their careers.

The nine-credit-hour program, provided sequentially over three semesters, included an introductory course, practicum, and advanced seminar. One year, the introductory course was offered as a distance education course, using the campus closed-circuit microwave television system.

The supervisory practicum, a minimum of 50 clock hours of experience, used a variety of formats: direct on-site observation of the supervisor

trainee by the university professor who directed the program, audio- and videotapes of interactions between the student and trainee, individual conferences between the trainee and the professor, and group discussions with all trainees. Just as the supervisor and student planned, observed, and analyzed and discussed clinical work, so the work of the trainee was planned, observed, and analyzed and discussed with the professor who observed and held a conference once every two weeks with each trainee. Once a month, all trainees met on campus for three hours to view and analyze videotapes, discuss problems, and plan objectives and strategies for achieving target competencies. In follow-up evaluations, the trainees expressed that the practicum was an essential component of the total preparation program.

A final component of the program was the advanced seminar. In this seminar, students studied existing research in supervision, and the focus changed to preparing the trainees to function as consultants for other supervisors of student interns in their district. Thus, the training was extended beyond the original students.

This type of program has many possibilities. It could be extended to supervisors in other settings. Additionally, graduate students may be inspired to take more than the beginning course after they obtain CCC. A number of universities provide a variety of offerings for their off-campus supervisors and this undoubtedly has benefits for all parties involved. For example, Kelman and Whitmire (1994) described a one-year project in which graduate students and their off-campus supervisors completed a series or workshops and related experiences that ultimately improved field-based practicum experiences.

Doctoral-Level Preparation

It appears that preparation in the supervisory process at the doctoral level has been available in several forms for some time but it is not clear how much or in what form. Courses, practica, independent study, and internships have been provided to some extent at this level as a part of some traditional doctoral programs. Beginning in 1972, however, a doctoral-level program, in which the main emphasis was preparation in the supervisory process, was funded by the U.S. Department of Education (DOE) at Indiana University under the direction of Jean Anderson (Anderson, 1981, 1985). The program was funded for 10 years and has been subsequently continued by the university. McCrea secured additional U.S. DOE funding from 1990–1993. Since 1972, 16 dissertations and numerous theses on the supervisory process have been completed. The program has been refined so that the following guidelines can be presented for others who are interested in developing a similar program:

- The objectives of a doctoral-level program should be (a) to prepare personnel who can teach other supervisors and (b) to prepare researchers in the supervisory process.
- The core content of a program should include at least the following: an introductory course that provides a framework and introduces the supervisory literature in speech-language pathology and audiology; an advanced seminar in which research in the supervisory process is studied extensively (this must include the 25+ dissertations that have been identified in SLP supervision); practicum experiences directed toward the development of the ASHA tasks and competencies (ASHA, 1985b); independent study as needed to fill in the areas not covered in coursework and practica; research experiences; dissertation.
- Programs for doctoral students should be individually planned, based on students' experience and needs. In addition to coursework, practicum, and research experience in supervision, each program should include a concentration in another area of speech-language pathology or audiology that the student will be able to teach in a university once they attain their degree. This is important, because the reality is that most university programs are not currently able to employ a person to teach *only* supervision courses. Although many programs desire someone who has had preparation in supervision, their budgets re-

quire that they find prospective employees who can teach in more than one area.
- The supervised practicum requirement, as described earlier, should be considered an essential part of the program. It is here where skill training takes place and where important research questions are identified. All of the ASHA competencies are relevant to students of the supervisory process at the doctoral level.
- Programs should include a strong research emphasis, both academic and experiential, because of the great need for research about the supervisory process. Research competencies to be achieved should be identified.
- Programs should meet all the basic requirements of the regular doctoral program in the university—research, dissertation, and qualifying examinations.
- Whenever possible, courses from other departments of the university that are relevant to students' goals should be included in their program; for example, from business management, counseling, education, higher education, special education, psychology, instructional technology, and so on.
- Because most doctoral students are preparing themselves to teach in universities, they should have an opportunity for teaching experience. This experience should be supervised by a faculty member with expertise in the content area. Many campuses also offer non-credit programs that prepare individuals for their roles as instructors and help them develop competencies for effective teaching.

In addition, a minor concentration consisting of coursework and practicum should be available for doctoral students who prefer to concentrate in another area but wish to obtain some information about and experience in the supervisory process.

Continuing Education

Another common, accessible mechanism for learning new information is continuing education. Ulrich (1985) suggested that the purposes of continuing education in the supervisory process may be to either increase knowledge *or* to develop skills in the tasks of supervision and that it is important for the leader to differentiate between the two objectives. The ASHA tasks and competencies may provide a foundation for continuing education. Formats range from lectures and panel discussions, peer interaction, and contemporary paradigms for distance learning such as teleconferences, web-based instruction, and directed independent study.

Continuing education takes place at conventions, conferences, seminars, special organizations of supervisors, and within organizations. Some colleges or university programs provide continuing education opportunities for off-campus supervisors who work with their students. A group of supervisors in an organization can gain a great deal from group study of the process. As an example, Susan Anderson (1993) reported on supervisory preparation at a 198-bed acute rehabilitation hospital in which a staff of 20 SLPs trains 10 to 12 students per year. They decided they needed a preparation program for supervisors, so a 16-week course and practica experience were developed. The six supervisors who participated developed competencies in four tasks: establishing and maintaining an effective relationship [1], observing and analyzing treatment and evaluation sessions [6], planning, executing, and analyzing supervisory conferences [8], and evaluation of clinical performance [9].

Hagler and McFarlane (1994) described an interdisciplinary approach designed to foster recognition that quality supervision requires specific expertise and knowledge. In a five-year period, a total of about 880 professionals across disciplines attended 22 one-day workshops. Workshop topics included: applying contemporary theory in clinical education; achieving maximum student potential—the supervisor as coach; learned pessimism and learned optimism—understanding and using exploratory style to optimize professional growth; and supervision of support personnel.

The new standards for the Certificate of Clinical Competence (CCC) in SLP mandate continued professional development for maintenance of one's CCC (ASHA, 2000a). The standard will take effect on January 1, 2005, and the renewal period will be three years. Thus, every three years, certificate holders must accrue three CEUs (30 contact hours) or two semester/three quarter hours of credit in order to renew their CCC. Many states already have continuing education requirements for renewing licenses and/or teaching credentials. Some states—for example, California—require supervision training for those who supervise speech-language pathology assistants (SLPAs).

Implications of Adult Learning Styles

The extensive literature on adult learning or adult education has been neglected by most speech-language pathologists and audiology supervisors and the people they supervise. In adult education, Knowles (1984) differentiated between *pedagogy,* the teaching of children, and *andragogy,* "any intentional and professionally guided activity that aims at a change in adult persons" (p. 50). The two are seen as somewhat similar to the continuum presented here, moving from dependency of the learner in pedagogy to self-directiveness in andragogy. Knowles suggested that an andragogical model of learning be based on several assumptions:

1. Adults need to know why they need to learn something before they begin the process
2. Adults have a concept of being responsible for their own decisions, which may lead to resistance to certain types of educational experiences
3. Because adults bring more experience to a learning situation, not only is there a greater need for individualization in teaching but often the "richest resources for learning reside in the adult learners themselves" (p. 57), providing educators can open their minds to new approaches
4. Readiness to learn is as important to adults as to children
5. Orientation to learning is life-centered; that is, task-centered or problem-centered, not subject-centered (in other words, adults learn best when they can perceive application of learning to their daily life)
6. Although adults respond to some external motivators like money and promotions, the

most potent motivation for learning is from internal pressures (increased job satisfaction, self-esteem, quality of life)

Knowles advocated such methods as organizing adult learning around needs and interests, life situations (not subjects), analysis of experience, and mutual inquiry, and allowing for differences in style, time, place, and pace of learning. In fact, the points he made are compatible with the continuum of supervision. Thus, the continuum is as relevant for the supervisor-in-training as it is for the clinician-in-training.

Knowledge of adult stages of development is also relevant to preparation of supervisors. Individual differences and needs are factors that should be known. Adult learners are often voluntary participants, which implies sacrifices of time and money (Haverkamp, 1983). On the other hand, they may be meeting mandatory requirements of an organization or a degree requirement, which influences attitudes.

Although group activities are recommended, if small-group techniques are used to involve learners more directly in their own learning, it must be realized that "few learners are adequately prepared to function in group learning efforts" (p. 8). Therefore, an orientation to group participation is often a useful tool if the instructor intends to use this methodology. Additionally, many individuals who attempt to lead groups are not very skillful (Haverkamp, 1983).

IS EDUCATION IN SUPERVISION EFFECTIVE?

As preparation in the supervisory process continues, the professions will need to ask themselves some searching questions. Any kind of educational program, pre-service or continuing education, costs time and money and effort on the part of the teacher and the learner. The effectiveness of the teaching–learning process needs to be demonstrated. Further, the wide variety of possible approaches must be investigated. We need to know if pre-service preparation is effective—in other words, if education at this level carries over

to the somewhat distant future when the supervisee becomes the supervisor. There is also a need to know if continuing education can be designed to meet the needs of adult professionals in a skill area such as supervision.

Particularly important at the present time, because many of the offerings appear to be continuing education, are certain questions about its effectiveness:

- What is the effect of convention presentations, with their wide variety from scientific reports to didactic, tutorial sessions?
- What is the value of a three-hour lecture or a six-hour workshop that may include a period of group discussion or experiential activities in changing attitudes that helps that attendees develop a philosophy about supervision or identify and modify skills?
- What is the impact of a professor who, in addition to an already overloaded schedule of teaching, supervision, and research at the university, drives across the state one night a week to teach a course to professionals who have also worked a full day?
- What is learned by the professional who has supervised for years, whose habits are firmly established, and who is taking a course merely to meet certification or organizational credit?
- Is the use of television, web-based instruction, and other new communication systems more effective than face-to-face instruction?

NEED FOR RESEARCH ON PREPARATION OF SUPERVISORS

With the adoption of the position paper on supervision (ASHA, 1985b), the need to prepare supervisors for their roles was officially recognized. With that comes the need for research, not only to validate the tasks and competencies contained in that document, but also to determine how to effectively and efficiently prepare supervisors to perform the tasks.

Dowling (1986) analyzed the task behavior of two supervisors enrolled in a doctoral program with emphasis on the clinical supervision approach

(Cogan, 1973; Goldhammer, 1969). She found their behavior to be different than that of supervisors in other descriptive studies of the conference (Culatta & Seltzer, 1976, 1977; Roberts & Smith, 1982; Smith, 1979). Conferences included more equality in the relationship; supervisors did not dominate and supervisees were not passive. Another difference was that conference behavior varied from one supervisee to another, demonstrating that supervisors did modify their styles. Although experimental studies need to be designed to determine if differences can be attributed to academic and practicum work, descriptive studies like this provide a foundation.

One study (Hagler, 1986) that used the "bug-in-the-ear" technique described earlier attempted to modify the amount of verbal behavior of supervisors during the conference by providing feedback through an electronic device that delivered immediate feedback to subjects. The findings show that supervisors were able to reduce their verbal behavior as a result of a verbal directive to "try to talk less," which was delivered via a bug-in-the-ear at two-minute intervals. Data provided to the subjects about the amount of verbal behavior and contingent social praise delivered in the same manner did not produce change. Generalization to other behaviors cannot be supported without further research, but, as the author states, the study does constitute a "first step toward systematic modification of a supervisor conferencing behavior, which may lead someday to strategies for teaching supervisory styles" (p. 67).

Hagler, Casey, and DesRochers (1989) examined the effects of feedback on facilitative conditions offered by supervisors during conferencing. They attempted to increase facilitative behaviors by providing supervisors with data about their use of concreteness, facilitative genuineness, respect, and empathic understanding and instructions for change. Analysis of two consecutive conferences, using McCrea's adapted scales, revealed no significant differences between experimental and control groups. They concluded that simple, written suggestions pertaining to each behavior has too little substance and impact to induce change. They suggested that subsequent studies train facilitative be-

haviors, including opportunities to role play and practice.

Using a multiple baseline across behaviors design, Strike-Roussos (1988) examined the effects of training supervisors to ask a variety of questions and to talk about the supervisory process during their conferences. A three-phase program for each of the two behaviors was implemented—each phase involved one-hour training sessions. Phase I was designed to teach supervisors to distinguish between the clinical versus the supervisory process and broad versus narrow questions. Phase II, in which subjects received verbal feedback about their use of a target behavior in actual conferences, and III, in which subjects engaged in self-analysis of a target behavior, were implemented only when a subject failed to reach criterion after training for the previous phase. The results revealed that the teaching methodology was effective in causing an increase in the amount of broad question asking and discussion of the supervisory process during conferences for the seven subjects.

In a post-hoc analysis of her 1988 dissertation study, Strike-Roussos (1995) examined questions for four subjects to determine whether the cognitive level of supervisees' responses matched the cognitive level of the questions. Eighty total conferences were analyzed.

> Data trends suggest that without specific education about the use of questions, supervisors tend to use predominantly Narrow questions, and that the frequency of higher-level questions increases in conjunction with education. More interestingly, the effectiveness of the higher-level questions in facilitating higher-level thinking by supervisees also improves after supervisors participate in an education program focused on question asking. (p. 17)

Dowling (1995) investigated if supervisee and supervisor questions and responses changed as a function of academic training. In a nine-hour module and subsequent 15-week regular academic course, 29 graduate students/"supervisors-in-training" participated in lecture-discussion, role play, and simulations. Simulated therapy and conferences were used to assess the trainees skills in decreasing conference talk-time, collecting at least three different pieces of data during observations for use in conferences, and one goal of their choosing. Supervisors' use of open–closed questions and supervisee's simple–elaborated responses were measured. Supervisory training resulted in a dramatic change in supervisors' use of open questions and supervisee-elaborated responses.

Dowling (1992, 1993, 1994) and colleagues (Dowling, Sbaschnig, & Williams, 1991) have examined the effects of graduate student supervisory training. At the beginning of a regular academic course (three credit hours) the "supervisors-in-training" baseline conference behaviors are measured, three professional goals are set, and progress is measured at the end of the semester. Findings have consistently demonstrated the value of pre-professional training in supervision in changing targeted behaviors and philosophies.

Research of this nature must continue. Demonstrating that supervisors who have been trained are more effective than those who have not will substantiate the need and provide the clout for mandating academic preparation and practicum for the important role of clinical supervisor.

OUTCOMES OF THE SUPERVISORY PROCESS

In addition to investigating the impact of training in the supervisory process, individual supervisors and supervisees will want to engage in self-study of the supervisory process. Competency 8.9 highlights the need for "ongoing *analysis* of supervisory interactions." Principles and methodologies for observing and analyzing the clinical process are covered in Chapters 6 and 7. Virtually everything stated there applies to observation and analysis of the supervisory conference. To review, observation and analysis must have a purpose and should be jointly planned by supervisor and supervisee. It must be objective and scientific. Its primary focus should be on gathering data to determine if objectives have been met. The data will be analyzed to show if change is needed. Observation and analysis are prerequisites to evaluation.

Differences between studying the clinical and supervisory process will be found in the questions to be answered, the types of behavior to be observed, the data to be recorded, the method of observation, the observation instruments used, the method of discussion with the supervisee, and the implementations of change.

STEPS IN SELF-STUDY

Self-study of the supervisory process will include all or some of the following steps:

■ The task of learning about what actually occurs in the interaction may begin with **unstructured,** open-ended listening to an audiotape or viewing of a videotape. Since most supervisees and supervisors have never done this, they may find themselves in the same place as beginning clinicians who are told to observe a tape without guidelines. What do they do? They probably see a mass of behavior for which they have no labels or guidelines.

Redundant behaviors, certain responses to each other that stand out, or even missing behaviors may be apparent. It may be easy to see who dominated the discussion, what topics were discussed most frequently or at greatest length, whether supervisees were involved in problem solving, and other salient behaviors. This first step should be unstructured, with the viewers remaining open and nonjudgmental. The temptation will be, as it is in viewing the clinical session, to make immediate judgments—"instant evaluations."

■ The next step is analogous to screening in the clinical process—**subjective** identification of certain behaviors, to which further, more specific attention will be given. For instance, the supervisee may be contributing very little to the conference even though it had been determined in the planning phase that she or he is well advanced along the continuum. The supervisor may interrupt frequently. The supervisee may engage in lengthy monologues. The supervisor may ask many questions. The supervisee may appear not to be answering the supervisor's questions. From these behaviors, selections can be made for further in-depth observation and analysis.

Another way to obtain preliminary information is to use an interaction analysis system (IAS) as a screening device. Certain systems are better for this purpose. As a result of their use, some patterns may emerge that might not be noticed through unstructured observation or that might be misperceived or misinterpreted during the subjective observation.

■ Once patterns to be further studied have been identified, the interaction can be observed in greater depth. As with the clinical process, data collection techniques include individually devised tally systems, verbatim or selective verbatim recordings, anecdotal reports, checklists, or interaction analysis systems. The type of behavior, the availability of appropriate systems, the goal of the observation, and the complexity of the interaction will determine the methodology.

■ After data are collected, they will be analyzed. Behaviors will be categorized, sequences identified, inferences proposed, and hypotheses stated.

■ Objectives will then be set for further study, for supervisor and supervisee behavior changes, and for subsequent data collection after the changes have been attempted.

OBTAINING FEEDBACK ABOUT THE SUPERVISORY PROCESS

If the supervisory process is to be discussed and analyzed by supervisor and supervisee, information must be gathered to form the nucleus of this discussion. Attitudes, perceptions, actual behaviors, needs—all go into the analysis.

In addition to the objective data obtained by the observation systems to be discussed next, there is a need to obtain subjective feedback about the conference. Rosenshine (1971) and Rosenshine and Furst (1973) have strongly urged the use of high-inference ratings (subjective ratings) along with low-inference category counts, which are more objective, as have Ingrisano and Boyle (1973) and Smith and Anderson (1982a).

> Low-inference systems are classification systems which code specific, notable supervisor and supervisee behaviors and require few inferences on the part of the coder who is analyzing one event at a time. High-inference systems are classifications which rate general supervisor and supervisee behaviors and require inferences on the part of the rater who is analyzing a series of events. (Smith & Anderson, 1982a, p. 243)

How is this feedback obtained? Three methods are useful to varying degrees: (1) general discussion with the supervisee, (2) the use of rating scales or evaluation forms, and (3) the collection of objective behavioral data through the use of interaction analysis systems.

General Discussion

Discussion about the supervisory process was presented as a part of the first component—Understanding. Such discussion continues throughout the entire interaction. What are supervisees' perceptions of whether their anticipations, needs, and goals are being met? Objectives for the supervisory process, set during the planning stage, should be reviewed periodically. New impressions of the supervisory process, gained through experiences, should be expressed.

One drawback of attempting to obtain feedback directly from the student is that it may be difficult, if not impossible, to obtain honest feedback from supervisees, especially if it is negative. Supervisors *do* give grades to supervisees, or write recommendations or evaluations. There are behaviors that are difficult to discuss with the supervisor. How do students tell supervisors that they talk too much? That they don't give supervisees a chance to use their own ideas? That they always tell them about the negative aspects of their clinical work, not the positive? Or a host of other complaints one hears from supervisees—some justified, some not?

Supervisors, too, may find it difficult to engage in this general discussion of supervisees' activities. They may not have any better understanding of the components of the supervisory process than the supervisees, and therefore may not know how to structure such a conversation. They may also not be able to deal face to face with their supervisees on sensitive issues.

The success of analysis of the conference depends on the individual situation. The manner in which the supervisory process is presented at the beginning of the interaction will influence ongoing discussion. Adequate information about the components of supervision and tasks and competencies will facilitate discussion. Discussions may come more easily as they progress along the continuum. The interpersonal skills of the supervisor will make a difference in the supervisees' ability and willingness to be open and frank. The specificity of the objectives set for the supervisory process may determine the productivity of the discussion—for example, if an objective has been to increase the amount of talk by the supervisee in the conference and, if data are available to quantify this talk, it will be easier for both.

The direction of such discussion will need to be considered carefully by the supervisor at first. Although it should be encouraged, it may come easily only after experience with the types of feedback discussed next or from a very experienced or secure supervisee. It is also important to deal with this feedback as *perceptions,* which may or may not be accurate. Their validity can be tested through the collection of data, but until that point, they must be dealt with as reality, at least for the perceiver.

Rating Scales

Rating scales or evaluation forms are high-inference scales that are a slightly more objective way of obtaining feedback about the supervisory interaction than general discussion. Such forms may be developed and used by the agency, or supervisors may develop their own. In Chapter 4,

it was suggested that such rating forms as those developed by Powell (1987, Appendix 4E) and Brasseur and Anderson (1983, Appendix 4F) are a good basis for the early discussion of the process and in setting objectives for supervisor and supervisee. They are also valuable guides for ongoing discussion.

Interaction Analysis Systems.   Although there is a place for the high-inference methods just reviewed, they can not be considered **objective** measures of what happened in the conference. The use of interaction analysis systems for observation and data collection of behaviors in the supervisory conference is perhaps more important than it is in the clinical session (Anderson et al., 1979). Although subjectivity is never completely eliminated, the use of such systems in conjunction with the other methods is necessary for study of the conference. From the collected data, inferences can be made and compared with the results of ratings. This is particularly important for the conference where there is so little information about variables that are effective.

Interaction analysis systems for the clinical process were discussed in Chapter 6. Those systems were an outgrowth of similar systems for recording interaction in the classroom, based on the idea that a better understanding of what happens in the classroom will help teachers do a better job. This concept has been transferred now to supervisory activity.

> Any situation in which people are interacting is amenable to behavioral analysis by categories appropriate to it. Once the goals of the projected interaction are stated, it should be possible to deduce the kinds of information needed to understand it better. (Blumberg, 1980, p. 114)

To review what was said about clinical interaction analysis systems, they are not evaluations. They are low-inference instruments for collecting data on behaviors within the conference, which can then be examined, analyzed, and categorized so that inferences can be drawn about the interaction of the participants and its effects on their learning.

Systems from the education literature and from speech-language pathology for analyzing the supervisory process will be discussed here in relation to their objectives, content, usefulness, methodology, strengths and weaknesses, validity, and reliability, and how closely they meet the criteria for interaction analysis systems proposed by Herbert and Attridge (1975), as discussed in Chapter 6.

Blumberg's System for Analyzing Supervisor–Teacher Interaction.   Originally printed in *Mirrors on Behavior* (Simon & Boyer, 1970a, 1970b, 1974), this system was developed to quantify supervisor/teacher interaction. It was used in Blumberg's studies of the supervisory conference (Blumberg, 1974, 1980). Based on analysis instruments for use in the classroom (Bales, 1951; Flanders, 1967, 1969), the basic assumption of the system is that learning in the conference and satisfaction with the supervisory process are directly related to the supervisee's level of independence and ability to participate in the conference. The system is designed to help supervisors get some insight into their behavior and its effect on the course of their interaction with teachers. Underwood (1973) indicated that it is equally appropriate for speech-language pathology supervisors.

The system is time-based; that is, behaviors are recorded every three seconds or when a change of behavior occurs within the three-second interval. It is a single-scoring system, meaning that only one category number is applied to a verbal behavior.

The system includes ten categories for supervisors, four for supervisees, and one that applies to both. Supervisor behaviors are: (1) support-inducing communication behavior, (2) praise, (3) accepts or uses teacher's ideas, (4) asks for information, (5) gives information, (6) asks for opinions, (7) asks for suggestions, (8) gives opinions, (9) gives suggestions, and (10) criticism. Supervisee behaviors are: (1) asks for information, opinion, or suggestions, (2) gives information, opinion, or suggestions, (3) positive social-emotional behavior, and (4) negative social-emotional behavior. The final

category, silence or confusion, applies to both participants.

Blumberg justified the unequal number of categories in his system by referring to Flanders's seven categories for teachers and two for pupils. Because it is the behavior of the supervisor that is responsible for setting the tone and atmosphere in the conference, he says, it is more important to learn about the supervisor's behavior.

The Blumberg system is easily learned and used. The directions are clear and specific and include a description of each category and a form for collecting data from a tape recording. He also included a unique method for transferring data to a matrix, which makes it possible to analyze data both qualitatively and quantitatively.

Data obtained from the use of the system are interpreted in view of each act as a response to the last act of the other person in the interaction or in anticipation of the next act of the other. Blumberg made this important point because he views behaviors as sequentially related rather than isolated. He also views the system as recording interaction from the point of view of the receiver of the behavior, not the giver; in other words, the effects, not the intention of the behavior.

Blumberg did not present reliability and validity data, but addressed reliability of observation by providing what he called "ground rules," which are helpful in training reliability in recording (Blumberg, 1980). Brasseur (1980a, 1980b), who used the system in a study, stated:

> The amount of training needed to use the Blumberg system depends upon the user's objective—self-study or research. For personal self-study, the categories are easy to learn and it is rather easy to establish consistency with oneself in assigning behaviors to given categories. Learning to tally every three seconds on a time-based system is sometimes difficult but can be dealt with by using a tape containing a series of beeps at three-second intervals and by lengthening the time interval or coding all behaviors during the learning process. For research purposes the time required for training would depend on the number of coders and the percentage of agreement to be obtained. (Brasseur, 1980b, p. 72)

The system relates exclusively to cognitive behaviors. It is possible, however, to make assumptions about the affective from some of the categories and especially from the use of the matrix, which identifies what Blumberg calls "steady state" areas of behavior such as "building and maintaining interpersonal relationships."

The content of the conference behaviors is not identified by the system; therefore, significance of behaviors cannot be fully interpreted. There are, however, many questions that can be answered that relate particularly to the questions of the balance of active/passive behaviors. It is possible, through analyzing the collected data, to determine the most frequently used behaviors and the ratios of various behaviors to each other. For example, how talking time is used—asking, telling, criticizing; what behaviors follow other behaviors; and identifying other categories that then allow for inference making, interpretation, and value judgment.

Certain strengths and weaknesses are found in this system, as in all of the systems to be described here. Reliability and validity data are not given. Categories are not exhaustive; they do not cover all possible behaviors nor are they mutually exclusive (although Blumberg's ground rules alleviate this problem). Categories are general.

The emphasis on supervisory behavior and the grouping of three behaviors for supervisees into one item, although justified by Blumberg, limits its value in studying the styles of supervision proposed here where the behavior of the supervisee is deemed equally important to that of the supervisor. Thus, supervisee behaviors should be divided into separate categories—for example, asks for information, opinions, or suggestions should be revised as: (1) asks for information, (2) asks for opinions, and (3) asks for suggestions. The same holds true for "gives information, opinions, or suggestions."

The system has many strengths, one being the matrix, which identifies steady-state areas and yields a method for analyzing data. It makes it possible to make inferences from the data and to plan for behavior modifications in future conferences. Another strength of the system is its relative simplicity and ease of learning. Its focus on direct-indirect (active/passive) behavior makes a real

contribution to the study of the collaborative methodology presented in this text.

The system is not intended to be used as an evaluation. It is recommended for self-analysis, peer analysis, or research. It enables users to identify patterns of behavior and to devise ways to modify those that are not consistent with one's goals for the supervisory process.

Underwood Category System for Analyzing Supervisor-Clinician. Underwood (1979), after utilizing Blumberg's system in her 1973 dissertation study, modified the system. Her unpublished version includes the following categories for supervisor behavior: (1) supportive, (2) praise, (3) identifies problem, (4) uses clinician's idea, (5) requests factual information, (6) provides factual information, (7) requests opinions/suggestions, (8) provides opinions/suggestions, (9) criticism. For supervisees, behaviors include: (10) identifies problem, (11) requests factual information, (12) provides factual information, (13) requests opinions/suggestions, (14) provides opinions/suggestions, (15) positive social behavior, (16) negative social behavior. Underwood then includes (17) silence or confusion as other behavior, which applies to both participants. The system contains a fairly detailed description of each category and some ground rules for making certain decisions about categorizing verbalizations, a scoring sheet, and two analysis sheets to assist in interpretation.

Purposes, procedures, uses, and strengths and weaknesses are comparable to those of the Blumberg system. Underwood's items are, in several instances, more specific than Blumberg's and she does include more supervisee categories. Her items for both supervisors and supervisees combine opinion/suggestions, and it might be beneficial to separate them because suggestions imply an evidence-based orientation while opinions infer a subjective, personal preference.

Like the Blumberg system, Underwood's system is relatively simple and easy to learn; it focuses on behaviors and it enables users to make inferences about direct-indirect styles. Although it is a cognitive system, again it is possible to make inferences and assumptions about effect from the data. Underwood did not attend to sequences of behaviors as Blumberg did; rather she stops with having users summarize data by computing percentages for individual categories.

The major weakness of the revised system is that the lack of reliability and validity information renders its use for research questionable. It is, nonetheless, an interesting and useful tool for self-study. It is contained in Appendix 9A.

Content and Sequence Analysis of the Supervisory Session. This system, developed by Culatta and Seltzer (1977), was the first published system for studying the supervisory process in speech-language pathology and has been used in several studies. The authors perceive the importance of isolating the interaction variables in the supervisory conference and grouping them into manageable categories. To do this, they modified the Boone-Prescott *Content and Sequence Analysis System* for recording clinician-client behavior (1972). The theoretical base for both systems is behavior theory (Roberts, 1980).

The *Content and Sequence Analysis System* provides for recording behavior on one dimension only and in the cognitive domain only. It is a frequency-based system, recording all verbal behaviors as they occur. The authors gave directions, defined the categories, and gave an example of each. Despite the title, users can record only the type of behavior, not the content of the interaction. Categories are divided equally and include for supervisors: good evaluation, bad evaluation, question, strategy, observation, information and irrelevant. Categories for supervisees include: good self-evaluation, bad self-evaluation, question, strategy, observation, information, and irrelevant. Just as in the Boone-Prescott system, a chart is provided for marking the behaviors and then connecting the marks to produce a graph.

In addition, although this is a frequency-based system, Culatta and Seltzer presented a unique methodology for changing from a time-free analysis, which may produce misleading information, to a graph that also charts the number of seconds spent in each behavior. They presented an example of the way in which the two methodologies may provide entirely different pictures of what actually happened. For example, the time-free analysis may show a relatively equal interchange between supervisor and supervisee while the addition of the time component may reveal that the supervisor used long verbal statements while the supervisee responded with "Uh-huh."

The system's main strengths are its practicality, its simplicity, and its clarity. It can be learned easily and a large amount of valuable data can be collected rather quickly. It is particularly useful as an early introduction to isolating behavior in the conference. It can serve as a screening instrument to identify behaviors that may be studied in greater length (Roberts, 1980). The data collected can be used to answer many questions: Most frequent categories used? Ratios of the behaviors? Balance of input (using the time-based methodology)? Sequence of behavior?

The system has several weaknesses, despite its usefulness. Its theoretical bias may not be congruent with all approaches to supervision. Therefore, it may not measure all appropriate behaviors (Roberts, 1980). Categories are broad and unidimensional. For example, the number of questions asked by each participant can be identified. This information is of relatively little use in interpretation, however, unless there is more specific information, such as type of content of the question or the supervisee's reaction to it. The same can be said for the strategy category. Categories do not describe all components of the conference or represent all possible interactions. Some are not mutually exclusive—one sample of behavior might be coded as a question, a strategy, or an evaluation. The authors give no ground rules for coding when confusion exists between categories. They also do not include a method for analysis of data, as in Blumberg's and Underwood's systems.

A major weakness is that the authors presented no reliability or validity information, nor information about the development of the system, except that it was based on the Boone-Prescott system. A study by Dowling and colleagues (1982) questioned the reliability and validity of the system and stated that it has serious limitations as a research tool. However, because of its ease of learning and the fact that it identifies the occurrence and sequence of process variables in the conference, they suggested that it is an appropriate tool for supervisors with limited time who wish to objectify their own supervisory behavior.

Although it is clear that the system should not be used for research purposes and that the findings of several studies that have used it are somewhat suspect, the system has merit, as indicated. It must also be said that the authors made a **major contribution** by calling attention to the need to subject the supervisory conference in speech-language pathology to analytical study. It is contained in Appendix 9B.

McCrea's Adapted Scales. None of the previous systems provide for recording data in the affective or interpersonal domain. The *McCrea Adapted Scales for the Assessment of Interpersonal Functioning in Speech-Language Pathology Supervisory Conferences,* contained in Appendix 9C, addresses this complex issue (McCrea, 1980).

Developed from the work of Carkhuff (1969a, 1969b) and Gazda (1974), these scales are based on the work of Carl Rogers (1957) and test his theories, which stated that if certain core facilitative conditions are present within a clinical relationship and are perceived by the client, the client will experience positive change. The original concepts were developed for use in mental health, but workers in other helping professions have assumed that these constructs are applicable, not only to psychotherapy, but to other interpersonal situations such as parent–child, student–teacher, and supervisor–supervisee interactions (McCrea, 1980).

The *McCrea Adapted Scales* provide data about the presence or absence of four interpersonal categories of supervisor behavior: empathic understanding, respect, facilitative genuineness, and concreteness, and one category of supervisee behavior: self-exploration, which is assumed to be analogous to self-supervision.

The system is frequency based as well as rating based, that is, the presence or absence of the behaviors is noted and then the behavior is rated according to its degree of facilitativeness on a scale of one to seven, with the higher ratings being facilitating and the lower nonfacilitating.

The categories are clearly described, as are each of the seven points on each rating scale. Very specific ground rules and procedures are given for use of the scale. Score sheets and an analysis sheet are included. The system is easily used and is not difficult to learn. McCrea (1980) estimated five to seven hours of training to use the system in self-study, more to reach agreement for a research project.

Although the reliability study for this scale appears to indicate that it can be used to observe and analyze interpersonal processes in supervision in speech-language pathology, reliability was demonstrated only for respect, facilitative genuineness, and concreteness. Because of the infrequent occurrence of empathic understanding and self-exploration, reliability could not be established. McCrea (1980) indicated, however, the likelihood that reliability could be achieved if those behaviors were present in greater numbers.

The system can be used in self-study or research to obtain baseline levels of interpersonal functioning and to measure attempts to modify behavior in the interpersonal processes within supervision.

Weaknesses of the system are in the ambiguity and subjectivity of the scales on which the system was based (Carkhuff, 1969a, 1969b; Gazda, 1974). Because of the system's base in Rogerian theory, the only supervisee behavior identified is self-exploration, defined as the ability to talk objectively about personal behavior and its consequences. This is an important behavior, however, in the facilitation of the continuum described here because self-supervision is perceived as a natural consequence of the ability to self-explore (McCrea, 1980).

Another weakness in the system is that it does not identify or categorize nonverbal behavior. A major portion of affect is carried through the nonverbal; therefore, data obtained from this scale can be assumed to be incomplete.

Despite these weaknesses, the system has strengths. It is the first system in speech-language pathology to record and analyze interpersonal behavior. It has a strong theoretical base in the works of Rogers, Carkhuff, and Gazda. It is contained in Appendix 9C.

Smith's Adaptation of the Multidimensional Observational System for the Analysis of Interactions on Clinical Supervision (MOSAICS). Smith (1978) adapted and validated the Multidimensional Observational System for the Analysis of Interactions in Clinical Supervision (MOSAICS) for use in speech-language pathology. The system, contained in Appendix 9D, provides an analysis of both content and process of the interaction in individual or group conferences.

The system is multidimensional, each unit of discourse (pedagogical move) being scored in six different dimensions. For example, each move is scored as follows: (1) according to the person doing the speaking—supervisor, supervisee, or observer, (2) according to type—structuring, soliciting, responding, reacting, or summarizing, (3) according to topic, which is in turn broken down into instructional and related.

If the move is instructional, a decision is made under the heading of generality—Is it general or specific? Then the focus of the discussion is coded—objectives, methods and materials, or execution. The third decision made is whether the move is in the domain of cognitive, affective, or disciplinary/social interaction. If the move is not instructional, it is coded under related areas, and here the choices are subject matter, supervision, general topics related to speech-language pathology or not related to speech-language pathology. The final category is the logical analysis area or substantive logical meanings. The move is again coded to analyze the instructional process and there are ten choices: defining, interpreting, fact stating, explanation, evaluation, justification, suggestion, explanation of suggestion, opinion, and justification of opinion (Smith, 1980b). Weller (1971) included more categories in his original system, but Smith did not incorporate all of them into her adaptation.

Although the system appears somewhat formidable, Weller (1971) provided extensive procedures and definitions for its use. Smith (1978), in her adaptation, rewrote certain definitions to fit speech-language pathology, clarified some of the rules for scoring, and developed a score sheet for recording behaviors.

Extensive suggestions were given by Weller (1971) about the interpretation of the data that can be gathered with the system. The most useful are the analysis of the teaching cycles or the sequence of the pedagogical moves and the critical ratios produced by manipulating certain data. The analysis procedures counteract what is probably the main weakness of the system—the massive amount of data obtained. Another weakness of the system is its complexity, which makes it appear to be difficult to learn, and, for research purposes, to obtain agreement among coders.

The strengths of the system are so great, however, that the weaknesses are almost inconsequential in a consideration of its use. Of all the systems presented here, it comes closest to meeting the standards set by Herbert and Attridge (1975). It is the only one which addresses content, and its multidimensional nature provided in-depth information. Categories are clearly described, exhaustive, and for the most part, mutually exclusive. Directions for use and analysis are clear. No transcript is needed for coding, that is, it can be coded directly from audio- or videotape. Weller's suggestions for data reduction through critical ratios and teaching cycle analysis make it possible to manipulate the data for in-depth interpretations.

The MOSAICS can be used for self-analysis, peer analysis, and for individual or group interactions. Its greatest advantage, however, is in its appropriateness for research. No other system described here approaches it in terms of its support as a research tool or its multidimensional nature. It provides a highly reliable and valid dependent measure for descriptive and experimental designs. It is contained in Appendix 9D.

USE OF INTERACTION ANALYSIS SYSTEMS

In discussing the use of interaction analysis systems in the clinical session, it has been stated that there is still uncertainty about the sampling process for studying clinical interactions. Likewise, the question applies to the supervisory conference. Some attempts have been made to determine whether or not sampling a segment of conferences is adequate to represent the entire conference.

Underwood (1973) stated that five-minute segments using the Blumberg system are representative of the total conference. Culatta and Seltzer (1977) utilized a five-minute segment of their system to analyze 10 conferences and gave as their support for this sampling the work of Boone and Goldberg (1969), Boone and Prescott (1972), and Schubert and Laird (1975). This is highly questionable support, since those are all clinical systems, not systems designed to analyze supervisory conferences.

Casey (1980) researched the validity of analyzing only a portion of conferences with *McCrea's Adapted Scales*. She asked what portions of the conference, if any, can be considered representative of the entire conference. Findings were that

> scores derived for respect, facilitative genuineness, and concreteness [the only categories that occurred frequently enough to be analyzed by McCrea (1980)] during (1) the beginning 5-minute segment, (2) the ending 5-minutes, (3) a random 5-minute segment from the middle of the conference, and (4) two random 2-and-1/2 minute segments from the middle of the segment are representative of scores derived from coding the entire conference with *McCrea's Adapted Scales*. (Casey, 1980, p. 65)

No such conclusions can be drawn for empathic understanding or self-exploration because of their infrequent occurrence.

Casey further stated that it is possible to generalize the results of her investigation to all systems used for supervisory conference analysis. This statement is based solely on the fact that all these systems are frequency based, not on the fact that they are all equally adequate instruments for analyzing conferences. Generalization cannot be made to clinician-client interaction from Casey's (1980) study.

Further, Casey cautioned that the time segments would not be valid for categories of behav-

iors which have a minimal frequency of occurrence during the segment. Minimal frequency is defined as between 20% and 25% percent of behaviors in the segment. This is an important point in view of the fact that some analysis systems include categories that have been found to occur infrequently in conferences, that is, questions, empathy, and others identified in various descriptive studies of the conference.

Hagler and Fahey (1987) investigated the use of short-segment samples of supervisory conferences with the MOSAICS system (Weller, 1971) and found five-minute samples to be generally valid representations of events of the entire conference. All of these studies contain some problems, which result in a reluctance to wholeheartedly recommend small-segment sampling for study. More work is needed in this area. Certainly it would further the study of the process if one could assume the representative nature of a small sample. Questions must be asked about the purpose of the study and the content and variability within the conference before depending on small samples.

REALITIES OF STUDYING THE CONFERENCE

The discussion of these methodologies for studying the supervisory process may seem overwhelming and impossible. They are neither. For purposes of self-study, they may be used to whatever degree is possible in terms of time and interest. If the only thing supervisors and supervisees can do to gain some insight about their interaction is to listen to audiotape and gain subjective impression of their behaviors—that is better than nothing.

For those who profess and interest in learning about themselves as supervisors, however, there is no better way at the present time than the methods suggested here. Those who wish more information are encouraged to start slowly, to use the simpler systems first to gain some insights, and then to devise a plan for ongoing study. Even studying one behavior will raise the consciousness level about what actually happens in the conference and this is *where the action is!*

SUMMARY

Historically, preparation in the supervisory process has not been considered necessary, nor has it been available to many supervisors in the past. The situation has been changing and the formal adoption of the 13 tasks performed by supervisors and the 81 competencies necessary to carry them out (ASHA, 1985b) gives further impetus for developing preparation programs in the supervisory process. A variety of models are available. Programs should be developed in conjunction with research that will demonstrate their effectiveness.

In addition to preparation, it is also important to study the supervisory process. Methodologies for self-study and for research are provided in this chapter but there is a need to develop better approaches. In the earlier discussion of observation and data collection in the clinical process, it was noted that new clinical methods, and consequently new approaches to data collection on clients, could influence the study of clinician behaviors as well. Similarly, such developments may influence the supervisory process. For example, discourse analysis offers possibilities for the study of the supervisory process. The need for formative outcome measures mandated by the new standards for CCC in speech-language pathology (ASHA, 2000a) will also likely lead to some new methods for studying the supervisory process. Continued attention to the development of reliable and valid techniques to study the supervisory process will also enable educators to refine preparation programs.

Underwood System for Analyzing Supervisor-Clinician Behavior

SUPERVISOR BEHAVIOR
1. Supportive
2. Praise
3. Identifies problem
4. Uses clinician's idea
5. Requests factual information
6. Provides factual information
7. Requests opinions/suggestions
8. Provides opinions/suggestions
9. Criticism

CLINICIAN BEHAVIOR
10. Identifies problem
11. Requests factual information
12. Provides factual information
13. Requests opinions/suggestions
14. Provides opinions/suggestions
15. Positive social behavior
16. Negative social behavior

OTHER BEHAVIOR
17. Silence or confusion

CATEGORY DEFINITIONS

Supervisor Behavior

Category 1: *Supportive*
Supervisor talk which enhances the supervisor-clinician relationship. This category does not include praise. Supervisor behaviors which encourage the clinician to continue talking (e.g., "mmhmm") are categorized *Supportive*. In instances where supervisor supportive behavior is followed immediately by another supervisor behavior, the supportive behavior is not scored. (e.g., "Mmhmm, that was a good idea." This sequence is scored 2; not 1, 2.)

Category 2: *Praise*
Supervisor behavior which connotes positive value judgment is categorized *Praise*. This may relate to the clinician's behaviors or thoughts. Supervisor praise of client or other person's behavior (e.g., "Her /r/ sounds good." Or "He (parent) is really helping her at home.") is categorized *Provides Opinions,* not *Praise.*

Category 3: *Identifies Problem*
Supervisor statements which help pinpoint a problem requiring some kind of solution. The word "problem" need not be in the statement.

Category 4: *Uses Clinician's Ideas*
Supervisor repeats, clarifies, extends or develops clinician's thoughts. Also, supervisor asks clinician to modify or develop her or his own ideas (e.g., How could you carry that idea further?) Often praise precedes this category.

Category 5: *Requests Factual Information*
Supervisor attempts to gain information. This category is factually oriented and not concerned with opinions. A response is scored Category 5 if the information being requested is about something that has already happened and there is only one right answer. The question, "How did you (Clinician) respond to her (client)?" is categorized *Requests Factual Information,* since what has already occurred is fact and cannot be changed. The question, "How would you respond to that behavior next time?" is categorized *Requests Opinions/Suggestions.*

Category 6: *Provides Factual Information*
Supervisor behavior much like Category 5, only the Supervisor is giving instead of asking for information. Any lecture-type behavior is included here.

Category 7: *Requests Opinions/Suggestions*
Supervisor attempts to learn clinician's feelings, thoughts, or ideas. This category includes supervisor behavior which asks the clinician to analyze, evaluate, or think about alternative procedures.

Category 8: *Provides Opinions; Suggestions*

Supervisor behavior much like Category 7 only the supervisor is giving instead of asking for analysis, evaluation, or alternative procedures. Included are supervisor's feelings, thoughts, ideas.

Category 9: *Criticism*

Supervisor behavior which connotes negative value judgment is categorized Criticism. This may relate to the clinician's behaviors or thoughts. Supervisor criticism of any person other than the clinician is categorized Provides Opinion, not Criticism. The supervisor's tone of voice and body language must be considered in determining whether or not a response fits into Category 9. An evaluative statement with a "but" in it often fits in this category.

Clinician Behavior

Category 10: *Identifies Problem*

Clinician behavior which helps pinpoint or shows recognition of a problem requiring some kind of solution. The word "problem" need not be in the statement.

Category 11: *Requests Factual Information*

Clinician attempts to gain information. This category is factually oriented and not concerned with therapy techniques. The question, "Is it OK to have therapy outside?" is categorized *Requests Factual Information.* "What would you have done in that situation?" is scored *Requests Opinion/ Suggestion.*

Category 12: *Provides Factual Information*

Clinician behavior much like Category 11, only the clinician is giving instead of asking for information.

Category 13: *Requests Opinions/Suggestions*

Clinician attempts to learn supervisor's feelings, thoughts, or ideas. This category includes clinician behavior which asks the supervisor to analyze or evaluate therapy techniques.

Category 14: *Provides Opinions/Suggestions*

Clinician behavior much like Category 13 only the clinician is giving instead of asking for analysis,

evaluation, or alternative procedures. Included here are clinician's feelings, thoughts, ideas.

Category 15: *Positive Social Behavior*

Clinician behavior which is the counterpart to Category 1. Statements which convey agreement by choice are categorized here, but those that indicate compliance related to supervisor's authority are *Negative Social Behavior.* In an instance where clinician positive social behavior is followed immediately by another clinician behavior, that positive social behavior is not scored (e.g., "Mmhmm, I don't think that would work with this client.") This sequence is scored 14, not 15. Positive Social Behavior is typically one word or a short phrase or sentence.

Category 16: *Negative Social Behavior*

Clinician behavior which tends to produce tension, convey defensiveness, or is disruptive. Compliance related to supervisor's authority and rationalizations are included here. Negative Social Behavior is typically one word or a short phrase or sentence.

Other Behavior

Category 17: *Silence Or Confusion*

This category is used when there is silence or both supervisor and clinician are talking at the same time, so that it becomes impossible to categorize behavior specifically. An exception would be when there is silence that seems to produce defensiveness (either Category 9 or 16). Any pause of four seconds or longer is scored as silence.

General Note about Scoring procedures:

If there is a topic change within any category, that category is scored again. This could occur any number of times.

GROUND RULES

In order to facilitate high reliability in scoring, Blumberg's guidelines are used:

1. View each act as a response to the last act of the other person or as an anticipation of the

next act of the other. The point is that we are dealing with sequentially related behavior and not that which occurs in isolation. Operationally, this means that interaction is recorded from the point of view of the recipient of the behavior, not the giver. This is so because we are interested in recording the *effects* of behavior, not the intentions of the person behaving.

2. Difficulty is apt to arise in differentiating behavior in the following categories: 1 and 2; 5 and 7; 6, 8, and 9; 15 and 16, and so on. In such cases the ground rule is, after replaying the sequence to understand the context, choose the lower numbered category of those that are in question.

3. The use of "Ohh-h" or "Hmm" by itself is taken to be encouragement and is in category 1. When "Uh huh" is followed by a rephrasing or use of the teacher's idea it is in category 4.

4. Start and end the tallying with a "15"—silence. It is assumed that the conference begins and ends in silence.

UNDERWOOD ANALYSIS SHEET

Supervisor-Clinician Conference Analysis

Date: _____   Supervisor: _____

Clinician: _____

SUPERVISOR CATEGORY COUNTS			CLINICIAN CATEGORY COUNTS	
Category	*# of Events*		*Category*	*# of Events*
2	_____		10	_____
3	_____		11	_____
4	_____		12	_____
5	_____		13	_____
6	_____		14	_____
7	_____		16	_____
8	_____			_____
9	_____			

Supervisor Significant Total (SST) _____ $= \dfrac{SST}{ST} =$ ___%

Clinician Significant Total (CST) _____ $= \dfrac{SST}{ST} =$ ___%

SIGNIFICANT TOTAL (ST = Supervisor Significant Total + Clinician Significant Total) = _____

_____

Category	*# of Events*
17	_____
1	_____
15	_____

GRAND TOTAL (GT = Total Events in Session) _____

SUMMARY DATA

Supervisor Talk: Clinician Talk $\qquad \dfrac{SST}{ST} : \dfrac{CST}{ST} = \underline{\quad\quad} \% : \underline{\quad\quad} \%$

Supervisor Supportive Behavior $\qquad \dfrac{Category\ 1}{GT} \quad \underline{\quad\quad} = \underline{\quad\quad} \%$

Supervisor Praise $\qquad \dfrac{Category\ 2}{ST} \quad \underline{\quad\quad} = \underline{\quad\quad} \%$

Supervisor Use of Clinician's Ideas $\qquad \dfrac{Category\ 4}{ST} \quad \underline{\quad\quad} = \underline{\quad\quad} \%$

Supervisor Use of Criticism $\qquad \dfrac{Category\ 9}{ST} \quad \underline{\quad\quad} = \underline{\quad\quad} \%$

Supervisor Request for Factual Infomation $\qquad \dfrac{Category\ 5}{ST} \quad \underline{\quad\quad} = \underline{\quad\quad} \%$

Supervisor Request for Opinions or Suggestions $\qquad \dfrac{Category\ 7}{ST} \quad \underline{\quad\quad} = \underline{\quad\quad} \%$

Factual Information Exchange $\qquad \dfrac{Categories\ 5+6+11+12}{ST} \quad \underline{\quad\quad} = \underline{\quad\quad} \%$

Problem Solving Behavior $\qquad \dfrac{Categories\ 3+4+7+8+10+13+14}{ST} \quad \underline{\quad\quad} = \underline{\quad\quad} \%$

*Direct Supervisory Behaviors $\qquad \dfrac{Categories\ 6+8+9}{Total\ Supervisory\ Behaviors} \quad \underline{\quad\quad} = \underline{\quad\quad} \%$

*Indirect Supervisory Behaviors $\qquad \dfrac{Categories\ 1+2+4+5+7}{Total\ Supervisory\ Behaviors} \quad \underline{\quad\quad} = \underline{\quad\quad} \%$

(*Additions made to original system by authors.)

ANALYSIS SHEET

Supervisor-Clinician Conference Analysis of Behavior Change over Time

Supervisor: _____   Clinician: _____

Dates: _____ to _____

	DATE: ____	DATE: ____	DATE: ____	DATE: ____
Supervisor Talk: Clinician Talk	_____ %	_____ %	_____ %	_____ %
Supervisor Supportive Behavior	_____ %	_____ %	_____ %	_____ %
Supervisor Praise	_____ %	_____ %	_____ %	_____ %
Supervisor Use of Clinician's Ideas	_____ %	_____ %	_____ %	_____ %
Supervisor Use of Criticism	_____ %	_____ %	_____ %	_____ %
Supervisor Request for Factual Infomation	_____ %	_____ %	_____ %	_____ %
Supervisor Request for Opinions or Suggestions	_____ %	_____ %	_____ %	_____ %
Factual Information Exchange	_____ %	_____ %	_____ %	_____ %
Problem Solving Behavior	_____ %	_____ %	_____ %	_____ %

From Underwood, J. (1973). Interaction analysis between the supervisor and the speech and hearing clinician (Doctoral dissertation, University of Denver, 1973). *Dissertation Abstracts International, 34,* 2995B. (University Microfilms No. 73-29, 608); Underwood, J. (1979). *Underwood category system.* Unpublished manuscript, University of Northern Colorado, Greeley, CO.

The Culatta and Seltzer Interaction Analysis System

CATEGORIES OF THE CULATTA AND SELTZER SYSTEM

SUPERVISOR

Category	Title	Definition
1	Good Evaluation	Supervisor evaluates observed behavior or verbal report of trainee and gives verbal or nonverbal approval.
Example:	Supervisor:	You did a good job in reinforcing the correct production of the X sound.
2	Bad Evaluation	Supervisor evaluates observed behavior or verbal report of trainee and gives verbal or nonverbal disapproval.
Example:	Supervisor:	You made a mistake by not reinforcing correct productions of the X sound.
3	Question	Any interrogative statement made by the supervisor relevant to the client being discussed.
Example:	Supervisor:	Why did you choose candy as a reinforcer?
4	Strategy	Any statement by the supervisor given to the clinician for future therapeutic intervention.
Example:	Supervisor:	I think you will probably keep his attention longer if you give him a piece of candy for a correct response.
5	Observation/ Information	Provision by the supervisor of any relevant comment pertinent to the therapeutic interaction that is not evaluating, questioning, or providing strategy.
Example:	Supervisor:	It appeared that when you sat on the floor the child gave you more correct responses.
6	Irrelevant	Any statement or question made by the supervisor which has no direct relationship to the supervisory process.
Example:	Supervisor:	Pittsburgh sure is a beautiful city in the fall.

CLINICIAN

Category	Title	Definition
7	Good Self-Evaluation	Clinician provides a positive statement about his own behavior or strategy.
Example:	Clinician:	Sitting on the floor was a really good idea with this child.

CLINICIAN

Category	Title	Definition
8	Bad Self-Evaluation	Clinician provides a negative statement about his own behavior or strategy.
Example:	Clinician:	Boy, it was dumb to sit on the floor with this child.
9	Question	Any interrogative statement made by the clinician relevant to the client being discussed.
Example:	Clinician:	Do you think I should sit on the floor with this child?
10	Strategy	Any statement or suggestion made by the clinician for future therapeutic intervention or justification of past therapeutic intervention.
Example:	Clinician:	I think in the next session he would pay more attention if I positioned him so that we maintained better eye contact.
11	Observation/Information	Any statement made by the clinician relevant to the therapeutic interaction that is not evaluating, questioning or suggesting strategy.
Example:	Clinician:	I notice that when he looks at me he can follow directions better.
12	Irrelevant	Any statement or question made by the clinician which has no direct relationship to the supervisory process.
Example:	Clinician:	It sure looks like the Steelers are going to win the Super Bowl.

PROCEDURES AND GROUND RULES FOR USING THE CULATTA AND SELTZER SYSTEM

1. Tape record the conference.
2. Select a random 5-minute segment to analyze.
3. Time the statements of both speakers and any silent periods.
4. Categorize each statement and place a mark in the appropriate place in the scoring grid—code every time there is a change in behavior.
5. Connect the marks in each square to get a picture of the types of utterance and sequence of behaviors.

GROUND RULES

1. Determine from the context if verbal lubricants (e.g., "um hmm," "OK," etc.) should be ignored or categorized as a good evaluation.
2. Consider any period of silence lasting 5 seconds or longer as a silent period.

CODING FOR CULATTA AND SELTZER SYSTEM

Name: _____   Date _____   Time _____

Supervisor_____   Trainee _____   Silence _____   Totals

1. Good Eval
2. Bad Eval
3. Question
4. Strategy
5. Obs/Info
6. Irrelevant Trainee
7. Good Self-Eval
8. Bad Self-Eval
9. Question
10. Strategy
11. Obs/Info
12. Irrelevant

Name: _____   Date _____   Time _____

Supervisor_____   Trainee _____   Silence _____   Totals

1. Good Eval
2. Bad Eval
3. Question
4. Strategy
5. Obs/Info
6. Irrelevant Trainee
7. Good Self-Eval
8. Bad Self-Eval
9. Question
10. Strategy
11. Obs/Info
12. Irrelevant

DATA ANALYSIS FORM FOR THE CULATTA AND SELTZER SYSTEM

SUPERVISOR CATEGORY	FREQUENCY (TOTAL NUMBER OF BEHAVIORS IN EACH)	PERCENTAGE OF TOTAL
1. Good Evaluation		
2. Bad Evaluation		
3. Question		
4. Strategy		
5. Observation/Information		
6. Irrelevant		

Total Participation

Time:

CLINICIAN CATEGORY	FREQUENCY	PERCENTAGE
7. Good Self-Evaluation		
8. Bad Self-Evaluation		
9. Question		
10. Strategy		
11. Observation/Information		
12. Irrelevant		

Total Participation

Time:

Reprinted with permission from Culatta, R. and Seltzer, H., (1976). Content and sequence analysis of the supervisory conference. *Asha, 18,* 8–12.

McCrea's Adapted Scales for Assessment of Interpersonal Functioning

Five categories of interpersonal functioning are scored according to the following rules:

PROCEDURES

1. Generally you will begin by making two passes through the segment of audio recording that you want to analyze. The first time you will record the speaker and the first few words of his or her utterance. This information is the unit of coding. The second time you will:

   a. Decide the category/categories for the utterance.
   b. Rate each category.

   You may make several passes through the data if necessary.

2. A set of formal scoring procedures is unavailable. Scorers may use their own methods for recording.

GROUND RULES

1. The utterance is the unit of observation. An utterance changes when the speaker changes or the topic of conversation changes.

2. Generally, the pattern of transcription will follow the CHANGE IN SPEAKER. However, there are some exception to this rule:

   a. Background "umhmms," "oks," etc. will not be transcribed.
   b. "Umhmm," "ok," "right" that stand out as separate because of a break in the primary speaker's speech *will not be transcribed* if they appear to be a social lubricant, a filler, acceptance that the message is being received. They *will be transcribed* when they appear to be meant as *positive reinforcement* or agreement; this will, in part, be determined by context or nonverbal cues.
   c. In extended utterances, segments will change when they do not relate to or focus upon the previous segment.
   d. When within-speaker off-topic interjections occur: transcribe the original statement, transcribe the off-topic interjection, *do not* transcribe the concluding statement but bracket it with the preceding two statements.
   e. In instances of parallel talk, transcribe each speaker's utterances separately. Do not try to keep track of the multiple overlaps in the transcript.
   f. When utterances are completely unintelligible, transcribe with an as unintelligible.
   g. When utterances are partially unintelligible, transcribe the audible portion and utilize a for the part that is not understood. This will allow coding and rating of the audible portion.

3. Rate each utterance. Level 5 represents a neutral statement, 6 and 7 add to the statement and below 5 subtracts from the statement.

$$\underline{1 \quad 2 \quad 3 \quad 4 \quad / \quad 5 \quad / \quad 6 \quad 7}$$
$$\text{subtracts} \qquad \text{neutral} \quad \text{adds}$$

4. The following are general clues to aid category selection:

   a. *Empathic understanding* is scored only when the supervisor deals with the supervisee's feelings.
   b. With the exception of tag questions, all supervisor questions are scored at some level of respect. Negative and positive

reinforcement of the supervisee is scored as *respect*.

c. *Facilitative genuineness* is scored when the supervisor is relating his or her opinion.

d. All supervisor statements are scored under concrete.

5. Score the supervisor utterances in as *many* categories as apply.

6. Supervisee self-exploration is scored only when the supervisee is discussing his or her own behavior or feelings. If a supervisee has no self-exploration, score the utterance as NA (i.e., not appropriate).

7. In rating behavior categories, utilize Time Rule, that is, in extended utterances when several rating of a behavior seem to occur, only apply the rating associated with longest segment of the utterance.

SUPERVISOR CATEGORIES

Concreteness: Concreteness means being specific. It is often complementary to empathy because one needs to be specific to show understanding.

Scale for Measuring Concreteness During a Supervision Conference

1 Supervisor statement, which is extremely vague, causes confusion and greatly detracts from the flow of discussion.

2 Vague statements by the supervisor, which have no focus on the topic being discussed.

3 Supervisor statements, which are vague but have focus related to the immediate past utterance.

4 Supervisor statements that have a previous focus and include some specific terms along with some vague terms. A new supervisor statement, which is general with some focus.

5 Supervisor uses no vague terms. No use of indefinite pronouns in place of nouns. Statements are specific.

6 Supervisor statements will be specific (like level 5) but will include example or reasons.

7 Supervisor statements must be specific with an example and rationale.

Facilitative Genuineness: Facilitative genuineness is expressing one's self naturally and openly. It is revealing one's own feelings and thoughts rather than acting strictly in terms of one's role as supervisor. To be genuine is to be honest, real, or authentic. In the early stages, a relationship only requires an absence of phoniness. The supervisor is silent or refrains from communicating his judgments. Facilitative genuineness is being open when it is helpful to the supervisee. However, higher levels of genuineness may require the supervisor to give negative feedback to the supervisee. When negative feedback is necessary, the supervisor tries to take out the hurt.

Scale for Measuring Facilitative Genuineness During a Supervision Conference

1 Supervisor's opinions are stated in a sarcastic or insulting manner.

2 An apparent discrepancy between the supervisor's intent and what he or she says.

3 Supervisor may teach about a disorder, technique, supervisory process, and so on. Supervisor reinforces client behavior and/or the therapy activity.

4 Supervisor as teacher but he or she includes some of his or her feelings.

5 Supervisor requests feedback from the supervisee or gives a suggestion directed toward the supervisee. Veiled negative evaluation.

6 Supervisor gives opinion that disagrees with supervisee's. Supervisor gives positive and negative evaluation. If negative evaluation is hurtful score level 5. Veiled positive evaluation.

7 Supervisor takes a risk and evaluates with justification.

Respect: Respect involves accepting the supervisee as a separate person with potentialities, apart from any evaluation of his behavior or thoughts; a supervisor may evaluate behavior or thoughts and still rate high respect if it is quite clear that his valuing of the supervisee is unconditional. The supervisor must believe in the supervisee's ability to deal with a problem constructively when given proper guidance. For example, the supervisor does not give the supervisee advice off the top of his head. By avoiding this and encouraging the supervisee to offer his own ideas, the supervisor conveys to the supervisee that he believes the supervisee has the ability to find his own solutions. Respect is rarely found alone in communication. It is frequently paired with responses in other dimensions.

Scale for Measuring Respect During a Supervision Conference

1 Supervisor relates a clear lack of respect for the supervisee in a sarcastic manner.

2 Supervisor may deliberately put the supervisee off by changing the topic of discussion or by communicating a statement with no focus to the previous one made by the supervisee.

3 Supervisor may ask the supervisee for clarification of an activity on a client. Also coded at this level are information and self-answered questions. Questions which seek rote or mechanical answers. Statements of the type "yes, but…" are level 3.

4 Supervisor may ask for clarification of the supervisee's behaviors or feelings. Questions which guide the clinician to a specific answer.

5 Supervisor provides clarification of supervisee's previous utterance. Supervisor mirrors supervisee's thought, ideas, and so on. Supervisor asks open-ended questions which ask the supervisee for analysis or opinion regarding therapy. Supervisor makes a suggestion.

6 Supervisor clarifies the supervisee's utterance and goes further to interpret the supervisee's evaluation. Supervisor gives positive opinion about supervisee's behavior.

7 Supervisor positively evaluates the supervisee and goes further to take a risk for the supervisee related to the positive evaluation.

Empathic Understanding: Basically, this behavior communicates understanding. It involves more than the ability to of the supervisor to sense the supervisee's private world; it involves both the supervisor's sensitivity to current feelings and his or her verbal facility to communicate this understanding in a language attuned to the supervisee's current feelings. The supervisor does not need to feel the same emotions but he must demonstrate an appreciation for and sensitive awareness to those feelings.

Scale For Measuring Empathic Understanding During A Supervision Conference

1 Supervisor denies the feelings reflected by the supervisee. Denial may be accompanied by a hurtful or sarcastic manner.

2 Supervisor ignores feelings reflected by the supervisee.

3 Supervisor communicates only partial awareness of the supervisee's feelings.

4 Supervisor recognizes the supervisee's feelings without accepting or refuting them.

5 Supervisor recognizes and accepts the supervisee's feelings. Exact repetition or reflection of supervisee's feelings.

6 Supervisor recognizes and elaborates upon the supervisee's feelings. This may include providing a label for the supervisee's feelings when the clinician him- or herself may not have labeled his or her feelings.

7 Supervisor recognizes, labels, elaborates on, and accepts supervisee's feelings.

SUPERVISEE CATEGORY

Self-Exploratory: The ability to objectively talk about one's own behavior and its consequences.

Scale for Measuring Self-Exploration During a Supervision Conference

1   Supervisee is dishonest about his or her feelings or behaviors.

2   Supervisee holds back or refuses to self-explore when the opportunity is presented.

3   Supervisee gives a limited direct response to the supervisor's question about his or her feelings.

4   Supervisee may report that his or her behavior had a certain effect on the client or the therapy activity (e.g., cause and effect relationships).

5   Supervisee analyzes the consequences of his or her behavior with no reporting.

6   Supervisee analyzes his or her behavior and relates his or her feelings about the behavior.

7   Supervisee analyzes his or her feelings or elaborates on his or her feelings about his or her behavior.

From McCrea, E. (1980). Supervisee ability to self-explore and four facilitative dimensions of supervisor behavior in individual conferences in speech-language pathology. (Doctoral dissertation, Indiana University, 1980). *Dissertation Abstracts International, 41, 2134B.* (University Microfilms No. 80–29, 239)

Smith's Adapted MOSAICS Scale

CATEGORIES

Speaker

S: Supervisor—The individual who has major responsibility for the conference.
C: Clinician—The individual who participates with the supervisor in the conference.

Pedagogical Moves

STR: *Structuring.* Structuring moves set the context for subsequent behavior by (1) launching or halting/excluding interactions between participants, focusing attention on a problem; or (2) indicating the nature of the interaction in terms of time agent, activity, topic, and cognitive process, regulations, reasons, and instructional aids. Structuring moves from an implicit directive by launching discussion in specified directions and focusing on topics and procedures. Structuring may occur either by announcing or stating propositions for subsequent discussion. In general, structuring serves to move the discussion forward.

SOL: *Soliciting.* Soliciting moves are intended to elicit (1) an active verbal response on the part of persons addressed; (2) a cognitive response (e.g., encouraging persons to attend to something); (3) a physical response. Soliciting moves may be questions, commands, or requests. Rhetorical questions are not counted as solicitations.

RES: *Responding.* Responding moves bear a reciprocal relation to soliciting moves and occur only in relation to them. Their function is to fulfill the expectation of the solicitation. Responses may be in the form of answers, statement of not knowing, etc. In general every solicitation must

be intended to elicit a response, and every response must be directly elicited by a solicitation.

REA: *Reacting.* Reacting moves are occasioned by prior structuring, soliciting, responding, or reacting moves but are not directly elicited by them. Pedagogically, these moves serve to modify (clarifying, synthesizing, or expanding) or to rate (positively or negatively) what has been said in the moves that occasioned them. Reacting moves may evaluate, discuss, rephrase, expand, state implications, interpret, or draw conclusions from a previous move.

RSM: *Summary reaction.* A summary reaction is occasioned by more than one previous move and serves the function of a genuine summary or review.

Substantive Areas (Content Analyses)

A. Instructional

   1. Generality

      S: *Specific.* Pedagogical moves that focus on the objectives, methods, or instructional interactions for the particular client(s) on which the supervision is based. These may be related to the client(s) in the past, present, or future.

      G: *General.* Pedagogical moves that focus on generalized objectives, methods, or instructional interactions. These may include generalizations, past experiences, or applications of theory from speech pathology and audiology or related fields (e.g. child development, linguistics, psychology).

   2. Focus

      O: *Objective and Content.* Expected therapy outcomes and the content or subject matter related to these outcomes.

M: *Methods and Materials.* Materials of therapy and strategic operations designed to achieve objectives.

X: *Execution and Instructional Interactions.* Interactions between clinician, client(s), and content therapy, either as the execution of a particular therapy plan or unexpected interactions and critical incidents.

3. Domain

C: *Cognitive.* Pertaining to cognition, knowledge, understanding, and learning. The cognitive domain is here restricted to cognitive interactions between client(s) and therapy.

A: *Affective.* Pertaining to interest, involvement, and motivation. Affective interaction between client(s) and therapy.

D: *Social and Disciplinary.* Pertaining to discipline, control and social interactions. Interactions between clinician and client(s) or client(s) and client(s).

B. Related Areas (Discussion that does not focus on the analysis of instruction)

SBJ: *Subject.* Discussion of content and subject matter where the intent is to have the clinician understand the topic of discussion.

SPR: *Supervision.* Discussion of topics related to supervision, the supervisory process, and training of clinicians.

GRL: *General Topics Related to Speech Pathology and Audiology.* Dis-cussion of topics such as school, other professionals, parent interactions, and referrals, which are only indirectly related to therapy interactions.

GNR: *General Topics **Not** Related to Speech Pathology and Audiology.* Discussion of topics unrelated to speech pathology and audiology such as the weather or sports.

Substantive-Logical Meanings (Logical Analysis)

A. Process Relating to the Proposed Use of Language

DEF: *Defining.* A statement of what a word means, how it is used, or a verbal equivalent. Definitions may be in the form of the characteristics designated by a term or specific instances of the class designated by a term.

INT: *Interpreting.* Rephrasing the meaning of a statement; a verbal equivalent which makes the meaning of a statement clear. Interpreting bears the same relationship to statements that defining does to terms.

B. Diagnostic Processes

FAC: *Fact Stating.* Giving an account, description, or report of an event or state of affairs which is verifiable in terms of experience or observational tests. Included are statements of what is, what was, or what will be, as well as generalizations and universal statements.

XPL: *Explaining.* Explanations or reasons which relate one object, event, action, or state of affairs to another object, event, action, or state of affairs, or which show relationship between an event or state of affairs and a principle or generalization. Included are conditional inferences, explicit instances of compare-and-contrast and cause-and-effect relationships.

EVL: *Evaluation.* Statements about the fairness, worth, importance, value, or quality of something.

JUS: *Justification.* Justification or vindication of an evaluation. Reasons for holding an evaluation; support or criticism for explicit or implicit opinions and evaluations.

C. Prescriptive Processes

SUG: *Suggestions.* Suggestions, alternatives, and possible actions and goals which might be used or could have been used in therapy.

SGX: *Explanations of Suggestions.* Reasons for offering a suggestion; relationships between suggestions and other objects, events, actions, states of affairs, principles, or generalizations.

OPN: *Opinions.* Directives or opinions of what should be done or ought to have been done in a given situation. A definite evaluative overtone is presumed.

OPJ: *Justifications for Opinions.* Justification or vindication of an opinion; reasons for opposing an opinion; support or criticisms for opinions.

SUMMARY OF MOSAICS SCORING

Speaker

S: Supervisor
C: Clinician

Pedagogical Moves

STR: Structuring, launching or halting move that directs the flow of discussion.

SOL: Soliciting, asking for a physical or verbal response.

RES: Responding, answering or fulfilling the expectation of a solicitation.

REA: Reacting, amplifying, qualifying, or making an unsolicited reaction.

RSM: Summary reaction to more than one move or genuine summary or review.

Substantive Areas (Content Analysis)

Instructional
  Generality
  S: Specific, pertinent to the specific client(s) being discussed
  G: General, pertinent to generalized objectives, methods, theory or related fields

Focus
  O: Objectives and content to be taught.
  M: Methods and materials, strategic and planned aspects of implementing objectives.
  X: Execution, critical incidents, tactical and unexpected interactions.

Domain
  C: Cognitive, pertaining to knowledge, learning, information, and understanding.
  A: Affective, pertaining to affective interactions—interest, motivation, attending.
  D: Disciplinary and social interactions.

Related
  SBJ: Content and subject matter to be learned by the clinician.
  SPR: Supervision and clinician-training.
  GRL: General topics related to speech pathology and audiology.
  GNR: General topics NOT related to speech pathology and audiology.

Substantive-Logical Meanings (Logical Analysis)

Processes Relating to the Proposed Use of Language
  DEF: Defining, definitions and verbal equivalents.
  INT: Interpretations and rephrasing.

Diagnostic Processes

FAC: Fact stating, accounts, descriptions, or reports.

XPL: Explanations, reasons, or relationships.

EVL: Evaluations.

JUS: Justifications, reasons for evaluations.

Prescriptive Processes

SUG: Suggestions, alternatives, and possible actions.

SGX: Explanations, reasons, and relationships for suggestions.

OPN: Opinions, directives of what should or ought to be done.

OPJ: Justifications for opinions, reasons, support and criticisms.

RULES FOR SCORING MOSAICS

General Rules

1. Listen to tape and score: speaker and pedagogical move.
2. Rewind tape, listen and score: instructional or related substantive areas.
3. Rewind tape, listen and score: substantive-logical meanings

Specific Rules

GENERAL CODING INSTRUCTIONS

A. Code from the viewpoint of an observer, with pedagogical meaning inferred from the speakers' verbal behaviors.
B. Grammatical form may give a clue, but it is not decisive in coding. For example, SOL maybe found in declarative, interrogative, or imperative form. Likewise, RES may be in the form of a question, indicating a tentative answer on the part of the speaker.
C. Coding is done in the general context of the discussion. When two people are speaking at once, or when a person makes an interruption which is not acted upon (the interrupted party continues speaking on the original topic), the interruption is not counted and coding continues in the basic context.
D. When one individual is making an extended pedagogical move which is periodically encouraged by grunts and statements such as "uh huh" and "go on," without actually changing discourse or pausing for longer than two seconds, these interruptions are not counted as separate pedagogical moves.

PEDAGOGICAL MOVES

A. STR moves from an implicit directive by launching discussion in specific directions and focusing on topics or procedures. The function of STR is either launching or halting-excluding, generally by the method of announcing or stating propositions. When a choice may be made between STR and REA, code STR for statements which move the discourse forward or bring it back on the track after a digression. For example, a new SUG or OPN is almost invariably found in a structuring move.
B. In general, internal or parenthetical shifts of topic or emphasis are not separately coded unless they constitute a relatively permanent change in the discourse. The discourse is coded in the overall context.
C. Checking Statements (e.g., "follow me?") are not coded as SOL within the context of another move unless some cue indicating a desired RES is present.
D. Implicit in any SOL is the concept of knowing or not knowing. Therefore, code RES for any of the range of possible responses, including invalid ones and those indicating knowing or not knowing alone (e.g., "I don't know").
E. A SOL which calls for a fact is coded FAC, but if the RES gives both a fact an explanation, the response is coded RES/XPL. In the same way, complex responses to solicitations of EVL, SUG, and OPN are coded as JUS, SGX, and OPJ.

F. A speaker cannot respond to his or her own solicitation. An immediate self-answer to a question indicates that it was a rhetorical question, which is not coded SOL in the first place. If a speaker answers his or her own question after an intervening incorrect answer, the correction is coded as a reaction to the incorrect answer. If the speaker answers his or her own question after a pause, the answer is coded as a reaction to the absence of an expected response.

G. When a reaction to a previous move is followed by genuine summary reaction (RSM), both moves are scored for the same speaker.

H. RSM frequently occurs when a unit of discussion is concluded by a speaker, who then turns to a new topic. The coder must determine when RMS ends and STR begins.

I. A reaction to a solicitation occurs only when the reaction is about the solicitation and not a response to the SOL.

J. A reaction may follow the absence of other reactions to a move such as STR. For example, a speaker may make a proposal and then react to the absence of any positive reactions from the other participants.

SUBSTANTIVE AREAS

A. Coding of Substantive Areas is in terms of the main context of discussion. However, in nondirective discussions shifts of substantive area are common. In order to code these shifts, which are an important aspect of supervision, the following rules are observed:

B. Code Instruction Areas in preference to Related Areas if a conflict arises. For example, if it is difficult to determine whether discussion of subject content (e.g., language) is in the context of objectives for the clients (SOC) or in the context of the understanding of the content by the clinician (SBJ), code SOC in preference to SBJ.

C. Code Instructional Domain (*C*ognitive, *A*ffective, *or D*isciplinary-social) first. This is the most general of the content dimensions, it tends to persist longest in the discourse, and

it is the most difficult to code out of context. If a conflict arises in coding, code *C*ognitive in preference to *A*ffective and *A*ffective in preference to *D*isciplinary-social.

D. Code Instructional Focus (*O*bjective and content, *M*ethods and materials, e*X*ecution) second. Significant shifts in these areas occur more frequently than changes in Instructional Domain. If a conflict arises in coding, code *O*bjectives in preference to *M*ethods and *M*ethods in preference to e*X*ecution.

E. Code Instructional Generality (*S*pecific or *G*eneral) last. Moves commonly shift from *S*pecific to *G*eneral and back again. For a single move, code the area which occupies the most time or emphasis in the move, and code each move separately. If a conflict arises, code *S*pecific in preference to *G*eneral.

F. Indicate the Substantive Area of each move even if is not explicitly referred to.

SUBSTANTIVE-LOGICAL MEANINGS

A. Only when DEF or INT are the main focus of the discourse are they coded as such. They are not coded when they are in the immediate context of other Substantive-Logical Meanings.

B. In a sequence of complex moves (XPL, SGX, OPJ, or JUS), individual simple moves (FAC, SUG, OPN, or EVL) are coded in the context of the complex moves. For example, in a series of explanations, a move stating a fact will generally be coded as XPL since one can consider the fact is intimately related to the interrelationships among the other explanations. However, when FAC represents a definite shift to a new topic or when it is in response to SOL/FAC, it is coded as FAC.

C. Complex moves (XPL, SGX, OPJ, and JUS) always involve relationships between their simple analogues (FAC, SUG, OPN, and EVL) and other factors, such as generalizations, other simple moves, etc. In the analysis of therapy particularly for objectives and methods, it is often difficult to determine when relationships are actually involved and when the move represents merely an extended description. As a general rule, these substantive-logical meanings are coded as complex whenever relationships are made to clients or specific therapy situations. In most other situations these moves are extended descriptions and codes as simple moves.

D.   When more than one Substantive-Logical process occurs within a single pedagogical move

and the overall context or emphasis is unclear, code according to the following order of priority; OPJ, JUS, SGX, XPL, OPN, EVL, SUG, FAC, INT, DEF. In effect, this means that complex is coded in preference to simple, prescriptive in preference to diagnostic.

SCORING SHEET FOR ADAPTED MOSAICS

NAME _____ DATE _____ TIME _____ to _____

Speaker S, C	Move STR SOL RES REA RSM	Substantive S, G, O, M, X, C, A, D, SBJ, SPR, GRL, GNL	Substantive- Logical OPJ, JUS, SGX, XPL, OPN, EVL, SUG, FAC, INT, DEF	Notes

Reprinted with permission from Smith, K. (1978). Identification of perceived effectiveness components in the individual supervisory conference in speech pathology and an evaluation of the relationship between ratings and content in the conference. (Doctoral dissertation, Indiana University, 1977). *Dissertation Abstracts International, 39, 680B.* (University Microfilms No. 78–13, 175)

CHAPTER TEN

ACCOUNTABILITY

Supervision may well be the oldest, most traditional
approach to quality assurance.
—Flower (1984, p. 297)

The growth of the professions of speech-language pathology and audiology has been characterized by a constant effort to provide better services for clients and better preparation for those who are planning to become speech-language pathologists or audiologists. There is ample evidence of this in what has become a rather vast literature for a relatively young profession. There is further evidence in the continually increasing standards set by the professional organization for certification of programs or individuals and the development of a variety of approaches to what has become known as "quality assurance"—how to assure that the clients served by the professions receive the best possible service.

As the professions have continued their concern for *clinical accountability,* certain formalized systems have been developed through ASHA and other agencies or organizations external to the professions, which focus on accountability and influence supervisory practices. The role of the supervisor with regard to clinical accountability will be discussed only briefly in this chapter, because numerous publications deal with processes and procedures for clinical accountability.

The thesis for this entire book has been on supervisors as facilitators of objective supervisee self-analysis or on joint-analysis as a teaching process that enables the participants to make changes in behavior to better meet objectives that have been set. It is argued that this is a learning process that will result in greater generalization by the supervisee than if the supervisor makes all the evaluations and suggestions. It is also a process that becomes an accountability procedure. Clinicians become self-analytical, able to measure their own progress, and as a result become accountable for their work with their patients/clients. This level of individual accountability is often carried out within larger accountability systems required by the professions as well as work settings.

ACCOUNTABILITY SYSTEMS WITHIN THE PROFESSIONS

Members of the professions who are clinical educators and provide supervision in any setting have dual roles, one as a service provider and one as a clinical educator. This means, then, that supervisors must be aware of the need to be accountable for their responsibilities as they fulfill both roles. Further, in their clinical educator role, supervisors have a dual responsibility to balance supervisee and client needs so that both achieve maximum outcomes within the context of the goals of the organization. For example, Rao (1990) describes a 24-step process used at the National Rehabilitation Hospital in Washington, D.C., which includes everything from continuing education needs, clinical fellowships, and peer evaluations to criterion-based performance evaluations for staff. Whitelaw and her colleagues (Whitelaw & Donohue, 1996; Whitelaw & Wynne, 1996) describe methods to insure increased collaboration between universities and off-campus practicum sites that ultimately yield increased clinical competence in students' performance in these practica.

The ASHA Position Statement on Clinical Supervision

The professions, through the Legislative Council, adopted the "Position Statement on Clinical Supervision in Speech-Language Pathology and Audiology" (ASHA, 1985b) (Appendix 3A). This statement identified clinical supervision as a distinct area of professional practice and specified 13 tasks and 81 supporting competencies fundamental to its competent execution. As such, these tasks and competencies need to be understood and implemented by those who function as supervisors of clinical activity in any setting, but most especially in training and CF settings. In addition, the Position Statement recognizes the notion that effective clinical supervision begins (but does not end) with the demonstration of "quality clinical skills" (p. 57).

The Council For Clinical Certification (CFCC)

Perhaps the most fundamental clinical accountability system within the professions are the requirements of the Standards Council (ASHA, 2000a), which established the standards for the Certificate of Clinical Competence in either speech-language pathology or audiology. These standards identify the Master's degree as the entry-level academic degree for professional practice in speech-language pathology and stipulate the necessary academic coursework and

practicum requirements that must be incorporated into the degree. These requirements are reviewed and upgraded periodically to reflect the current Scope of Practice in Speech-Language Pathology and Audiology as well as Preferred Practice Patterns in communication disorders and are a concrete statement by the professions about what are the minimum education and training standards requisite for the provision of competent services to communicatively disordered persons.

In addition to the standards for coursework and practica, the Council also stipulates minimum standards for supervision of students during their practica experiences in speech-language pathology: a minimum of "25% of the student's total contact with any patient/client" must be supervised by a speech-language pathologist with a current CCC. "These are minimum requirements and should be adjusted upward if the student's level of knowledge, experience, and competence warrants." In audiology, supervision must be sufficient "to ensure the welfare of the patient and the student in accordance with the ASHA Code of Ethics" (ASHA, 2000a).

These requirements focus on the administrative aspects of the supervisory process and have been a part of the standards since their inception; however, the revision of the standards which will begin implementation in most training programs in the fall of 2003, and which will require formative and summative assessments of supervisees across the breadth of their clinical training, implies clinical education processes that are consistent with the continuum model of supervision that is the foundation of this book:

- The amount of supervision must be appropriate to the student's level of knowledge, experience, and competence.
- The process of assessing students' *developing* knowledge and skill must be completed *throughout* the applicant's program of study.
- Such assessments must evaluate *critical thinking, decision making, and problem solving skills* (ASHA, 2000a).

The mandate for skill in implementing evidence-based practice (Standard III-G) is also consistent with the foundation of this book in that evidence-based practice is dependent on the **scientific method** and necessitates the application of research **data** (scientific evidence) to clinical decision making.

The Code of Ethics

The purpose of the Code of Ethics (ASHA, 2001a) is the "preservation of the highest standards of integrity and ethical principles which are vital to the responsible discharge of obligations in the professions." Fully three of the four Principles of Ethics contained in the Code speak to this obligation in regard to the supervisory process:

- Principle I—Individuals shall honor their responsibility to hold paramount the welfare of persons they serve professionally.
- Principle II—Individuals shall honor their responsibility to achieve and maintain the highest level of professional competence.
- Principle IV—Individuals shall honor their responsibilities to the professions and their relationships with colleagues, students, and members of allied professions. Individuals shall uphold the dignity and autonomy of the professions, maintain harmonious interprofessional and intraprofessional relationships, and accept the professions' self-imposed standards (ASHA, 2001a).

Given the intent as well as the content of the previous two documents, it is clear that the Code of Ethics compels those engaged in the supervisory process to develop and maintain current skills both as a clinician and as a clinical educator.

ACCOUNTABILITY IN SERVICE DELIVERY SETTINGS

Accountability in service delivery systems is most often directed toward quality assurance for clinical services through activities such as facility or program accreditation, peer review, record system audits, case management presentations, and most

recently, through the ASHA National Outcomes Measures Project. Sometimes, these activities may also include a focus on accountability of individuals through self-assessment, continuing education, and in some settings, the use of single-subject approaches for determining the effectiveness of procedures.

ACCOUNTABILITY SYSTEMS EXTERNAL TO THE PROFESSION

A number of external forces affect all aspects of our society as well as our professional service delivery. Among the more salient are: (1) changing demographics, (2) ongoing health care changes, (3) continual education reform, (4) rapid technological advances, (5) mandates for continuous quality improvement and cost containment, and (6) liability and litigation issues. Each of these yields a number of related challenges which must be successfully managed to insure professional viability.

Demographics

Lubinski and Frattali (2001) identify four factors with regard to the increasing and changing population. First is the growing number of persons with disabilities. At the present time, "disabilities affect one fifth of all Americans, and the proportion is likely to increase in the coming decades" (Lubinski & Frattali, 2001, p. 4). Second is the number of clinically complex cases. The prevalence of clients with co-morbidities and multiple disabilities present assessment and intervention challenges.

Third is the aging of Americans. The Baby Boomers, those born between 1946 and 1964, comprise about 30% of the current U.S. population. This group is beginning to retire and will obviously have an impact on the demand for health care and related services. Conversely, the newest generation, the Baby Boom Echo (those born between 1977 and 1997) also comprises about 30% of the current population and it will present some rather immediate challenges to the education system. Wolf (2000) discusses the fact that this generation, rather than being influenced by television, as were the Boomers, is the Net Generation. Their reliance on computers and the Internet, including rapid and continued access to the latest information as well as a high amount of interaction, will drive changes in education and ultimately the workforce.

Simultaneously, there has been an explosion in minority populations over the last 25 years (Wolf, 2000). The influx of people from Asia, Africa, the Caribbean, Central and South America, and the Pacific Islands yields a current minority population of about 24 percent. Within the next 50 years, it is projected that there will be no majority population in the U.S. "Members of minority groups lag behind their majority counterparts in almost all health measures from life expectancy to chronic disease rates (Wolf, 2000, p. 78). Minority populations have also had an impact on the schools.

Health Care

The 1990s was a decade marked by drastic cuts in health care and utilization of managed care has become the norm. As the Baby Boomers age, they are expected to influence health insurance trends. In Canada and Europe, increasing privatization is a trend that will undoubtedly influence health care in our country. Technological advances are influencing service delivery and the Internet is increasing the level of education of consumers. The Human Genome Project and other research in genetic mapping will yield powerful opportunities for change—particularly an increased focus on prevention.

Education

The reauthorization of IDEA and Goals 2000 (1994) initiatives have influenced school practices. The general education curriculum and functional behavior assessments impact IEP objectives and implementation. Mirroring population trends, students are more culturally diverse and some have limited English speaking skills. Speech-lan-

guage pathologists are combining classroom-based service delivery with the traditional pullout approach. ADA legislation has provided individuals with disabilities access to technology that facilitates effective communication.

Technology

Technology plays a significant and vital role in service delivery. Procedures for swallowing assessments, vocal tract imaging, infant hearing screening, cochlear implant rehabilitation, and AAC are but a few of the technological advances that influence the practice of speech-language pathology and audiology. In addition, information technology has had an impact both on consumers and service providers. Telehealth practices are increasingly more evident. Web-based teaching is providing self-paced, self-directed learning opportunities for increasing numbers of students and practitioners.

Quality Improvement and Cost Containment

The Joint Commission on Accreditation of Healthcare Organizations (JCAHO) and The Rehabilitation Accreditation Commission (CARF) mandate quality improvement for organizations they accredit. Quality improvement programs enable service providers to demonstrate treatment effectiveness and to contribute to the knowledge base about clinical outcomes. Spahr (1995) reported that cost containment has changed how we operate in all settings. Universities, schools, and health care settings all are demanding that workers do more with less resources. Cost containment means fewer, less expensive, and multi-skilled personnel (Spahr, 1995).

Liability and Litigation

"Professional liability results when a professional's conduct is negligent in the course of treating a client and such conduct results in some injury to the client" (Kooper, 1994, p. 166). In today's litigatious society, it is inconceivable to practice without liability insurance. As the professions continue to engage in invasive and technologically complex procedures, risks increase. The ability to demonstrate competent practice, to have current evidence to support practices, to document procedures and outcomes, and to demonstrate accountability are imperative. Further, professionals must keep abreast of current state and federal laws and legislation that govern practice in their immediate work environment. ASHA's governmental affairs website provides an excellent resource for this.

SUPERVISOR ACCOUNTABILITY

Almost 20 years ago Douglas (1983) stated that a "major consideration in clinical accountability is the effectiveness and efficiency of treatment" (p. 116). The statement is just as true today as it was then, perhaps even more so. An application of this principle to supervision would assume that the effectiveness and efficiency of supervision would be the main consideration in accountability regarding the supervisory process. The meaning of effectiveness in supervision can be extrapolated from the definition of the supervisory process found in Chapter 1: ensuring optimal service to clients as well as professional growth and development in supervisors and supervisees. Efficiency is the skill with which supervisors utilize the procedures of supervision. More specifically, effectiveness in supervision is based on whether or not what the supervisors does makes a difference in the subsequent behavior of the supervisee and ultimately, in the change in their client.

Accountability for Supervision through Research

One of the first in our professions to question the efficacy of supervision was Nelson (1974), who presented a paper at an ASHA convention entitled, "Does Supervision Make a Difference?" Nelson assigned 24 inexperienced students to three different conditions—individual supervision, group supervision, and no supervision—and then rated

supervisees on 24 competencies. Her data indicate that the individual and group subjects were rated higher than those who had no supervision. Thus, Nelson concluded that supervision *does* make a difference. Some other early studies examined the effects of different methodologies of supervision. Hall (1971), Engnoth (1974), Goodwin (1977), Dowling (1977), and Nilsen (1983) searched for answers about supervision efficacy and, despite methodological problems, these studies were instrumental in raising questions such as whether conference length or individual versus group conferences, or immediate versus delayed feedback, impact certain clinician behaviors.

Underwood (1973), on the basis of descriptive data gathered with the Blumberg analysis system and ratings of perceptions of conference effectiveness, proposed guidelines for effective conferences. These include:

- There should be more clinician than supervisor talk.
- Silence should be followed by clinician talk.
- Supervisors should minimize asking for and giving information and spend more time asking for clinician opinions, ideas and suggestions.

Smith (1978) studied both the content and perceived effectiveness of components of conferences, using Weller's MOSAICS and her Individual Supervisory Conference Rating Scale (Smith & Anderson, 1982a) as dependent measures. Results revealed that both direct and indirect supervisor behaviors were perceived to be effective and that supervisors, supervisees, and trained raters perceived an effective conference differently. Both Underwood and Smith had findings similar to the earlier studies of Blumberg and his colleagues, reported earlier in this text.

The basic questions that must be answered are:

- Does supervision make a difference?
- Is one methodology better than another?
- What variables in the conference make a difference in subsequent behavior of supervisees?

- Which tasks and competencies (ASHA, 1985b) are important for facilitating supervisee growth at various points on the continuum?

A few studies have begun to address these issues. The effectiveness of commitments by supervisees to carry out specific activities in subsequent sessions was examined by Shapiro (1985b). As reported earlier, a commitment is, in essence, a form of a contract and beginning clinicians demonstrated better follow through with written commitments, while more advanced clinicians needed only verbal commitments to effect desired outcomes. Thus, commitments are an effective supervisory method.

Gillam, Strike and Anderson (1987), using a single-subject design, conducted a study to determine if supervisees would alter their clinical behaviors as a direct consequence of supervision conducted in accordance with the clinical supervision model (Cogan, 1973; Goldhammer, 1969). Three behaviors—informative feedback, number of explanations per activity, and clinician responses to off-task utterances—were targeted for change. Results indicated that supervisees changed the targeted clinical behaviors as a function of data-based discussions with their supervisor, jointly developed observation and data analysis strategies, and written conference agreements.

Schill & Glick (1994) evaluated the impact of portfolio review on students' ability to self-evaluate. Twelve randomly selected undergraduate clinicians were divided into two groups. Both constructed portfolios and one group had a midterm review with a partner and two supervisors. Results revealed that portfolio development was a viable method to use to assist clinicians in self-evaluation. Both groups demonstrated positive attitudes about the use of portfolios but the group who had a review were more positive than those who did not.

These studies emphasize the need for increased research in the supervisory process. It is encouraging to note that many supervisors are teaming with colleagues who may be more knowledgeable than they in research techniques to conduct studies. Research is certainly a compelling way to demonstrate accountability.

Individual Supervisor Accountability

Who supervises the supervisor? The answer, unfortunately, is probably "No one." The literature contains virtually nothing about organizational structure in relation to the practice of clinical supervision. Little is known about what educational programs or service delivery settings expect or require from their supervisors in regard to the **clinical education** aspects of their positions. Most likely, if supervisors are evaluated, it is probably an administrative evaluation or one that focuses on subjective perceptions of the global behavior of supervisors. It is not one that will provide insight into the issues of supervisory effectiveness and efficiency. These evaluations probably do not consider specific behaviors of supervisors in their interactions with supervisees, nor is growth in supervisees measured or taken into consideration as judgments about supervisors' effectiveness are made.

Evaluations generated from supervisees cannot be assumed to be sufficient data for evaluation of supervisors, although they do have some relevance. Supervisees may not have sufficient understanding of the supervisory process to know what to expect or evaluate, thus rendering the value of their feedback somewhat questionable. Supervisees, as seen in the descriptive data, seldom challenge or confront their supervisors, even though they may disagree or complain in private. Further, unless complete anonymity is assured, the chances of honest feedback, even perceptual, may be questioned.

The competencies proposed by the ASHA Committee on Supervision (ASHA, 1982), and again by the Position Statement on Clinical Supervision (ASHA, 1985b), suggest a reasonable basis for the construction of a supervisor evaluation tool. Glaser and Donnelly (1994) reported on the development of a competency-based evaluation tool that encompassed all 13 tasks identified in the position statement. They defined two to three behaviors that exemplified each task and then field tested the tool across 22 supervisors and 95 students in Ohio. Some organizations and facilities appear to be using competency-based evaluation tools, although nothing of this kind has been validated and published. As a result, this continues to be a very necessary area for research.

Supervisor Accountability through Self-Assessment

Given the lack of validated guidelines for their clinical education activities and with none on the horizon, supervisors must draw on other resources to obtain some sense of the results of their own behavior. In previous chapters, a great deal was said about planning, observing, and analyzing clinician behavior. The data on clinician behavior as it relates to what has been discussed during the conference are one measure, perhaps, of a supervisor's effectiveness. Shapiro's (1985b) methodology to determine if commitments were actually carried out is an example of one form of accountability. Do the results of the conference show in the subsequent clinical session(s)? The supervisor who wishes to measure his or her effectiveness in this manner can devise any number of data collection techniques that will help identify some answers to that question.

Supervisors may also utilize the competency list (ASHA, 1985b) for self-assessment. Casey (1985, 1988) developed a *Supervisory Skills Self-Assessment,* contained in Appendix 4G. In this procedure, supervisors answer two questions about each competency: (1) How important is this competency for effectiveness to my program? and (2) How satisfied am I with my ability to perform this skill? and then record their present and ideal score.

For example, the supervisor may score him- or herself high on the importance of competency 8.3—the ability to involve the supervisee to jointly establish a conference agenda—but low on satisfaction with the way it is performed. This lack of satisfaction may be related to the fact that the supervisor is aware from the conferences themselves or on the basis of a videotape or audiotape that the supervisee usually has few ideas

about what she or he wants to discuss in the conference and, therefore, participates very little. The supervisor may further decide that it appears that the supervisee is not analyzing the clinical session adequately; thus, she or he has nothing to bring to the planning conference. The supervisor may then decide on certain procedures—to demonstrate the analysis process for the supervisee in the next two conferences with data collected by the supervisee, to make specific assignments for observing certain behaviors in certain categories, or any of many other ways to teach the analysis process. Thus, the supervisor can set an objective and determine whether or not it was accomplished on the basis of the outcomes achieved, that is, supervisees' subsequent ability to identify issues for the conference agenda and participate effectively within it. Further appropriate follow-through for total accountability would be to determine change or lack of it in the clinical process.

Studying the supervisory process in one's own behavior is the first step to accountability in the clinical teaching aspect of the supervisory process. It should be seen as an opportunity for supervisors to develop their own quality assurance mechanisms rather than having accountability measures imposed on them by those who have little understanding of the dynamics of clinical teaching and education. Studying the manner in which one might implement the dynamics of the supervisory process in one's own practice is also the platform upon which an individual supervisor can build her or his own program of lifelong learning.

Liability and the Supervisory Process

Vicarious liability is a term that is frequently used in the legal discussion of supervision and refers to supervisory situations when a person of authority is responsible for the actions of those under his or her supervision (Newman, 2001). Several aspects of the supervisory relationship are relevant to this determination of supervisory responsibility:

- Supervisor's power to control the supervisee
- The situation in which the problem occurred
- The supervisor's ability to reasonably predict the outcome of the interaction between the supervisee and the patient/client

Even though the supervisor may not participate in an evaluation or a treatment session when a problem occurs because minimal observation standards are being met (25%–50%), the supervisor is nonetheless responsible, legally and ethically, for being aware of supervisee interactions with the patient on an ongoing basis.

Newman (2001) suggests several strategies to help ensure that the supervisee is appropriately monitored and controlled.

- Provide education and training prior to the provision of any assessment or intervention protocol
- Take an active role in all aspects of clinical management of patients with whom supervisees work
- Provide the minimum level of direct supervision required by the ASHA standards or by state licensure laws, whichever is most conservative
- Be aware that supervision in excess of defined guidelines may be viewed as suspect
- Document why more supervision than required is provided. Although provision of higher percentages of supervision is commendable, in litigation, higher percentages of supervision may be viewed as an indication that a supervisee's performance was considered questionable and required increased involvement of the supervisor
- Maintain a consistent percentage of supervision across supervisees in facilities where supervision is provided at a higher percentage rate than the suggested minimum (p. 10)

It isn't directly stated, but use of supervision in the above suggestions seems to refer to the time spent in direct observation of the supervisee with the patient/client. Earlier in this book, observation was identified as just one part of the supervisory process. The authors of this book are of the opinion that it is not just the amount of supervision that is important, but the content of the process that is equally, if not more, important to the question of liability and ethics in the supervisory process. It's not just that problems are identified, but how these problems are managed after they are identified that is pivotal. The model and process of supervision described in this book suggest a supervisory process that is oriented toward identifying, analyzing, and solving problems of supervisee professional growth and change. As such, these strategies can also be brought to bear if ever issues of supervisor liability are raised.

LEADERSHIP, ADMINISTRATION, AND MANAGEMENT

Supervision outcomes are affected by an organization's mission, goals, policies, and procedures that define expectations and standards of performance. Organizational structure, including the hierarchy of administrators, impacts how work is conducted and how accountability is addressed and checked.

An administrator, at whatever level within an organization (e.g., unit manager, division head, program coordinator, executive director, department chair, CEO), must have the ability to work with individuals to accomplish the established goals and objectives of the unit(s) for which he or she is responsible. The basic management functions inherent in administration include planning, organizing, motivating, and controlling. Planning involves refining and establishing specific goals and objectives for the unit and developing implementation plans. Organizing involves integrating resources (human, capital, equipment, etc.) in the most effective manner to accomplish goals. Motivating is a critical factor for affecting the level of employee performance, which in turn influences how successfully the organizational goals will be met. Controlling involves providing feedback on results, conducting follow-ups to compare accomplishments with planned outcomes, and making appropriate adjustments when outcomes differ from expected results.

An effective administrator must have good human relations skills, the technical knowledge and skills necessary to perform specific management tasks, and the conceptual abilities to understand the complexities of the overall organization/system. Regardless of the administrative unit for which one is responsible, the goal of an administrator is to improve or increase the efficiency and effectiveness of his or her unit, while simultaneously striving to improve the quality of services for consumers and the quality of work life for employees. To achieve this primary goal, an administrator should be prepared and able to assume a variety of roles—for example, trainer/educator, collaborator in problem-solving, fact finder, process specialist, conflict negotiator, mediator, and catalyst. Skills in teaching, problem assessment, relationship building, bargaining, negotiating, conflict resolution, and behavior modification are among those needed to execute these roles.

Leadership was discussed in Chapter 2 but a few key distinctions between an administrator or manager and a leader seem relevant here. Rassi, Rao, and Hicks (1995) emphasized that leadership encompasses the process of directing or influencing group or individual activities toward goal achievement. Further, it embodies the **perception** held by individuals or group members that another individual(s) or group member(s) is (are) in a position to determine behavior patterns or improve outcomes for others. Thus, an administrator may be a leader—or merely a manager or whatever title is ascribed to a particular position. Other members of an organization may, in actuality, be leading a group.

"People seek to be led, not managed" (Rassi, Rao, & Hicks, 1995, p. 84). Leaders are individuals who empower others within the organization. Thus, a savvy administrator is one who knows how to organize, deputize, and supervise—one who recognizes the diverse strengths and weaknesses of group members and who empowers those with the expertise to be "the leader" for a particular task or function. Twenty-first century leaders must be able to assume the roles of designer, teacher, and steward. Employing a **systems approach,** leaders must be able to test mental models, balance inquiry and advocacy and recognize gaps in espoused views and practices, and avoid solutions that merely treat a symptom rather than the actual problem (Rassi, Rao, & Hicks, 1995).

Levert (2000) maintains that successful 21st century leaders will be those who can effect change—who can take people from where they are to where they need to be. Although not all change is good and leaders must avoid unproductive change, change is an inevitable part of life. As Plato said, "Nothing endures but change." Internal and external forces are precipitating changes in the way people work in both educational and healthcare professional settings, as well as in the way professionals are being prepared in the academic world. The probability of success in dealing with change will be enhanced if we recognize, as did Hem and Haw in *Who Moved My Cheese* (Johnson, 1998), the "handwriting on the wall":

- Change Happens—They keep moving the cheese
- Anticipate Change—Get ready for the cheese to move
- Monitor Change—Smell the cheese often so you know when it is getting old
- Adapt to Change Quickly—The quicker you let go of old cheese, the sooner you can enjoy new cheese
- Change—Move with the cheese
- Enjoy Change!—Savor the adventure and enjoy the taste of new cheese
- Be Ready To Change Quickly and Enjoy It Again and Again—They keep moving the cheese

While the roles and responsibilities of an administrator, the generic term for a person in an authority position, will vary as a function of the setting in which they work, all administrators must deal with the inevitable changes precipitated by internal and external forces. Understanding the differences between leadership and management and recognizing the importance of empowering other people in a group will yield more effective and efficient functioning and undoubtedly a more satisfied, motivated work force.

SUMMARY

Supervisors are involved in accountability procedures at various levels. They are responsible for ensuring that clients receive the best possible service; they are also responsible for growth and development of supervisees at varying levels of development and in varying settings. They are also responsible to uphold the standards and ethics of the professions in regard to both patients/clients and to supervisees in their role as a supervisor. Recent attention to and development of accountability measures for clients and clinical work are helpful to supervisors, but they must, however, continue to seek better accountability methods for themselves.

CHAPTER ELEVEN

SUPERVISION ACROSS SETTINGS

*Clinical supervision is a necessary and desirable component
in any truly comprehensive clinical program.*
—Kleffner (1964, p. 20)

The focus in each of the preceding chapters in this book has endeavored to indicate the applicability of Anderson's continuum model of supervision across the varying levels of experience. It is true that the bulk of supervision in speech-language pathology and audiology does take place in college or university training programs. Supervision has historically been assumed to be the very necessary and important process by which students are trained and inducted into the profession. But in point of fact, supervision is of no less importance in service delivery settings than it is in training sites.

The continuum of supervision has been designed specifically to illustrate its appropriateness and applicability to all settings. The varying nature of the styles of supervision and the assertion that supervisees and supervisors move back and forth on the continuum, unrelated to amount of experience or setting, is basic to understanding the function of the supervisor and supervisee in the process at all levels and in all settings.

Although the profession has defined, through ASHA requirements and guidelines, the need for supervision in educational programs, including off-campus practicum, the Clinical Fellowship Year (CFY), and now, the utilization of speech-language pathology assistants, less interest has

been documented about supervision in other settings. Kleffner (1964) maintained that no one is "so adept, so experienced, and so insightful" (p. 20) that he or she could not gain from supervision, clinical consultation, or peer review. That is exactly the point made in this book in relation to the Self-Supervision Stage of the continuum and its accompanying Consultative Style. Despite the assumption that the attainment of the CCC indicates the ability to work independently and with a degree of professional autonomy in providing clinical services, in professions changing as rapidly as speech-language pathology and audiology, it is foolhardy to assume anything other than a continuing need for professional growth and development. No strong action has ever been taken by ASHA to encourage the employment of supervisors with specific clinical education responsibilities in service delivery settings other than the requirements for Professional Standards Board certification, which itself has now been sunsetted.

SUPERVISION IN SERVICE DELIVERY SETTINGS

Organizational requirements for supervisors or their tasks in service delivery settings are not well documented in the literature. What is found is related mainly to administration or program management. It is probable that these administrative responsibilities occupy even more time now because of the demands in implementing IDEA in school settings and responding to the requirements of regulatory and accrediting bodies in healthcare, such as the Joint Commission on Accreditation of Hospitals and the Commission on Accreditation of Rehabilitation Facilities.

Supervision or Administration?

Everyone is aware of the immense amount of administrative detail currently required in any organization. It cannot be denied or ignored if the program is to continue. Without preparation in the clinical teaching role, some professionals with program leadership responsibilities may feel more secure in completing the program management tasks as opposed to undertaking the face-to-face interaction required of the clinical teaching role. Such interactions may be especially difficult with personnel who are not operating at the Self-Supervision Stage. Further, some program supervisors still seem to persist in the stereotypic belief that they must provide the correct answer to all questions posed by staff members. If they realize they do not have it, they may avoid encounters that reveal that fact. Additionally, some supervisors may be threatened by supervisees who possess information they do not have and avoid face-to-face interactions. As a result of these dynamics and others like them, it is likely that most of what is called supervision in service delivery settings is related to the administrative aspect of the role and not the clinical teaching function that directly supports the professional growth of staff members.

The Continuum in the Service Delivery Setting

The continuum of supervision is as applicable in service delivery settings as it is in the educational program. It seems overly optimistic to assume that all professionals will have reached the same level of clinical ability by the time they enter the workforce or that their continuing professional development will proceed at the same rate. All program supervisors know that there is great unevenness in their staff. Thus, any or all of the components of supervision discussed in this book are appropriate to all settings. Certainly, interaction between supervisor and supervisee will stand a better chance of being satisfactory if there is mutual understanding of each individual's perceptions of the role or expectations of the other, if activities are planned, and if the interaction is analyzed objectively.

Professional Development in the Service Delivery Setting

There are other ways than one-to-one interaction between supervisor and supervisee to promote professional growth and development; however, they do not negate the responsibility of the supervisor for the one-to-one interaction with the supervisee. This is the essence of accountability, and ultimately, it will be the supervisor who is accountable for the work done by the clinician. Perhaps one of the most important skills for the supervisor to develop is the diagnostic process for supervisees discussed under Planning. Hersey and Blanchard (1982) emphasized that change must begin with the identification of problems. In turn, problems cannot be solved until they are documented and analyzed. The utilization of the continuum of supervision is essential in this process.

The works of Cogan (1973), Goldhammer and colleagues (1980), and Acheson and Gall (1980), although historical, are useful reading for a program supervisor. Even though they were originally written for the supervision of teachers, much of the information is applicable to any work setting at any time. Certainly, the general attitude of colleagueship and objectivity that they emphasize are as important in one setting as another. An example of a method for utilizing the clinical supervision approach in a school system, described by Tanck (1980), is just as relevant now as it was when it was first published and could be applied to speech-language pathology and audiology programs in any setting. The plan was implemented by supervisors and supervisees in a school district who worked as a group to develop a cooperative approach to the improvement of instruction. The group selected nine teaching techniques considered to be applicable in all teaching situations, such as introducing a lesson, giving directions, and providing feedback. Each of these techniques was operationalized by listing the specific behaviors deemed to contribute to the effective accomplishment of the technique. Thus, criteria were established for self-evaluation by the supervisee as well as feedback from the supervisor, leading ultimately to the formal evaluation into which each provided input. Based on Cogan's cycles, the supervisory process was then divided into the preobservation conference, preparation for observation, observation, postobservation analysis, postobservation conference, and postconference analysis. The selected teaching techniques were the subject of observation, self-analysis by the teacher, and analysis by the supervisor. The nine techniques selected were observed first. Checklists for analysis were devised. Only after completion of joint analysis and the reaching of agreement on the level of competence of the supervisee, did the dyad go on to other teaching techniques.

This plan has several advantages and would be easily adaptable in any setting. It is probably used informally or unknowingly in some form by supervisors who have already identified for themselves the most important techniques, and therefore, concentrate on those in their own observation. The Mawdsley (1985b) system of data collection and analysis contained in Appendix 6A is somewhat similar to this approach. One advantage of the plan is that supervisees know what is expected of them and what will be observed, and they are involved in its analysis. There is less uncertainty and probably less anxiety about supervision in response to such a procedure. The most important characteristic of this system is that the focus is on the improvement of instruction (i.e., delivery of assessment and/or treatment services in speech-language pathology and audiology), through objective observation and joint analysis, not just evaluation from the supervisor.

SUPERVISION OF THE OFF-CAMPUS PRACTICUM

The off-campus practicum experience varies greatly across educational programs. It may begin early in the student's preparation or be reserved for an "externship" experience late in the program. It may consist of a few hours per week or an intensive full-time affiliation over an academic term. The assignment may be geographically close to campus or at such a distance that the only contact is by FAX/letter, telephone, or e-mail. Some programs maintain a minimal on-campus clinic and depend primarily on off-campus clinical programs and their employees for their practicum assignments.

Issues in the Off-Campus Practicum

Particular issues exist in varying degrees in off-campus practicum assignments, which require continuing communication between on-campus and off-campus personnel. These dynamics will become even more important as the new standards for the accreditation of academic programs (ASHA, 2000a) go into effect and require formative assessment of graduate students/supervisees. Training programs which utilize off-campus practica placements to help graduate student clinicians/supervisees acquire certain clinical skills that cannot be developed on-campus (e.g., opportunity to develop entry level skill in assessment of deviant swallows) will need to help off-campus supervisors understand the importance of their role and contribution to the student formative assessment process. University supervisors who are responsible for liaison between the two settings are and will be key figures in this communication. They may serve one or a combination of several functions:

- They may serve only as liaison for administrative purposes, such as assignment of students or processing of paperwork required by the university or the practicum site.
- They may serve in a consultant role to the off-campus supervisor, providing guidance, formal or informal teaching about the super-

visory process, or consultation in relation to the work of the student supervisee.

- They may monitor the off-campus supervisor's activities, in effect "supervising the supervisor."
- They may directly supervise the student supervisee in places where the two sites are close enough to make this possible.

Whatever the type of assignment or the structure of supervisors' roles, there will be a variety of issues that both the university supervisor and the off-campus supervisor must face. Among the more common are:

- Selection of appropriate sites and supervisors
- Maintaining accountability while balancing supervisee and client needs
- Unrealistic expectations for students' knowledge and skill level by the off-campus supervisor
- Students who are inadequately prepared for the experiences they will have in the service delivery setting
- Lack of communication between the university and off-campus site
- Lack of definition of roles for all participants
- Lack of assumption of responsibility for supervision by the off-campus supervisor (perceiving the student as a helper and not engaging in supervisory activities)
- Grading and evaluation
- Loss of autonomy by the off-campus supervisor because of the university supervisor's direct supervision

A few of these will be discussed in detail.

Selection of Site Supervisors.   The selection of off-campus supervisors is an important and sometimes difficult process. Criteria are sometimes vague or nonexistent, and are usually subjective beyond the need for the supervisor to hold a current Certificate of Clinical Competence.

It is helpful if the university program can set criteria for site selection. Certain requirements can be stated, especially for conference time. Organizations willing to accept the responsibility of shar-

ing in the preparation of professionals must be willing to provide adequate time and experience. If they cannot, this should be made clear to the university and the student(s) should not be assigned to the site. Formal agreement or contracts that specify the content and procedures for the assignment may be necessary in some instances. Again, ongoing and open communication is essential.

Balancing Supervisee and Client Needs.   The issue of balancing the needs of student supervisees and clients has been discussed earlier in this book. It is, perhaps, a greater problem for the inexperienced supervisor than the experienced, but it must be considered by all involved in the practicum. Much of the confusion that exists over this issue could be alleviated during the planning component of the supervisory process. It is also an important part of the understanding component, since it is often related to a lack of understanding of supervisee needs and communication about them.

Unrealistic Expectations by Site Supervisors. Unrealistic expectations by site supervisors about the knowledge and skill level of the student supervisee often creates dissatisfaction. This may be related to their inexperience in the supervision of practicum students, inflexibility, lack of knowledge about the supervisee's place on the continuum or how to determine it, or lack of information from the university about the student. University supervisors may find themselves serving as mediators in such situations. Site supervisors must understand that the student is still completing his or her education, and is not a "finished" professional. Here again, an understanding of the continuum and the student's place on it are of utmost importance.

Students Who Lack Adequate Preparation. The dissatisfaction of some supervisors with the level of the students who come to them may be justified. Universities have a responsibility to carefully monitor the ability of the students who are assigned to off-campus practica. It is unfair to off-campus supervisors to expect them to assume responsibility for developing knowledge and skills that should have been attained through coursework and on-campus experiences. The new formative standards required by the 2005 standards will provide training programs the opportunity to more closely monitor the student development of competency across a wide spectrum of clinical skills and their application. If training programs identify areas of need, then it is incumbent upon them to formulate action plans (Bartlett, 2001; Whalen, 2001) to enhance the competency of the student before an off-campus placement is pursued. Similarly, if training programs work in concert with off-campus sites from the beginning of students' practica experiences, then the training program and its off-campus supervisors must work closely together to assess clinical competency throughout the students' training, including the development of action plans to support those students who are having difficulty.

Definition of Roles of Supervisors.   Some speech-language pathology and audiology programs, for reasons of budget, distance, or time, cannot provide adequate or possibly any supervision from the university. Others provide so much that the on-site supervisor loses a sense of autonomy. An understanding must be established of the differentiation in roles between on and off-campus supervisors. This becomes particularly important in terms of grading and evaluation procedures, especially as training programs move toward implementation of the new academic program accreditation standards.

Supervision by the Off-Campus Supervisor.   A continuing source of concern in relation to the off-campus experience is the type and amount of supervision provided by the off-campus practicum in contrast to that provided on-campus. Often, supervisors are reluctant to turn over new clients to students they perceive as novices. Indeed, the current Medicare-Part B regulations prohibiting students from seeing clients without the immediate presence and participation of the supervisor encourages this dynamic. The university viewpoint, Medicare notwithstanding, is that students have been closely supervised at the beginning of their training and are now ready to

demonstrate their skill and problem-solving in a less closely observed and monitored experience. Further, although students may not be familiar with procedures specific to every site, they are capable of delivering services or they should not have been assigned to the off-campus experience in the first place. Nevertheless, because the site supervisor is ultimately responsible for the quality of service to the patient/client as well as observance of regulatory requirements, they can be expected to provide close observation and supervision of students in many settings. The challenge in these instances is to find ways to accommodate the intense supervision but not encourage dependency upon the supervisor by the supervisee. Here again, discussion during the planning stage can facilitate the accommodation of both the supervisor's need for intense supervision as well the student's need for increasing independence.

Role and Responsibility of University Supervisors

University supervisors of off-campus practica or externships have a very difficult and varied role. They can be perceived as interlopers by the site supervisor. They are often the mediator of problems or miscommunication between the supervisee and the site supervisor. However, their most important role is to assist the off-campus supervisor in developing their skills in the supervisory process. In this role, they can assist the supervisors in data collection methods, analysis as opposed to evaluation, and understanding the dynamics of the continuum.

University supervisors themselves sometimes contribute to problems that may arise. They may not be objective. Their methods may also be outdated or inappropriate to the setting and the dynamics of the situation. They may not be skillful communicators. They may have no preparation in supervision themselves, making it difficult for them to assist the off-campus supervisor in developing supervisory skills when it seems necessary. Sometimes they may not thoroughly understand the dynamics of the service delivery site and, as a result, may not be fully aware of the needs of site supervisors or students. They may be as threatening to some supervisors, especially those who are new to the experience, as they are to some students. They may be perceived as living in an "ivory tower," at least professionally, where they know little of the "real world."

Advantages of the Off-Campus Experience

Despite the negatives listed here, the fact is that probably most off-campus practicum experiences are positive, successful experiences. They are often perceived by students to be the most important part of their total preparation. Students have the opportunity to integrate what they have learned. They gain experience across variations in sites and service delivery options. They gain some sense of independence from the relative safety and familiarity of the educational program.

One great advantage for students is the opportunity to work with other professionals who may not be so readily available on-campus: social workers, principals, physicians, physical and occupational therapists, teachers, and many others. Interaction with other speech-language pathologists and audiologists is also a valuable experience. Depending upon the responsibilities they are given by the supervisor, students often mature perceptibly during the practicum.

Experience in more than one setting, which is currently required by ASHA program accreditation standards, and certainly implied by the 2005 standards, has value. It introduces the students to the dynamics of various settings and helps them understand the demands of professional practice in each of them before they become independent professional practitioners during the Clinical Fellowship (CF).

The "bottom line" is that university programs are undeniably dependent on their off-campus colleagues for a portion of the training of their students. Constant changes in delivery systems make it imperative for students to have as many experiences as possible. Universities will never be able to, nor should they attempt to, simulate all the organizational structures in which

their students will seek employment. Thus, if students are to receive adequate training, there must be continued cooperation between the universities and service programs. These linkages will become even more important and substantive with the 2005 ASHA standards and the need for off-campus experiences and the skills developed there to be included in the formative evaluation of students. The implications of this dynamic for training programs is a significant one and will need to be thoughtfully addressed in collaboration with the service delivery settings/off-campus sites.

Recommendations for the Off-Campus Experience

- The basic concept of the continuum and the cycle of supervision must be continued into the off-campus site.
- Supervisors in off-campus sites should receive preparation in the supervisory process.
- University supervisors of the off-campus practicum should be chosen with care for their own clinical and supervisory ability, ability to deal with other professionals, capability to assist others in developing their supervisory skills, and ability to provide feedback to the university program about the performance of students in off-campus assignments. These supervisors serve dual roles, becoming representatives of the university to the service sites and also communicating the concerns of practicing clinicians and of students back to the program.
- Every program should have a manual, or at the very least a set of guidelines, for off-campus practica assignments. Expectations of the university should be clearly defined. These should include clear communication of the philosophy, goals, evaluation procedures, and the interaction the off-campus supervisor can expect with the university.
- Some method should be devised to provide recognition to off-campus supervisors for the role they play in the total educational program.

SUPERVISION OF THE CLINICAL FELLOWSHIP

Discussion of the Clinical Fellowship experience began as early as 1964, when a conference was held to discuss the guidelines for an internship year (Kleffner, 1964). The proceedings of the 1964 conference on this internship year devoted a great deal of attention to the supervision provided to the CF. The supervisor was identified as a the key figure in the experience, which was seen as the "final proving ground for clinical competence" (p. 10). Over a decade later, ASHA (1978b) stated that one of the principles underlying the requirement of the CF was that "Academic training alone is not sufficient for preparation to function as an independent, competent, professional person. Therefore…the Clinical Fellowship Year, if properly planned and monitored constitutes a useful and necessary transition from trainee status to status as a mature, professional person" (p. 333).

The 1964 conference participants also made a strong recommendation for extending knowledge and skill in supervision and stated, "There is a clear need in speech pathology and audiology for training for supervisors" (Kleffner, 1964, p. 5). One of the needs identified by the ASHA Committee on Supervision (1978b) was to attend to several problems related to the supervision of the CF: standards and guidelines for evaluation, role definition and guidance for supervisors, a method of monitoring the activities of CF supervisors, more accountability, and a need for providing information about supervisory techniques. In response to these early pleas for preparation of supervisors and for better quality of supervision, the professions, over time, have developed specific requirements to help organize and structure the supervision of the CF but have not similarly developed experiences to support the clinical education/supervisory process skills of members of the profession who might supervise CFs.

Standards for the Clinical Fellowship

ASHA requirements for the CF experience have evolved over the years, including, at one point, a proposal to abolish it (ASHA, 1987). Many of the reasons given in support of the proposal were related to supervision issues: difficulty in finding supervisors, inadequacy of the supervision provided, and lack of evidence of the value of the supervision. One of the most obvious changes that has occurred is the renaming of the term Clinical Fellowship Year (CFY) to Clinical Fellowship (CF) in recognition of the fact that for most students the period of time for completion of the experience is something other than a calendar year, that is, 36 weeks of full-time employment after the completion of the Master's degree.

Currently, the requirements for supervision of the CF include (ASHA, 2000a):

- Completion of 36 supervisory activities, 18 of which must be on-site observations of direct client contact. One hour of observation equals one contact and no more than six on-site observations can accrue in one day.
- At least six on-site observations must occur in each third of the experience and must be of the clinical fellow providing direct assessment and treatment services to patients/clients.
- In addition, 18 other monitoring activities must be completed during each of the three segments of the clinical fellowship. These activities may be completed through correspondence, review of audio/videotapes, evaluation of reports, and phone calls and conferences with clinical fellow and her or his colleagues.
- The completion of Clinical Fellowship Skills Inventory at least once during each of the three segments of experience, to evaluate the clinical fellow's clinical skills. Each evaluation must be discussed with the clinical fellow and signed and dated by both the fellow and the supervisor.

A review of these standards, while they are more explicit about the amount of supervision that needs to be provided during the CF experience, indicates that they focus exclusively on administrative aspects of the supervisory process. They do not speak at all to the clinical education role of the CF supervisor.

As long as the CF continues to be required, and regardless of the regulations for its completion, supervisors need to be aware of the their responsibilities beyond those implied in the regulations. They need to see themselves as professional mentors, if not clinical educators. The continuum model of supervision should be the basis for determining the appropriate supervisory style with which to implement this aspect of the role of the CF supervisor. Presumably, the Consultative Style or the upper levels of the Collaborative Style will most frequently be used with CFs who are in the Self-Supervision Stage or the more advanced levels of the Transitional Stage of the continuum (Chapter 2). Without formal training in the supervisory process readily available, CF supervisors will need to create professional development opportunities for themselves as they develop and refine the skills to enhance their practice. In addition, self-study combined with feedback from the CF will be important to the supervisor of the experience. The chapter on preparation in the supervisory process and of supervisors could be helpful to readers who undertake self-study as a mechanism for their continued professional growth as a supervisor.

SUMMARY

Organizational structure, differing levels of supervisees, goals of organization, objectives of the program, and other variables may create differences in procedures across settings, but do not negate the need for clinical teaching nor the fact that the principles remain the same. Supervisors and supervisees may have changing needs and their procedures may change as they progress along the continuum, but the basic objective of professional growth and development for both remains at the core of the supervisory process.

CHAPTER TWELVE

THE SUPERVISION OF SPEECH-LANGUAGE PATHOLOGY ASSISTANTS

Another option for meeting the service delivery needs in a more cost-effective manner is the use of appropriately trained speech-language pathology assistants who must be supervised by fully qualified speech-language pathologists.

Paul-Brown and Goldberg (2001, p. 4)

The environments in which speech-language pathologists work are experiencing significant and, it seems, ongoing changes. These changes are subsequently increasing the need for speech-language pathology services across the lifespan and for personnel to provide them. This increase in need is occurring at the same time that financial resources to develop and support services in response to it are decreasing (Uffen, 1998). As a result, those responsible for the organization and management of service delivery programs in speech-language pathology must find ways to extend appropriate and effective service to patients and clients in more cost-effective ways.

The use of appropriately trained speech-language pathology assistants (SLPAs) who are supervised by certified speech-language pathologists is one way to "increase the frequency of service to clients while maintaining service quality and controlling cost" (ASHA, 2001c). However, in a 1999 ASHA survey (ASHA, 2000b) 73.4% of responding speech-language pathologists indicated that they had no experience with assistants and 11.1% indicated that assistants were helpful but that there were "limitations on their effective use." Five and one-half percent of speech-language pathologists stated that assistants were an asset in clinical service delivery activities. Indeed, Hagler, Warren, and Pain (1993) reported that Canadian speech-language pathologists noted a 77% increase in service to clients as a result of the use of support personnel. Similar findings were found in the provision of audiological services with a 64.5% increase in service to clients. The authors caution, however, that their study did not address the very important issue of quality as a result of the increased use of support personnel.

BACKGROUND

ASHA's activity regarding support personnel began over 30 years ago in 1967, when the Committee on Supportive Personnel was created to develop guidelines for the use of personnel other than certified members of the profession. These guidelines were first published in 1970 (ASHA, 1970) and were revised in 1981 (ASHA, 1981). They provided only general direction about the education and training, utilization, and supervision of assistants. The guidelines indicated that assistants should have at least a high school diploma, receive on-the-job training, and be supervised 10% of the time. Later, in 1988, the committee published a second report which focused on the use of support personnel in meeting the needs of underserved populations; this report stressed the need for support personnel to have "thorough knowledge and understanding of the culture and language of the persons with whom they work clinically" (ASHA, 1988, p. 55).

The Ethical Practices Board published an issues in ethics statement in June 1979, which was later revised (ASHA, 1994), concerning the supervision of support personnel. The statement provided guidance in the ethical responsibilities of the supervising professional and stressed the dependent role of the support person. The statement was clear about the fact that "communication aides could not independently diagnose, treat, or advise clients of disposition" (ASHA, 1994, p. 24).

The impact of health care financial reform, scientific and technological advances, an expanding scope of practice, and rapidly growing public school caseloads on practice patterns became more dramatic in the decade of the 1990s. In 1992 a new task force was formed by ASHA to review all aspects of the support personnel issue, recommend an official ASHA statement, and develop new guidelines that were consistent with the contemporary service delivery environment. The task force examined the issue of support personnel from a number of perspectives (ASHA, 1992), including: effects on caseload, supervisory responsibility, and professional positions. Its findings indicated that the use of support personnel re-

sulted in larger caseloads in the schools as well as the opportunity to increase the frequency and intensity of speech-language services to children. The task force also reported that the ratio of support person(s) to supervisor ranged from 1:1 to 1:3. Finally, the report indicated that the use of support personnel did not result in any substantial decrease in the availability of positions for professionals. Subsequent to this report, ASHA approved a position statement which recognized the use of speech-language pathology assistants and authorized the establishment and credentialing of different categories of support personnel (ASHA, 1995). The revised ASHA Code of Ethics (2001a) stipulates that members of the profession must not misrepresent the credentials of assistants, technicians, or support personnel and must inform those they serve of the name and credentials of persons providing service; that certified professionals will not delegate any tasks within their scope of practice to assistants or other support personnel; and finally, that certified professionals may only delegate tasks to assistants and support personnel when that individual is adequately trained.

ASHA has also approved guidelines for training, credentialing, use, and supervision of speech-language pathology assistants, which replace the 1981 guidelines (ASHA, 1996). Recently, "Background Information and Criteria for Registration of Speech-Language Pathology Assistants (ASHA, 2000a), "Criteria for Approval of Associate Degree Technical Training Programs for Speech-Language Pathology Assistants" (ASHA, 2000b), and a technical packet on speech-language pathology assistants (ASHA 2000c) have also been published. Finally, "Knowledge and Skills for Supervisors of Speech-Language Pathology Assistants" (ASHA, 2001c; Appendix 12A) was approved by the 2001 ASHA Legislative Council and, together with the previous four documents (Code of Ethics, Guidelines, registration document, and AA Degree programs), provides specific and comprehensive standards for the profession regarding the training, credentialing, use, and supervision of speech-language pathologists and support personnel. It must be noted, however, that ASHA's policies for credentialing and registration of assistants may differ from those which have been developed by licensing boards and other state regulatory bodies within some individual states. Paul-Brown and Goldberg (2001) summarized these differences across the 36 states that currently regulate support personnel. When differences occur between ASHA policies and standards and those of states or employers, it is incumbent on the certified professional to be aware of the difference(s). If state policies are more liberal than those of the profession, the certified professional is required by the Code of Ethics to observe those of the profession.

SCOPE OF RESPONSIBILITY

"Guidelines for the Training, Credentialing, Use and Supervision of Speech-Language Assistants" (ASHA, 1996) suggests a curriculum and competencies for SLPAs. More pertinent to the purpose of this book, however, are the bases for the supervisory process in the utilization of assistants. The foundation for this consideration begins with the scope of responsibilities for both SLPAs and supervisors of assistants, which is also contained in the ASHA Guidelines (1996) and which defines the broad parameters of the work of both assistants and their supervisors.

Scope of Responsibilities of Speech-Language Pathology Assistants

The scope of responsibilities of assistants is limited and language used in the document makes it clear that SLPAs work *to assist* the speech-language pathologist. The scope includes the following activities:

- Assist the speech-language pathologist with speech-language and hearing screenings (without interpretation)
- Follow documented treatment plans or protocols that have been developed by the supervising speech-language pathologist
- Document client performance (e.g., tallying data for the speech-language pathologist to use; preparing charts, records, and graphs)

and report this information to the supervising speech-language pathologist
- Assist with informal documentation as directed by the speech-language pathologist
- Assist with clerical duties such as preparing materials and scheduling activities as directed by the speech-language pathologist
- Perform checks and maintenance of equipment
- Support the speech-language pathologist in research projects, in-service training, and public relations programs
- Assist with departmental operations (scheduling, record keeping, safety/maintenance of supplies and equipment)
- Collect data for quality improvement
- Exhibit compliance with regulations, reimbursement requirements, and speech-language pathology assistant's job description (ASHA, 2000c; Paul-Brown & Goldberg, 2001)

At the same time there are activities which the assistant may *not* implement:

- Perform standardized or nonstandardized diagnostic tests, formal or informal evaluations, or interpret test results
- Participate in parent conferences, case conferences, or any interdisciplinary team without the presence of the supervising speech-language pathologist or other ASHA-certified speech-language pathologist designated by the supervising speech-language pathologist
- Provide client or family counseling
- Write, develop, or modify a client's individualized treatment plan in any way
- Assist with clients without following the individualized treatment plan prepared by the speech-language pathologist or without access to supervision
- Sign any formal documents (e.g., treatment plans, reimbursement forms, or reports; the assistant should sign or initial informal treatment notes for review and co-signature by the supervising professional)
- Select clients for services
- Discharge a client from services

- Communicate with the client, family, or others regarding any aspect of the client status or service without specific consent of the supervising speech-language pathologist
- Represent him- or herself as a speech-language pathologist (ASHA, 1996; Paul-Brown & Goldberg, 2001)

Scope of Responsibilities of the Supervising Speech-Language Pathologist. Similarly, the scope of responsibilities for speech-language pathologists who might supervise an assistant are equally explicit:

- Complete initial supervision training prior to accepting an assistant for supervision and upgrade supervision training on a regular basis
- Participate significantly in hiring the assistant
- Inform clients and families about the level (professional vs. support personnel), frequency, and duration of services as well as supervision
- Represent the speech-language pathology team in all collaborative, interprofessional, and interagency meetings, correspondence, and reports (This would not preclude the assistant from attending meetings along with the speech-language pathologist as a team member or drafting correspondence and reports for editing, approval, and signature by the speech-language pathologist.)
- Make all clinical decisions, including determining client selection for inclusion/exclusion in the caseload and dismissing clients from treatment
- Communicate with clients, parents and family members about diagnosis, prognosis, and treatment plan
- Conduct diagnostic evaluations, assessments, or appraisals and interpret obtained data in reports
- Review each treatment plan with the assistant at least weekly
- Delegate specific tasks to the assistant while retaining legal and ethical responsibility for all client services provided or omitted
- Prepare an individualized treatment plan and make modifications prior to or during implementation

- Discuss the case with, or refer the client to, other professionals
- Sign all formal documents (e.g., treatment plans, reimbursement forms, and reports; the supervisor should indicate on documents that the assistant performed certain activities)
- Review and sign all informal progress notes prepared by the assistant
- Provide ongoing training to the assistant on the job
- Provide and document appropriate supervision to the assistant
- Ensure that the assistant only performs tasks within the scope of responsibility of the speech-language pathologist assistant
- Participate in the performance appraisal of the assistant (ASHA, 1996)

This review of the duties and responsibilities of both the certified supervisor and the speech-language pathology assistant makes it clear that the use of an assistant is to extend, not replace, the services of a speech-language pathologist. Assistants only work under the direct supervision of a speech-language pathologist who retains all legal and ethical responsibility for the client.

UTILIZATION AND TRAINING OF SPEECH-LANGUAGE PATHOLOGY ASSISTANTS

When a service delivery setting makes the decision to incorporate speech-language pathology assistants into its cadre of service delivery personnel, it should consider how the assistant(s) might be used and construct a job description that is consistent with this planning. Further, the setting should endeavor to hire assistants who have completed their training from an ASHA-approved SLPA technical training program. This will help ensure that the assistant will enter the setting with the general and technical education as well as the minimum competencies needed to function appropriately. Most importantly, hiring assistants who have graduated from an approved SLPA training program will ensure that the supervising speech-language pathologist will remain consistent with the intent of the Code of Ethics (ASHA, 2001a).

Since the primary responsibility for the assistant in any setting rests with the supervising speech-language pathologist, it is imperative that the potential supervisor be included in the hiring process of the assistant. In most settings, it is doubtful that the speech-language pathologist will make the offer to hire directly to the assistant, but she or he should certainly be included in the review of applications for the position and in the interview process as well. The success of any partnership is not just determined by the skill of the individuals who contribute to it, but by their ability to work together comfortably and well. This, in turn, is often determined by intangible aspects of behavior that can only be identified through face-to-face contact during the interview. Once the interview process is completed, the speech-language pathologist who will supervise should rank order candidates and give his or her recommendations to the individual or office that will make the actual job offer.

Once an assistant joins the speech-language pathology team, the supervisor must then decide how the assistant will be utilized, that is, what tasks or activities the assistant will be assigned. This crucial and pivotal decision should be based in part upon the job description for the position, but in instances where the description was broadly cast and written, it will also depend upon the decision of the supervising speech-language pathologist. The supervisor will need to consider multiple factors to make this decision, which might include the nature of the caseload for which the supervisor has responsibility, that is, the disorders presented in it, their severity, the disposition of the client toward working with an assistant, as well as the skills of the assistant and the dynamics of the service delivery setting itself. Indeed, there may be some situations in which it is not appropriate for an assistant to have direct client contact even though the scope of responsibility for assistants suggests that direct contact is

an activity in which assistants may engage. In these situations, it makes sense for the assistant to carry out the clerical and equipment-based functions necessary to support the practice of the speech-language pathologist and the services provided by the setting.

Despite their general education and technical training, assistants should also be provided additional orientation and training specific to the setting in which they will work and to the tasks they will implement. Although settings may provide a general procedural orientation to all new employees, the task-specific orientation will be carried out by the supervising speech-language pathologist. A case study at the end of the chapter will present a training example for an assistant who will provide direct client service.

SUPERVISION OF SPEECH-LANGUAGE PATHOLOGY ASSISTANTS

The dynamics of the process of supervision of speech-language pathology assistants are much the same as those associated with the process identified by Anderson (1988) in her Continuum Model of supervision. What is different, however, is the nature of the responsibilities that assistants will implement and the conditions under which they will work. An assistant will never work without supervision, either direct or indirect. Whereas Anderson's model was first developed to support the process of supervision in Master's degree training programs and professional service delivery settings, the cycle of supervision that Anderson postulated, as well as the tools that support it, are just as relevant to the supervision of assistants.

Supervision Standards for Speech-Language Pathology Assistants

Minimum standards for supervision of speech-language pathology assistants are clearly stipulated in the "Guidelines for the Training, Credentialing, Use, and Supervision of Support Personnel in

Speech-Language Pathology (ASHA, 1996) and involve both direct and indirect supervisory activities. *Direct* supervision is defined as on-site, in-view observation and guidance by the speech-language pathologist, while an assigned activity is performed by the assistant. *Indirect* supervision means those activities, other than direct observation and guidance, conducted by a speech-language pathologist. These may include demonstrations, record review, review and evaluation of audio or video-taped sessions, and/or interactive television (ASHA, 2001c). These standards are predicated upon the assistant's length of employment in a given setting. During the first ninety days of work, supervision must include a *minimum* total of 30% direct and indirect supervision, all of which is documented:

- No less than 20% direct supervision which accounts for 20% of client contact time.
- Indirect supervision may make up the remaining 10% of supervisory activity.
- Each client assigned to the assistant must have direct contact with the supervising speech-language pathologist at least once every two weeks.
- The supervising speech-language pathologist must review data on clients seen by the assistant each week.

After the first 90 days of work, the amount of supervision may be adjusted, dependent upon the assistant's competency and need; however, a *minimum* of 20% supervision must be maintained throughout the period of employment, 10% of which is direct. In addition, no supervisor may be responsible for, that is, supervise, more than three assistants within the same time period.

How Much Supervision Is Necessary?

Client quality of care is the primary concern of the supervising speech-language pathologist in every instance in which an assistant is utilized to contribute to the service delivery mission of a facility or private practice. The most significant concern, however, probably arises around those instances in which assistants provide direct treatment services to clients per a treatment protocol designed by the supervisor. Part of the resolution of this concern is determining how much supervision is appropriate and/or necessary for each client interaction carried out by the assistant. This is a pivotal decision because of its implications not only for the quality of service to the client but for the supervision of the assistant as well.

Hagler and McFarlane (1997) suggested a strategy for determining which tasks involving direct client contact require high levels of supervision and which require less intense supervision. The variables in their strategy are the degree of client contact, the complexity of the client contact, and the degree of interpersonal interaction required by the client contact. Based on these dimensions, Hagler and McFarlane (1997) suggest levels of supervision (amount and nature) for four levels of task.

TASK	AMOUNT OF SUPERVISION	TYPE OF SUPERVISION
A. Extensive contact that is highly complex or technical or requires high levels of interpersonal interaction.	20% to 80%	Direct only
B. Extensive contact that is minimally complex, minimally technical and requires minimal interpersonal interaction.	20% to 60%	Minimum of 5% direct or a combination of direct/indirect

| **C.** Without extensive contact that is highly complex or technical and requires high levels of interpersonal interaction. | 10% to 40% | Minimum of 5% direct or a combination of direct/ indirect. |
| **D.** Without extensive contact that is minimally complex, minimally technical, and requires minimal interpersonal interaction. | 0% to 20% | Indirect only or a combination of direct and indirect. |

It is important to note that the levels of supervision suggested by this strategy are not the same as those stipulated by ASHA (1996a). The analysis of the variables involved in assigning the assistant to a particular task enables the supervisor to determine the viability and practicality of an assignment in light of supervision needs. A case study example at the end of this chapter will give readers an opportunity to try and apply this strategy.

Given the range in the ratio of assigned assistants to supervisor (1:1 to 1:3) and the flexibility implied by Hagler and McFarlane's (1997) analysis of tasks to determine quantity/type of supervision, it is important for the speech-language pathologist to educate those responsible for making personnel assignments about the need for balance in assignment of assistants to supervisors. For example, a supervisor who has decided to use assistants to support the clerical aspects of their service delivery program could probably appropriately supervise three assistants; on the other hand, a supervisor who has assistants working directly with clients in both complex as well as less complex and interpersonally challenging situa-

tions probably should not assume responsibility for three assistants. Each speech-language pathologist will need to make this determination for her- or himself depending on the dynamics of their caseload and, realistically, the competency of the assistant.

KNOWLEDGE AND SKILLS FOR SUPERVISORS OF SPEECH-LANGUAGE PATHOLOGY ASSISTANTS

In November 2001, the Speech-Language Pathology Assembly of the ASHA Legislative Council voted to accept the document "Knowledge and Skills for Supervisors of Speech-Language Pathology Assistants" (ASHA, 2001c; Appendix 12A). This document was prepared by a working group composed of members from ASHA Special Interest Division 11-Administration and Supervision, ASHA national office staff, and speech-language pathologists with expertise in the supervision of assistants. It recognized the importance of supervision in the competent and ethical use of assistants and defined the knowledge and skills necessary for supervisors to demonstrate in their work with assistants.

The knowledge and skills identified in the document are consistent with the 13 tasks of supervision identified in the 1985 Position Statement on clinical supervision as well as the responsibilities for both supervisors and assistants identified in the "Guidelines for the Training, Credentialing, Use and Supervision of Speech-Language Pathology Assistants" (ASHA, 1996). The knowledge and skills document also implies the notion that supervision is a distinct area of practice that was recognized by the Position Statement on clinical supervision (1985b) and delineated by Anderson (1988) in her continuum model of supervision. The document also makes it clear that the ASHA-certified supervisor retains legal and ethical responsibility for all aspects of case management and service delivery, while at the same time helping assistants refine their skills with the scope of their responsibilities and assigned tasks.

The Cycle of Supervision

Anderson's cycle of supervision (1988), described extensively in this book, also has great utility as a basis for structuring the supervision of speech-language pathology assistants. The standards for supervision that appeared earlier in this chapter are more administrative in nature and do not address the content of supervision that must be implemented by the supervisor in their work with an assistant.

Understanding. This is the component of supervision that contributes to the formation of the relationship between the supervisor and assistant and helps them build an interpersonal rapport. It is also the component in which the information is gathered to identify the needs and expectations of both the supervisor and assistant toward not only *what* they will do in work together be like but *how* they will work together. With only minor modification, the strategies and tools suggested in Chapter 4 can be used to help gather this information.

Planning. This component addresses how the work between the speech-language pathologist and the assistant will be accomplished. Goals for the assistant will be established from job responsibilities within their scope of responsibility, such as clerical duties, equipment maintenance responsibilities, and specific client assignments, including their treatment goals and protocols. The parameters for supervision will also be established, including amount, schedule, type, and strategies/tools to be used.

In addition, the supervisor and assistant should review the tools that will ultimately be used in evaluation of the assistant's performance. In many instances, this evaluation will be competency-based. *Practical Tools and Forms for Supervising Speech-Language Pathology Assistants,* published by ASHA in 1999, contains a sample tool for verifying competency in regard to participating or assisting in the management of orofacial-myofacial disorders. While this particular disorder may not represent the needs of other supervisors and caseloads, the delineation of competencies associated with it provides a *model* for supervisors who work with other disorders as they attempt to construct similar tools to meet the needs of the assistants whom they supervise and the tasks that they are assigned. The Skills Proficiency Checklist (Appendix 12B) is another tool that permits the supervisor to identify specific skills important to the accomplishment of assigned tasks and then, in concert with the assistant, to rate the degree to which the competency is demonstrated.

It is imperative that, like other supervisees, assistants understand the parameters of their assigned tasks and the expectations upon which they will be evaluated. Using tools such as these in the understanding or planning component of the cycle provides a baseline of competency at the beginning of an assignment, which can then be compared to results in later administrations.

The supervisor should also establish goals for her- or himself in this phase that will ensure that she or he provides supervision that meets the needs of the assistant. The challenge of supervision that is posed by the supervision of assistants may suggest to supervisors that they need to structure a plan for their own development and growth as they integrate the requisite knowledge and skills for supervisors into their own practice.

Observation. The purpose of observation is to provide objective data that will help both the supervisor and the assistant understand if the goals for assigned tasks and direct client contact that were set in the planning phase have indeed been met. Chapter 6 detailed strategies and tools that might be helpful in implementing the observation phase of the supervisory process and include tallying and charting behaviors, verbatim transcripts, selected verbatim notes, and interaction analysis systems. The nature and scope of observation activities should be addressed during the planning phase.

In addition, observation is one of the most powerful ways to begin to understand one's own behavior. Given the fact that, after 90 days of employment, assistants need only to be directly supervised four hours per week (10% of a 40 hour week), it is imperative that they understand methodologies for monitoring their own behavior and its consequences. For example, structured observation of audio or videotaped interactions with assigned clients is a good way to build this insight and understanding. Further, the data from these observations provide important discussion information for the conferences that take place between supervisors and assistants about their work. Observational data can also provide indirect monitoring capability for the supervisor in an effort to bridge the gap between periods of direct supervision and to identify problems that might occur between those periods that might require a more rigorous supervision schedule and/or change in assignment of tasks to the assistant. The Direct Observation Follow-Up Contract (Appendix 12C) provides a tool that supervisors and assistants can use to identify and plan for enhancement of the assistant's direct service provision to clients.

Analysis. In the analysis phase observational data and feedback are categorized, examined, and interpreted in relation to the change or lack of it that has occurred relative to goals established in the planning phase and to the performance of the activities and tasks that have been assigned to the assistant. Chapter 7 addresses this phase of the cycle in depth. Analysis should always be based on objective information that has been collected in an organized and, hopefully, a shared fashion. Once the data have been distilled, they can be used to draw conclusions about the behavior of the assistant and make rational judgments about the teaching/learning process between the supervisor and assistant. Once the analyses are completed, the supervisor and assistant can draw conclusions, make inferences, and formulate hypotheses about what should happen next.

The assistant should always be involved in analysis. Initially, the supervisor may need to teach these skills and gradually increase the assistant's responsibility for self-analysis. During the early stages of their work together, a supervisor may complete an analysis and share it with

the assistant during a conference. Once the assistant understands analysis techniques, joint analysis of raw data during conferences becomes possible. As the assistant's skills increase, the supervisor may give the assistant raw data to analyze prior to the conference. Later, the assistant should be able to assume some responsibility for data collection and self-analyses; at this stage, the supervisor and supervisee complete separate analyses to share during the conference. The SLPA Self-Evaluation of Treatment Session (Appendix 12D) is a tool that contains 17 statements about aspects of direct client interaction that require the assistant to identify their level of agreement or disagreement with them. The level of disagreement that is selected should always be based on analysis of objective data. Even though this tool is designated as a tool for the assistant to use, it could also be used jointly by the supervisor and assistant to confirm their shared understanding of activities or to identify areas of misunderstanding.

Integrating. The previous components of the cycle of supervision require integration through some form of communication. Typically, this communication is verbal and takes place during a conference. The conference will be enhanced if an agenda that has been collaboratively structured by the supervisor and the assistant is used. The agenda may include discussion of procedural issues, specific discussion of data and their analyses, personal concerns, and general information that is relevant to the development of the participants.

Given the authors' view that a modified continuum perspective is a viable methodology for the supervisory process with assistants, it is important the conference content reflect this notion. That is, if growth is to occur on the part of the assistant within their scope of responsibilities and their assigned tasks, then there must be a shift between the supervisor and the assistant in responsibility for the substantive content of the conference and how it is implemented. The conference should not just focus on evaluations of the assistant by the supervisor but should develop into opportunities for joint problem-solving in an effort to enhance the assistant's knowledge and skill within their scope of responsibility.

PREPARATION FOR THE SUPERVISORY PROCESS

There is a significant body of literature that underscores the value of training for members of the profession who function as supervisors. Indeed, The "Guidelines for Training, Credentialing, Use, and Supervision of Speech-Language Pathology Assistants" (ASHA, 1996) recommend that speech-language pathologists who supervise assistants have at least two years of experience after the completion of the CF and complete at least one preservice course (a minimum of one semester credit hour or 15 contact hours) in supervision or one continuing education unit in activities or courses pertaining to supervision. This is in direct response to the complexity as well as the subtlety of the supervisory process and is consistent with the notion that supervision is a distinct area of professional practice that requires specific skills to implement it. Strong clinical skills and the Certificate of Clinical Competence alone do not directly translate into the ability to supervise in a manner that is consonant with the "Knowledge and Skills for Supervisors of Speech-Language Pathology Assistants" (ASHA, 2001c).

The difficulty in preparing for the practice of supervision is that currently, there is a paucity of formal coursework or continuing education. ASHA is currently organizing teleconferences that will focus on the supervisory process and its application with assistants. State associations should similarly be proactive for their members who might be involved in utilizing assistants to meet the demands of their caseload or work setting. Training programs should incorporate information into their curricula that will prepare their graduates to responsibly assume the role of supervisor. Chapter 9 suggests ways in which this

might be accomplished. In addition, given the shared responsibility for the supervisory process that this book suggests, the authors also recommend that assistant training programs consider incorporating information about the process into their curricula. The foci of this training should be helping the assistant understand their role in the supervisory process and their responsibility for helping implement it, using strategies and tools as a means of continuing their own skill refinement, growth, and development. Once an assistant begins work, the SLPA Individual Learning Plan (Appendix 12E) is a form (which can be modified as needed) that will help the assistant plan for their own continuing education needs.

ACCOUNTABILITY

The need to demonstrate accountability for the utilization of assistants is primarily the responsibility of the supervisor. Data and information that are generated by the assistant may be used in this process but it is the supervisor who will be responsible for compiling it, assuring its accuracy, and submitting it. The reasons for documenting the use of assistants include consumer protection, responsible management practices, accountability to employers, and protection to professionals if litigation or ethical practice concerns arise (ASHA, 1999). Indeed, the "Knowledge and Skills for Supervisors of Speech-Language Pathology Assistants" (Appendix 12A) identifies four specific knowledge areas supported by three skills that address the issue of accountability in the use of assistants.

Different state licensure laws may have requirements for documentation of the use of assistants. This paperwork, such as, verification of training, status of competency at the beginning of the work period and so on, may help meet the procedural need for documenting the use of assistants, but in reality, if there are ever questions or concerns raised about the use of an assistant or the supervision of them, the supervisor needs to be able to document specific supervisory practices and activities that were implemented in support of the assistant. Supervisors should be prepared, at a minimum, to document:

- The weekly activity of the assistant, which would account for all of the assistant's time
- A weekly summary of the supervisor's direct and indirect observation/supervision of the assistant
- The coordination of goals and documentation for each client assigned to the assistant

Forms to help in the gathering and organizing of these data and information can be found in Appendices 12F, G, H, and I at the end of this chapter. The authors also suggest that, in addition to the amount of time spent in supervision of the assistant, supervisors be prepared to document the content of their supervision. Again, Chapters 7 and 8 will help readers understand strategies and tools that will be useful in this process, but fundamentally, supervisors need to be able document that they were knowledgeable about the quality of the assistant's work and took steps to remediate it if it became of concern. This information will also be necessary if ever questions of due process are raised by an assistant in response to any job action. Supervisors need to be able to document that they complied with both the procedures and the process of responsible supervision.

SUMMARY

The supervision of assistants expands the role of the speech-language pathologist beyond that of a direct service provider. The broadened role requires that members of the profession who might supervise assistants understand the complexities of the process and be prepared to meet its demands. This chapter summarizes the major issues in the supervision of assistants, including the scope of responsibility for both the supervisor and the assistant, the utilization and training of an assistant, the supervision of the assistant, and the preparation of both the supervisor and the assis-

tant for their work together. Lastly, the supervisor's need to be accountable for the use of an assistant is discussed.

CASES FOR DISCUSSION

1. SLPA training and supervision example:

   The speech-language pathologist has determined that the SLPA can be utilized to assist several groups of children refine their sound production abilities. The SLP has previously helped the children establish the sounds in their sound systems; the SLPA will now follow through with a treatment plan constructed by the SLP and provide structured practice in the production of sounds in increasingly more complex linguistic contexts.

   DISCUSSION QUESTIONS:
   1. What kinds of information should the SLP consider in assigning this task(s) to the SLPA?
   2. What should the training of the SLPA for this task(s) "look" like, that is, what information should it contain and how should it be implemented with the SLPA?
   3. Identify strategies/tools that the SLP might employ to help ensure quality of care, efficiency, accountability, and continued growth of the SLPA.

2. Determination of level of supervision for SLPA provided services:

   Hagler and McFarlane (1997) suggest a strategy for determining the intensity of supervision that is needed for SLPAs based on the complexity of their task, degree of client contact, and the degree of interpersonal interaction required between the assistant and the client.

   Below are seven cases that are described by the above parameters. Decide what intensity of supervision (amount and type) is indicated according to the Hagler and McFarlane strategy and ASHA mandates.

   1. 25-year-old male, TBI-Rancho Level 3; compound fracture of left tibia and fibula;

fracture of left humerus; hairline fracture of mandible. Recently-married spouse is very involved and supportive.

Nature of Tasks:	Cognitive, swallowing, and communication Tx
	Family education
	Data collection
Frequency of Tx:	Prior authorization for 4 weeks, 2 hours/day

2. 75-year-old male aphasic; left cerebral artery CVA; good comprehension/memory for short utterances; automatic utterances but limited expression of novel utterances. Highly motivated. Supportive family.

Nature of Tasks:	Receptive and expressive language Tx
	Family education
	Data collection
Frequency:	Prior authorization for 4 weeks; 1 hour/day

3. 33-year-old female-mild TBI

Nature of Tasks:	Completion of computer-mediated problem-solving software
	Compilation of data
Frequency:	2×/day for .50 hour

4. Group of four children with sound production errors; good self-monitoring abilities.

Nature of Tasks:	Maintenance of Tx goals
	Covweek for .75 hour

5. Group of 1st grade children with delayed phonological awareness skills.

Nature of Task:	Identification of rhymes
	Segmentation of words into constituent phonemes
	Compilation of data
Frequency:	2×/week for .75 hour

6. Quadraplegic cerebral palsied 4th grader; essentially nonspeaking; normal nonverbal intelligence. Moderate feeding and swallowing issues. Oriented to new AAC device.

Nature of Tasks:	Extension of use of AAC device/strategies into classroom
	Feeding, swallowing management
	Education of teacher and parents
	Compilation of data
Frequency:	1×/day for 1 hour

ASHA Knowledge and Skills for Supervisors of Speech-Language Pathology Assistants

This Knowledge and Skills document is an official statement of the American Speech-Language-Hearing Association (ASHA). The ASHA Scope of Practice (2001) includes providing supervision of speech-language pathology assistants (SLPAs) as one of a speech-language pathologist's professional roles. The ASHA Preferred Practice Patterns (1997) are statements that define universally applicable characteristics of practice, inducing those related to supervision. ASHA requires members who practice independently in speech-language pathology to hold the Certificate of Clinical Competence in Speech-Language Pathology. ASHA members and certificate holders must abide by the ASHA Code of Ethics (2001a), which includes Principle of Ethics I-Rule D: "Individuals shall not misrepresent the credentials of assistants, technicians, or support personnel and shall inform those they serve professionally of the name and professional credentials of persons providing services"; Rule E: "Individuals who hold the Certificate of Clinical Competence shall not delegate tasks that require the unique skills, knowledge, and judgment that are within in the scope of their profession to assistants, technicians, support personnel, or any nonprofessionals over whom they have supervisory responsibility. An individual may delegate support services to assistants, technicians, support personnel, or any other persons only if those services are adequately supervised by an individual who holds the Certificate of Clinical Competence"; Principle of Ethics II-Rule D: "Individuals shall delegate the provision of clinical services only to (1): persons who hold the appropriate Certificate of Clinical Competence; (2) persons in the education or certification process who are appropriately supervised by an individual who holds the appropriate Certificate of Clinical Competence; or (3) assistants, technicians, or support personnel who are adequately supervised by an individual who holds the appropriate Certificate of Clinical Competence"; and Rule E: "Individuals shall prohibit any of their professional staff from providing services that exceed the staff member's competence, considering the staff member's level of education, training, and experience (p. 2–3).

This document was prepared by the Working Group on Supervision of Speech-Language Pathology Assistants, which is composed of representatives from the Steering Committee of ASHA's Special Interest Division 11: Administration and Supervision (Elizabeth McCrea, chair; Laura Billetdeaux, Judy Brasseur, Deborah Carlson, Leisha Eiten, Anita Halper, and Wren Newman); ASHA National Office staff in the clinical speech-language pathology practice unit who specialize in clinical issues in speech-language pathology (Diane Paul-Brown, coordinator; Amy Knapp); and other speech-language pathologists with expertise in the supervision of assistants (Jeanne Mullins; Lisa O'Connor). The ASHA monitoring vice president was Alex P. Johnson.

PREAMBLE

Dramatic changes have occurred over the last decade in the manner in which speech-language pathology services are delivered due to the challenges of health care finance reform, public school caseloads, scientific and technological advances, and an expanding scope of practice for members of the profession. As one response to these challenges, the profession's governing bodies now recognize the role of SLPAs who can support ASHA-certified speech-language pathologists (LC 1–95). Assistants are individuals who, following academic coursework, clinical practicum, credentialing, and perhaps voluntary registration by ASHA, can perform tasks prescribed, directed, and supervised by ASHA-certified speech-language pathologists (ASHA, 1996; ASHA, 2000).

The use of credentialed and supervised SLPAs is one way to increase the frequency of services to clients while maintaining service quality and controlling cost. The decision to shift responsibility for some aspects of speech-language pathology service delivery to assistants should be only made by ASHA-certified speech-language pathologists and only when the quality of care to patients/clients will not be compromised. In addition to direct patient/client contact, SLPAs may also assist service delivery by preparing materials, performing clerical duties associated with program or case management, or working on other appropriate assignments that fall within their defined scope of responsibilities (ASHA, 1996). Whatever tasks are assigned to the SLPAs, implicit in the decision to use them is the ethnical commitment by the ASHA-certified speech-language pathologist to provide appropriate supervision in order to ensure quality of care. It must be clear to all parties involved that the use of an SLPA is not meant to replace the work of a speech-language pathologist but, rather, to effectively extend it.

Using an SLPA as an interpreter/translator requires additional knowledge and skills that are not addressed in this document. ASHA's Multicultural Issues Board is developing guidelines to address this need.

INTRODUCTION

In 1985 the ASHA Legislative Council adopted the position statement Clinical Supervision in Speech-Language Pathology and Audiology (ASHA, 1985b). This document formally recognized the importance of the supervisory process in the clinical education of speech-language pathologists and audiologists as a fundaments mechanism to ensure quality service to clients. The position paper also outlined 13 tasks that are basic to effective clinical supervision and identified supervisor competencies that implement each task.

The importance of supervision in the competent and ethical use of SLPAs requires that the profession now identify and define the knowledge and skills necessary for supervisors of SLPAs. This document identifies the knowledge and skills that are consistent with the 13 tasks of supervision identified in the 1985 position statement, as well as those tasks identified in the ASHA Guidelines for the Training, Credentialing, Use, and Supervision of Speech-Language Pathology Assistants (ASHA, 1996). These tasks make it clear that the ASHA-certified supervisor retains legal and ethical responsibility for all aspects of case management and service delivery while at the same time helping assistants refine their skills within their scope of responsibilities and assigned tasks.

Role of the Supervisor

Direct and indirect supervision of SLPAs by speech-language pathologists expands the speech-language pathologists' role as a service provider to include responsibility for the work of support personnel (ASHA, 1996). This broadened role demands that members of the profession who might supervise SLPAs understand the complexity of the supervisory process and be prepared to meet its challenges. The knowledge and skills delineated in this document are the first steps in that preparation.

Terminology

Clinical Supervision: Clinical supervision refers to the tasks and skills of clinical teaching related to the interaction between the client and the service provider.

Direct Supervision: Direct supervision means onsite, in-view observation and guidance by the speech-language pathologist while an assigned activity is performed by support personnel.

Indirect Supervision: Indirect supervision means those activities other than direct observation and guidance conducted by a speech-language pathologist. These may include demonstrations, record review, review and evaluation of audio- or videotaped sessions, and interactive television.

Knowledge and Skills

Supervisors of SLPAs have the knowledge and skills to:

1. Select and assign appropriate patients/clients to the SLPA.

   KNOWLEDGE REQUIRED:

   a. Understand the ASHA Guidelines for the Training, Credentialing, Use, and Supervision of Speech-Language Pathology Assistants (ASHA, 1996), including:
      - Ethical and legal responsibilities of the ASHA-certified speech-language pathologist
      - Scope of job responsibilities of the SLPA
      - Exclusive responsibilities of the ASHA-certified speech-language pathologist
      - Appropriate amount of direct and indirect supervision
      - Ratio of supervisors to SLPAs
      - SLPA access to supervisor

   SKILLS REQUIRED:

   a. Assess the patient/client's disorder and concomitant needs in order to determine if use of an assistant is appropriate.
   b. Determine those tasks that the SLPA has the training and expertise to perform.
   c. Assign tasks to the SLPA that are within the scope of the SLPA's job responsibilities and are consistent with his/her knowledge and skill.

2. Determine the nature of supervision that is appropriate for each SLPA.

   KNOWLEDGE REQUIRED:

   a. Understand supervisory processes and practices, including strategies for direct and indirect supervision.

SKILLS REQUIRED:

a. Determine the amount of supervision required based on the needs of the client, the experience of the SLPA, the service delivery setting, the task assigned, and other pertinent factors.
b. Design and implement supervisory procedures that ensure patient/client confidentiality and quality of care.
c. Determine when it is necessary to alter the amount and type of supervision in response to changes in client/patient status and/or service delivery models, use of equipment, or assigned tasks.

3. Establish and maintain an effective relationship with the SLPA.

   KNOWLEDGE REQUIRED:

   a. Understand components of an effective supervisory relationship with the SLPA.
   b. Understand the dynamics of various learning styles.
   c. Understand diverse styles of interpersonal communication.

   SKILLS REQUIRED:

   a. Facilitate the SLPA's understanding of assigned tasks and the supervisory process.
   b. Accommodate a variety of learning styles in the supervision of the SLPA.
   c. Use effective interpersonal communication skills to maximize communication effectiveness in the supervision of the SLPA.
   d. Facilitate problem-solving of tasks assigned by the SLP.
   e. Maintain a professional and supportive relationship that allows for both supervisor and SLPA growth.
   f. Interact with the SLPA in an objective manner.
   g. Establish joint communications regarding expectations and responsibilities in assigned tasks and the supervisory process.
   h. Evaluate the SLPA and the effectiveness of the supervisory process.
   i. Guide the SLPA in developing appropriate interpersonal skills (e.g., collaborative

teamwork and conflict resolution), with patients/clients, family members, staff, and others.

4. Teach the SLPA to follow screening protocols:

   KNOWLEDGE REQUIRED:

   a. Understand speech-language screening tools and protocols, including how to administer them and document the results.

   SKILLS REQUIRED:

   a. Teach the SLPA to administer and score appropriately the assigned screening tools including:
   - differentiation of correct versus incorrect responses
   - accurate completion of protocols
   - accurate collection/scoring of patient/client screening data

   b. Direct the SLPA in managing assigned screening protocols and documentation.
   - Seek the supervisor's guidance if the administration of screening tools is in question
   - Report any difficulty encountered in screening
   - Schedule screenings
   - Organize screening tools

   c. Assist the SLPA in accurately communicating screening results, without interpretation to the SLP, including descriptive behavioral observations that enhance the clarity of results.

5. Demonstrate for and participate with the SLPA in the clinical process.

   KNOWLEDGE REQUIRED:

   a. Understand best practices in speech-language pathology, dynamics of patient/client-clinician relationships, clinical techniques, clinical materials and equipment, and behavioral management techniques.

   SKILLS REQUIRED:

   a. Demonstrate best practices for the SLPA.

   b. Demonstrate an effective client-clinician relationship.

   c. Demonstrate a variety of clinical techniques.

   d. Demonstrate the use of client-specific materials and equipment.

   e. Instruct the SLPA in the performance of tasks as outlined and demonstrated by the speech-language pathologist and to implement activities that use procedures prescribed by the speech-language pathologist.

   f. Assist the SLPA in developing skills to maintain patient/client on-task behavior.

   g. Teach the SLPA how to provide appropriate feedback regarding the accuracy of the patient/client response.

   h. Teach the SLPA to use feedback and reinforcement that is consistent, discriminating, and meaningful to the patient/client.

   i. Instruct the SLPA in giving directions and instructions that are clear, concise, and appropriate to patient/client's age and level of understanding.

   j. Instruct the SLPA in applying behavior management techniques and basic instructional strategies (e.g., asking questions, giving directions, providing positive reinforcement of desired behaviors) that are specific to the patient/client.

   k. Teach the SLPA how to provide appropriate cuing strategies to assist the patient/client in approximating accurate responses.

6. Direct the SLPA in following individualized treatment plans that have been developed by the speech-language pathologist.

   KNOWLEDGE REQUIRED:

   a. Understand communication disorders and the design of individualized treatment plans.

   SKILLS REQUIRED:

   a. Instruct the SLPA in understanding a patient/client's disorders and communication needs.

   b. Develop an individualized treatment plan for each client for the SLPA to follow:
   - Direct the SLPA to execute clinical goals and objectives in the specified sequence.

- Instruct the SLPA in description and data collection to measure patient/client behavior change.
- Instruct the SLPA in documenting patient/client outcomes.
  c. Teach the SLPA how to describe patient/client progress.

7. Direct the SLPA in the maintenance of clinical records.

KNOWLEDGE REQUIRED:

a. Understand clinical record keeping procedures.
b. Understand principles and procedures for maintaining client confidentiality.

SKILLS REQUIRED:

a. Assist the SLPA in maintaining accurate clinical records.
b. Assist the SLPA to effectively document clinical interactions, including:
   - Individual treatment plans and protocols
   - Patient/client performance
   - Other information on patient/client charts
c. Assist the SLPA in organizing records to facilitate easy retrieval of information concerning clinical interactions.
d. Assist the SLPA in following policies and procedures to protect the confidentiality of clinical records.

8. Interacts with the SLPA in planning and executing supervisory conferences.

KNOWLEDGE REQUIRED:

a. Understand components of both the supervisory process and supervisory conferences.
b. Understand strategies for observation and analysis of supervisory conferences.

SKILLS REQUIRED:

a. Establish a regular conference schedule.
b. Plan a supervisory conference agenda.
c. Involve the SLPA in a joint discussion of previously identified clinical or supervisory data or issues.

d. Adjust supervisory style and interact with the SLPA in a manner that facilitates the SLPA's self-exploration and problem-solving within assigned tasks.
e. Adjust supervisory conference content based on the SLPA's level of training and experience.
f. Encourage and maintain SLPA motivation for continuing self-growth and development of job skills.
g. Assist the SLPA in making commitments for changes in job skills.

9. Provide feedback to the SLPA regarding skills.

KNOWLEDGE REQUIRED:

a. Understand the skill level of the SLPA.
b. Understand the tools used for evaluation of SLPA clinical skills.
c. Understand effective supervisory communication styles.

SKILLS REQUIRED:

a. Develop and use clinical skill evaluation tools.
b. Assist the SLPA in the description and measurement of his or her progress and achievement of job skills.
c. Assist the SLPA in developing strategies for self-evaluation and documentation of job performance.
d. Use supervisory feedback to modify interactions with patients/clients.

10. Assist the SLPA in developing skills of verbal reporting and assigned informal written reporting to the SLP.

KNOWLEDGE REQUIRED:

a. Understand standards and strategies for effective oral and written communication.

SKILLS REQUIRED:

a. Assist the SLPA in identifying appropriate information to be included in oral reports.
b. Teach the SLPA how to present verbal and written information in a logical, concise, and sequential manner.

c. Instruct the SLPA in the use of appropriate professional terminology.

11. Assist the SLPA in effectively selecting, preparing, and presenting treatment materials and organizing treatment environments.

KNOWLEDGE REQUIRED:

a. Understand appropriate treatment materials for specific populations.

SKILLS REQUIRED:

a. Assist the SLPA in choosing appropriate materials from an approved materials list to be used to implement the assigned treatment plan.

b. Assist the SLPA in effectively organizing the clinical setting to meet the needs of the client and obtain optimal patient/client performance.

c. Assist the SLPA in selecting materials that are age and culturally appropriate as well as motivating.

d. Assist the SLPA in efficiently preparing and selecting treatment materials in a timely manner.

12. Share information regarding ethical, legal, regulatory, and reimbursement aspects of professional practice.

KNOWLEDGE REQUIRED:

a. Understand ethical, legal, regulatory, and reimbursement aspects of professional practice.

b. Understand the scope of practice in speech-language pathology.

SKILLS REQUIRED:

a. Communicate professional codes of ethics and conduct (e.g., ASHA, state licensure boards, other professional legal bodies) to the SLPA.

b. Communicate an understanding of legal and regulatory requirements and their impact on the practice of the profession (e.g., licensure, IDEA, ADA, Medicare, Medicaid) to the SLPA.

c. Communicate an understanding of reimbursement policies and procedures of the work setting to the SLPA.

d. Communicate due process policies and procedures in the work setting to the SLPA.

e. Articulate clearly the speech-language pathologist's scope of practice and exclusive responsibilities of the SLPA.

13. Model and facilitate professional conduct.

KNOWLEDGE REQUIRED:

a. Understand appropriate professional standards and conduct.

SKILLS REQUIRED:

a. Assume ethical and legal responsibility for all patient/client care.

b. Analyze, evaluate, and modify own behavior.

c. Model ethical and legal conduct.

d. Meet and respect deadlines.

e. Provide current information regarding professional standards.

f. Assist the SLPA in demonstrating appropriate conduct, including:

- Respect/maintain confidentiality of patient/client information
- Dress appropriately for the work setting
- Use appropriate language for the work setting
- Recognize own job limitations and perform within the boundaries of training and job responsibilities (e.g., refer the patient/client family and other professionals to the speech-language pathologist for any information regarding screening and treatment).

g. Assist the SLPA to effectively address patient/client attitudes and behaviors.

14. Direct the SLPA in the implementation of research procedures, in-service training activities, and public relations programs.

KNOWLEDGE REQUIRED:

a. Understand research projects and their procedures, in-service training activities, and public relations programs.

SKILLS REQUIRED:

a. Teach the SLPA how to complete assigned research tasks.
b. Teach the SLA how to complete assigned in-service training responsibilities.
c. Teach the SLPA how to complete assigned public relation program activities.

15. Train the SLPA to check and maintain equipment and to observe universal precautions.

KNOWLEDGE REQUIRED:

a. Understand operational procedures for equipment, including performance checks and maintenance.
b. Understand universal precautions policies and procedures.

SKILLS REQUIRED:

a. Instruct the SLPA in maintaining and performing assigned checks of equipment.
b. Assist the SLPA in the completion of universal precautions protocols.

16. Assist the SLPA in using appropriate language (oral and written) when interacting with patients/clients and others.

KNOWLEDGE REQUIRED:

a. Understand appropriate oral and written language skills to use when interacting with patients/clients and others.

SKILLS REQUIRED:

a. Model and instruct the SLPA with regard to the awareness of and sensitivity to cultural and linguistic needs of each client.
b. Model and instruct the SLPA to adapt language according to the patient/client's age,

culture, and linguistic, cognitive, and educational level.
c. Model and instruct the SLPA to be courteous and respectful at all times.
d. Model and instruct the SLPA in maintaining appropriate pragmatic skills, such as eye contact, body language, facial expression, and conversational turn-taking, as well as topic initiation, maintenance, and closure.

17. Establish a system of accountability for document use and supervision of the SLPA.

KNOWLEDGE REQUIRED:

a. Understand accountability systems for documentation of supervision of the SLPA.
b. Understand supervision requirements for the SLPA.
c. Understand due process rights and procedures.
d. Understand conflict resolution strategies, including referral, as appropriate.

SKILLS REQUIRED:

a. Document the type and amount of supervision provided to the SLPA.
b. Develop conflict resolution strategies that protect due process of the SLPA and patient/client quality of care.
c. Prepare summary reports regarding use of the SLPA, including accessibility of services to patients/clients, utilization cost-benefit analysis, and quality of service measures to administrators, patients/clients, and payers.

REFERENCES

American Speech-Language-Hearing Association. (1985). Clinical supervision in speech-language pathology and audiology. *Asha, 27,* 57–60.

American Speech-Language-Hearing Association. (1988). Utilization and employment of speech-language pathology supportive personnel with underserved populations. *Asha, 30,* 55–56.

American Speech-Language-Hearing Association. (2001a). *Code of ethics.* Rockville, MD: Author.

American Speech-Language-Hearing Association. (1996). Guidelines for the training, credentialing, use, and supervision of speech-language pathology assistants. *Asha, 38* (Suppl. 16), 21–34.

American Speech-Language-Hearing Association. (1997). Preferred practice patterns for the profession of speech-language pathology. *Asha,* 38 (Suppl. 16), 21–34.

American Speech-Language-Hearing Association. (2000). *Council on Professional Standards in Speech-Language Pathology and Audiology: Background information and criteria for registration of speech-language pathology assistants.* Rockville, MD: Author.

American Speech-Language-Hearing Association. (2001). *Scope of practice in speech-language pathology.* Rockville, MD: Author.

Dowling, S. (2001). *Supervision: Strategies for successful outcomes and productivity.* Boston: Allyn & Bacon.

Hagler, P., & McFarlane, L. (1997). *Collaborative service delivery by assistants and professionals (rev. ed.).* Edmonton, Alberta, Canada: Alberta Rehabilitation Coordinating Council.

Horton, A., Kander, M., Longhurst, T., & Paul-Brown, D. (1997). *Preparing and using speech-language pathology assistants.* Rockville, MD: American Speech-Language-Hearing Association.

Suggested Readings

Anderson, J. L. (1988). *The supervisory process in speech-language pathology and audiology.* Austin, TX: Pro-Ed.

Reprinted with permission from ASHA: American Speech-Language-Hearing Association. "Knowledge and skills for supervisors of speech-language pathology assistants." 2001.

APPENDIX 12B

SKILLS PROFICIENCY CHECKLIST

SLPA: _____

Supervising SLP: _____

		Self-Rating			Supervising SLP Rating		
SKILL OR PROFICIENCY	DATE	PROFICIENCY LEVEL	DATE	PROFICIENCY LEVEL	HOW LEARNED	DEMONSTRATED	

Competence Levels
1. Little or no experience.
2. Some experience, requires practice/assist.
3. Proficient with occasional supervision.
4. Proficient with independent performance.

How Learned
Observation
On the job training
Class
Video
Policy/Procedure
Other

Demonstrated
Direct observation
Test
(written/verbal)
Certificate/License
Discussion with
Supervisor
Other

Direct Observation Follow-Up Contract

DIRECT OBSERVATION FOLLOW-UP CONTRACT

Speech-Language Pathology Assistant: _____

Supervising SLP: _____

Date of session observed: _____

Patient/client observed: _____

Description of behavior/skill that needs improvement: _____

_____

_____

_____

_____

_____

Action plan and time frame: _____

_____

_____

_____

_____

_____

Follow-up date: _____

Was proficiency achieved in this skill area? _____

Within the expected time frame? _____

Comments:

SLPA Self-Evaluation of Treatment Session

SLPA SELF-EVALUATION OF TREATMENT SESSION

Medical Setting

Note: This form may be used in conjunction with the Direct Observation Skills Brief Checklist.

Date/Time of Session: _____

		Disagree			*Agree*
1. I maintained an appropriate relationship with the patient throughout the session.	1	2	3	4	5
2. I was self-confident in this session.	1	2	3	4	5
3. I considered the patient's needs in selecting my materials and interacting with this patient.	1	2	3	4	5
4. I considered the patient's cultural values in selecting my materials and interacting with this patient.	1	2	3	4	5
5. I used language appropriate for the patient's age and education.	1	2	3	4	5
6. I was courteous and respectful with this patient.	1	2	3	4	5
7. I was punctual for the session.	1	2	3	4	5
8. I was prepared for the session.	1	2	3	4	5
9. I was dressed appropriately for this session.	1	2	3	4	5
10. I used time efficiently during this session.	1	2	3	4	5
11. I completed the assigned tasks during this session.	1	2	3	4	5
12. I accurately determined correct vs. incorrect responses.	1	2	3	4	5
13. I provided appropriate feedback to the patient.	1	2	3	4	5
14. The treatment environment was appropriate for this patient.	1	2	3	4	5
15. I was aware of my professional boundaries during this session.	1	2	3	4	5
16. I documented the results of the session appropriately.	1	2	3	4	5
17. I shared the results with my supervisor.	1	2	3	4	5

Comments:

SLPA Signature: _____

SLPA Individual Learning Plan

SLPA INDIVIDUAL LEARNING PLAN

SLPA: _____

Supervising SLP: _____

Date of Plan _____

For Period Extending _____ to _____

Annual Required Training (includes CEU, licensure, certification, and/or regulatory requirements)

Course	*Expected Date*	*Estimated Hours*

Recommended Training Subsequent to Performance Appraisal

Course	*Expected Date*	*Estimated Hours*

Personal Learning Objectives

Course	*Expected Date*	*Estimated Hours*

_____   _____

SLPA Signature   *Date*

_____   _____

Supervising SLP Signature   *Date*

Reprinted with permission from: *Practical Tools and Forms for Supervising Speech-Language-Pathology Assistants,* p. 59. American Speech-Language Hearing Association. Copyright 1999.

SLPA Weekly Activity Log

SLPA WEEKLY ACTIVITY LOG

Sample

Week Ending: _____

SLPA: _____

Supervising SLP: _____

Patient	Monday	Tuesday	Wednesday	Thursday	Friday	Sat./Sun.
Joe	30 min + S	30 min	30 min	30 min	30 min	
Harry	15 min	30 min	Cancel	30 min + S	45 min	
Rhonda		60 min + S		60 min		
Michael	30 min + S		30 min		30 min	
Louise		45 min (dc)				
Phil	60 min	15 min	60 min + S	45 min	30 min	
Marilyn	15 min	15 min + S	15 min	30 min	30 min	
Al	30 min + S		30 min		30 min	
Debra	45 min	45 min + S	45 min	30 min	30 min	
James	15 min	15 min	30 min + S	15 min	45 min	
Total treatment time						
Total direct supervision						
Documentation time	60 min	60 min	60 min	60 min	60 min	
Meeting with supervisor				90 min		
Other meetings/ conferences	60 min		30 min			
Observation of sessions		60 min		60 min		
Equipment maintenance	30 min	30 min	30 min	30 min	30 min	
Clerical tasks	60 min	45 min	90 min	30 min	60 min	

S indicates Supervised session

SLPA Weekly Activity Record

SLPA WEEKLY ACTIVITY RECORD

SLPA: _____

Supervising SLP: _____

Week ending: _____

Total hours worked this week: _____

Activity	*Time Spent*
1. Direct patient treatment/intervention	_____
2. Observation of other sessions	_____
3. Meeting with supervising SLP	_____
4. Other meetings/Conferences (list)	_____
_____	
_____	
_____	
5. Equipment/materials maintenance	_____
6. Documentation	_____
7. Clerical activities	_____
	= 100%
A. Total time directly observed by the SLP	_____
B. Total treatment time provided this week	_____
Percent of time directly observed by the SLP (A/B)	_____

Reprinted with permission from *Practical Tools and Forms for Supervising Speech-Language-Pathology Assistants,* p. 47. American Speech-Language Hearing Association. Copyright 1999.

Supervisor Log of Direct and Indirect Observations

SUPERVISOR LOG OF DIRECT AND INDIRECT OBSERVATIONS

Week ending: _____

SLPA: _____

Supervising SLP: _____

Patient	*Monday*	*Tuesday*	*Wednesday*	*Thursday*	*Friday*	*Sat./Sun.*

Other activities						
Billing						
Equipment maintenance						
Documentation						
Meetings/In-services						
Other clerical						

* Indicate DO for direct observation + time
* Indicate IDO for indirect observation + time

Comments:

Speech-Language Pathology

SPEECH-LANGUAGE PATHOLOGY

Daily/Weekly Documentation and Goal Coordination

Patient Name: _____   Referring Physician:_____

SLP: _____   SLPA:_____

Treatment Frequency: _____   Diagnosis: _____

Week Ending: _____

Treatment/Intervention Goals (1 unit = 15 minutes)

Goals:	Monday	Tuesday	Wednesday	Thursday	Friday	Sat./Sun.
1.						
2.						
3.						
4.						
5.						

Total Daily Units

Daily Notes

Date:

Signature_____   Signature _____

Date:

Signature_____   Signature _____

CHAPTER THIRTEEN

CASE PROBLEMS

In order to provide a mechanism for problem solving and a practical way to apply the theoretical information presented in the component chapters, several cases are presented here. Different work settings are included so that readers will hopefully find at least one with which they can identify. Although the settings have been varied, the issues in each of the cases could be modified to apply to any setting. For example, the controlling supervisor in Case V could be a supervisor of interns in a medical setting or a supervisor of assistants. Readers are encouraged to shape the cases to fit into their own repertoire of experiences.

It is important to remember that although the context may change, the continuum perspective, the components of the process, and the tasks of supervision are the same and remain constant across settings and degrees of experience. Supervision of students and staff takes place in almost every professional setting. Despite differences in setting and clinical specialty, everyone who supervises has much in common professionally. Anderson's model of supervision (1988) provides substantive insights about the dynamics of the supervisory process, the roles and responsibilities of both the supervisor and supervisee, and the procedures to implement them.

Application. For the cases, readers are asked to consider what aspects of the understanding, planning, observing, analyzing, and integrating components are applicable to each. Some questions and ideas are posed to help facilitate problem solving.

For each of the cases that will be introduced (Joann—the Master's student, Sarah—the failing intern, Don—the employee in acute care, Mary—the employee in a rehabilitation setting, Mia—the student with a controlling supervisor, and the supervisor in a rural school district), specific aspects of behavior and situation that contribute to the problem must be identified and objectified. **Planning will be the first step in solving these problems.**

Observation and data collection strategies that have been identified in Chapter 6 can be utilized in this effort. Once all the aspects of the problem(s) have been pinpointed, they should be prioritized by supervisor and supervisee to determine which need to be addressed sequentially or concurrently and which will make the biggest positive difference for the supervisee and, ultimately, the client. Once this determination has been made, specific behavioral goals that can be observed and measured should be structured; these goals may focus on specific aspects of supervisee clinical skill, verbal and/or nonverbal behavior, ability to comply with organizational requirements, and so on. After the goals are identified, an *action plan* for both the supervisee and supervisor to address them should be constructed, implemented, and monitored. Bartlett's Supervisory Action Plan in Appendix 5C would be a helpful tool to use.

Supervisors should consider their skill and behavior in relation to each of the supervisees and the difficulty(s) they are experiencing. Some insight in this regard may be gleaned from the information shared by the supervisees during the understanding component of the model. Supervisors should *also* be prepared to target goals for themselves during this planning component that will concentrate not just on supporting the supervisee but on how they provide this support as well. Data should be obtained to document progress toward these goals.

CASE I, MASTER'S STUDENT

Joann is a second semester Master's candidate with 85 hours of previous supervised clinical experience. This semester, part of her clinical assignment includes a 7-year-old child who has quadriplegic cerebral palsy and significant oral motor programming difficulties. He is essentially non-speaking but as far as can be determined, he has normal cognitive abilities for his age.

Joann has had all the appropriate academic prerequisites to manage this child, including a course in AAC; however, she is having difficulty implementing her therapy with him. On paper her plans and materials appear appropriate, but each day, sometime within the first therapy activity, her client begins to become restless and move off-task. Joann is aware that this is happening, but she does not know why and therefore has not been able to make changes in her treatment implementation which will support her client's positive participation with her.

After observing for two sessions, you as the supervisor have determined to your satisfaction that the primary issue is Joann's apparent inability to tolerate silence. Because of his motor difficulties, the client requires a significant amount of time to execute his response(s) to Joann's treatment stimuli. During this time, the air is "full of silence." Joann appears to become uneasy and begins to reprompt the client, altering the stimuli because she is uncomfortable without an immediate response. In return, the client becomes angry and frustrated with this repeated (and to him, unnecessary) structuring of his treatment.

Applications

Understanding. A basic question is how can the supervisor objectively identify the problem

for/with Joann? Once Joann understands the dynamics of her difficulty, what should the supervisor do to support her ability to make the necessary changes in her clinical skill development with this client?

Observing. How much experience did Joann have observing her clinical sessions via audio or videotape during her first semester of grad school? What procedures has she used previously? She is bound to be a bit anxious about her forthcoming sessions given that her client has exhibited some frustration and anger. To assist her "in selecting and executing data collection procedures" (competency 6.2), it may be helpful to begin with observation strategies that Joann has used and/or to share data that you, her supervisor, have collected. What particular methods do you think would be most helpful to her? A time-based system, such as the ABC (Appendix 6C) would allow for the analysis of response time and the relationship between response time and a correct or incorrect response. It would also enable Joann to see what impact her behavior has on that of her client. What theoretical or pedagogical literature might be helpful to supplement observation data? Perhaps some demonstration therapy might be helpful. How would you jointly determine this?

Analyzing. How much experience did Joann have analyzing her clinical sessions via audio or videotape last semester? What procedures has she used previously? To assist her in "analyzing and interpreting data objectively" (competency 6.4), it may be helpful to begin with analysis strategies that Joann has used or to share those that you, her supervisor, have completed. Again, you will need to identify methods that will foster professional growth and independence. What theoretical or pedagogical literature might be helpful to provide in conjunction with the analysis—that is, what might facilitate accurate interpretation? Perhaps joint analysis would be a good first step. How will you decide?

Integrating. If you have engaged in joint analysis of her session prior to your conference, that will provide a major agenda topic. If not, joint analysis during the conference may be your first task. Some carefully crafted questions should facilitate Joann's critical thinking and problem solving.

CASE II, FAILING INTERN

Sarah is a graduate student clinician in speech-language pathology, assigned to an off-site placement in an acute care rehabilitation setting. She expects to complete her graduate program at the end of the current term and has accepted a CFY position in a rehabilitation program. Throughout the 5 day/week, 10-week placement, Sarah has had a number of problems. Her on-site supervisor observes that Sarah is often late for appointments, fails to complete paperwork, shows poor documentation skills, has difficulty relating to patients and families, and struggles to make clinical decisions and to master clinical assessment tools. During conferences, the supervisor has given Sarah constructive suggestions, and they have agreed on specific goals such as being on time for all clients, completing daily paperwork before leaving the facility, and preparing for sessions ahead of time.

Over the past few weeks, Sarah has shown some improvement but continues to need direction to select therapy materials, to set daily goals for patients she has been managing for several weeks, and to administer familiar assessment tools accurately.

The supervisor consults with the university practicum coordinator to outline her concerns. The university coordinator notes that Sarah's performance has been uneven throughout her enrollment in the program and that other supervisors have expressed similar concerns. The university coordinator points out that Sarah is scheduled to graduate this term and that a less-than-satisfactory grade could create problems.

Copyright 1997, 1998, 1999 American Speech-Language Hearing Association

Applications

Understanding.   Some information is critical to appropriate resolution of the situation. Specifically, what were the expectations of the facility, the supervisor, the university, and Sarah for this assignment? Are there external reasons contributing to her difficulties (e.g., illness, other responsibilities, family problems, financial difficulties)? To what extent did Sarah discuss her strengths and her needs with the off-campus supervisor, including objectives she selected for her own professional growth and supervisory strategies that she finds helpful? Were goals for the practicum established prior to beginning it? What ethical issues need to be considered? What are implications of passing or failing Sarah?

Faculty and supervisors had to be questioning the reason that Sarah was exhibiting so much difficulty, given the pattern described in this case and the fact that it deviates from the norm—that is, it is not characteristic of the average graduate student. What are the causes of her behaviors? Lack of motivation, personal problems interfering with her clinical performance, illness or a learning disability? Physical and psychological etiologies and solutions should have been explored.

What are the expectations of the facility, the supervisor, the university, and Sarah for this assignment? The supervisor should share the rehabilitation facility's policies and procedures and clearly articulate her own personal expectations. Knowing her learning style and the things she needs to work on, Sarah should be able to share her expectations for the internship—what she will be able to do by the end of the term and how her supervisor can help. Previous clinical evaluations should enable Sarah and her supervisor to identify target areas for professional growth. The university coordinator should assist the on-site supervisor in formulating reasonable objectives, timelines for completion, and performance criteria to measure competence. Further, the university should have a policy that delineates steps: for satisfactory performance, being awarded clock hours or being allowed to work in off-campus settings, repeating an internship or completing additional practica on-campus before being allowed off-campus, and so on.

Jointly developing an action plan with objectives, procedures, time lines, criteria, and so on is essential. Bartlett's format (2001), described in Chapter 5, provides a useful tool for ensuring a precise plan and making sure "everyone is on the same page." For example, a student like Sarah may begin her placement observing and shadowing the supervisor and observing other clinicians, as well. A next logical step would be acting as co-clinician with her supervisor. Then, Sarah might assume responsibility for part of the caseload, increasing the number of patients as she demonstrates proficiency in case management.

For each professional technical skill that Sarah needs to master, a clear plan must be formulated. For example, with regard to assessment tools, specific tests should be listed, timelines for demonstrating her ability to administer and score them should be indicated, and inter- and intra-rater agreement checks and criteria should be noted. Performance standards must be stated in observable, measurable terms. Further, evaluative or subjective words such as *appropriate,* must be operationally defined.

Observing.   What varieties of data collection procedures has the on-site supervisor employed? Has Sarah been actively involved in self-observation? What formative evaluations, based on data collected during previous clinical assignments, have been shared with Sarah? What has the campus coordinator done during this current assignment to maintain contact and assist both the student and the on-site supervisor? How have these efforts been documented? In this case, there are obviously more issues than those involving professional growth. There are ethical and legal issues resulting in a multitude of potential problems that the program faces. Data or lack of data will significantly influence the outcomes in Sarah's case.

Analyzing.   What varieties of analyses have the on-site supervisor employed? Has Sarah been actively involved in the process? What formative evaluations, based on observation and analyses during previous clinical assignments, have been shared with Sarah? What has the campus coordinator done during this current assignment to maintain contact and assist both the student and the on-site supervisor? How have these efforts been documented? In this case, there are obviously more issues than those involving professional growth. There are ethical and legal issues resulting in a multitude of potential problems that the program faces. Data, analyses, and appropriate documentation to reflect that these have been shared with Sarah will significantly influence the outcomes (e.g., student grievance, litigation, extending Sarah's master's program, etc.).

Systematic data collection for each objective specified in Sarah's remediation plan is a must. At first, the university and on-site supervisors should be responsible for data collection and analysis, but gradually Sarah must be eased into this process with joint efforts so that she can develop the problem solving skills needed to be able to independently function effectively. The observation tasks and analysis tools that Sarah needs to become proficient in using must be clearly delineated, as should the criteria for mastery.

Integrating.   The Sarahs of the world are rare, but unfortunately do exist. If the continuum model and the process described in the components had been applied, the situation described in Sarah's case could have been avoided. The fact that Sarah's previous supervisors expressed similar concerns about basic personal qualities such as being punctual and completing paperwork, which are fundamental "work ethic" kinds of expectations in *any* setting, should have been a major warning to the Clinic Director. Coupled with her "difficulty relating to patients and families," an interpersonal skill that is essential for persons in helping professions, we have to wonder why Sarah even wants to be a SLP. These are skills that are expected of students and professionals at all levels. Lastly, Sarah's level of competence with professional tasks such as selecting therapy materials and accurately administering assessment protocols indicates that she is at the Evaluation-Feedback end of the continuum. She needs serious help in developing self-analysis and problem solving skills in order to function effectively in an autonomous manner.

It also seems reasonable to assume that she has not been very active in her own professional growth, that is, she has not participated in the supervisory process. If she had been active in previous practica, she would have identified her problem areas and likely have requested more experience in the university clinic to achieve basic competencies before undertaking an internship. Even if she found herself being placed off-campus for some reason, she should have been able to communicate her strengths and weaknesses to her off-site supervisor at the beginning of the term, prioritize professional development goals, and participate with her supervisors (both the university coordinator and her on-site supervisor) in formulating specific objectives for acquiring entry-level competencies. What kinds of things should have occurred in the supervisory process?

Frequent planned individual and group conferences will be important for evaluating Sarah's progress and for providing a vehicle for learning and facilitating Sarah's movement along the continuum. Written commitments from Sarah would appear to be necessary (Shapiro, 1985b) to insure follow through on goals and suggestions that surface during conferences.

CASE III, EMPLOYEE IN AN ACUTE CARE HOSPITAL

Don has been a dream staff member in an acute care hospital. He is very conscientious, almost perfectionistic. He has little tolerance for anything that is less than perfect and his professional interactions with his clients reflect this attention. He makes use of continuing education to learn the "New Stuff" and upgrade his skills. His written documentation is flawless.

As the pressure for productivity has built in Don's hospital, a problem has begun to arise. Given his attention to thoroughness and detail in every aspect of his professional life, Don cannot generate the clinical documentation (to his satisfaction) that is required by his caseload without working nights and weekends. He is on a fast track to burnout and now you, as the manager of speech-language pathology, need to assign two more cases to him.

As the manager/supervisor for speech-language pathology, you ponder how to help Don manage the increasing demands of his position.

Applications

Understanding.   How can Don's manager assist him in developing realistic expectations for performance? How can the manager diplomatically clarify the hospital's expectations for billable units and documentation? What kinds of resistance might surface and what interpersonal skills could be most effective in managing Don's resistance?

Observing.   Don's perfectionistic tendencies make it likely that he has been involved in observing himself and collecting data. Here is a case where it might be beneficial to have him observe colleagues—particularly their strategies for scheduling, sample assessment and progress reports, and other aspects of program management. In an effort to assist him in modifying his work behaviors, you have to contemplate the forces and sources of Don's resistance to changing the status quo in order to guide his observations appropriately.

Analyzing.   It is highly probable that Don has been involved in self-analyses. Again, some outside data might be a good basis for comparative analyses. For example, Don could access data from ASHA's NOMS to compare his treatment outcomes to national outcomes. He could be directed to access Omnibus Survey data to compare the time he spends completing paperwork to that of typical SLPs in acute care settings. Are there other sources that might be helpful in his case? Would it be appropriate to direct him to some of the literature on burnout? In an effort to assist him in modifying his work behaviors, you have to contemplate the forces and sources of Don's resistance to change in order to appropriately guide his analysis and interpretation of data.

Integrating.   Don seems like the perfect candidate for group conferences. Having peers who can share some tips and short cuts for documentation might be helpful. Vicarious learning might also prove effective in modifying Don's behavior. In addition, he needs to formulate a professional development plan that targets decreasing the time required to complete documentation—separating the essential from the desirable. Task 7, "assisting the supervisee in development and maintenance of clinical and supervisory records," and its five associated competencies, particularly the "documentation requirements of various accrediting and regulatory agencies and third-party funding sources" (7.5) should be the primary focus for the supervisor.

CASE IV, EMPLOYEE IN A REHABILITATION FACILITY

Mary has recently been hired by your rehabilitation contracting company to be an SLP in a long-term care/rehabilitation facility. You are the regional supervisor for this contractor. Mary completed her CFY a year ago and has been working in an acute care hospital. Her resume indicates "clinical experience with dysphagia." You participated in Mary's interview which preceded her hiring, and although you recognized that Mary is relatively inexperienced in long-term care, you were comfortable with her hire.

Mary has been on the job six weeks when you get a call from the director of rehabilitation for the facility who expresses great concern with Mary's management of patients with dysphagia. Mary appears to be making changes in the thickness of patients' liquids without the appropriate diagnostic evaluation of the swallow. Nothing un-

fortunate has occurred to this point, but clearly, this situation needs to be addressed immediately.

As the supervisor, you are concerned about how to help Mary make immediate changes in her clinical management of patients with dysphagia in a manner that does not seem "negative" or "punitive" but is constructive for Mary and allows her to feel as if she is positively supported by management.

Applications

Understanding.   To what extent were Mary's expectations and those of the facility discussed when Mary was hired? Was she assigned a mentor? What ethical issues need to be considered?

Observing.   Obviously, Mary needs to be directed to collect data for her dysphagia patients. Are there particular techniques that you think would be most helpful? What other strategies might you employ to ensure safe and ethical practice? What are some of the things that might prevent Mary from accurately recording data? How could you assist her in collecting reliable, valid data?

Analyzing.   As with observation, Mary needs to be directed to analyze the data she collected for her dysphagia patients. Are there particular techniques that you think would be most helpful? What other strategies might you employ to ensure safe and ethical practice? What are some of the things that might prevent Mary from *accurately* analyzing data? How could you assist her in accurately analyzing and interpreting data? How can you assist her in revising client management plans based on data obtained and analyzed (competency 6.5)?

Integrating.   If the director of rehabilitation has accurate, valid perceptions and Mary is not appropriately evaluating patients with swallowing problems, your immediate concern has to be the welfare of the patients. In this instance, you would need to be directive in a conference with Mary and stipulate the policies and procedures that must be followed in serving swallowing patients in this facility. Using your best interpersonal skills, and identifying the need for a better "orientation" period, you should be able to allow Mary to save face and feel supported by you and the management.

If the director has misperceived what has been occurring, then you and Mary can use the data you have collected and analyzed to demonstrate that evaluation procedures are appropriate and safe. The two of you will collaborate and decide how to share the information with the director. The interpersonal interaction in the conference will be supportive and facilitative, with both of you being sensitive to the needs and feelings of each other and of the director.

CASE V, CONTROLLING SUPERVISOR

Mia is a second year graduate student who is in the sixth week of her second off-campus practicum—a public school placement. Before the current semester, she had accrued approximately 100 clock hours and previous practicum evaluations were very positive. Her on-site supervisor has supervised university graduate students for several years and has always been a bit reluctant in turning over her caseload.

In a meeting with interns, you, the university clinic director, learn that Mia is distressed. Mia shares that during the first three weeks of the semester, she received no feedback. Twice during that time, she heard a generic, "You're doing fine." In the past three weeks, as Mia has gradually assumed the caseload, her supervisor interrupts therapy to point out what Mia is doing wrong or needs to do differently. On occasion, she has taken over the session and instructed Mia to watch.

Mia states, "Her sole focus is on what I do wrong and I don't know what I'm doing right, if anything." Not only does the supervisor's observation style and strategy for giving feedback undermine her credibility with the students, it also makes Mia feel like a failure. "One day in the lunchroom with all the teachers around, she listed the things I had done wrong that morning. I suddenly lost my appetite."

Mia wants advice on how to manage this situation so it is a win-win for her and her supervisor. She has been afraid to say anything because she didn't want to rock the boat. You had a routine phone conference with Mia's supervisor last week; she reported, "Everything is going according to schedule. You've sent me another terrific intern!" Thus, her perception of this experience is that all is well.

The other students are also interested in how best to deal with this kind of situation. They want to know how to avoid conflict and how to let the supervisor know that her style causes a great deal of anxiety without sounding confrontational. This type of problem could occur with any of them during subsequent off-campus placements, during their clinical fellowship year, or during a probationary term of employment.

Applications

Understanding.   What are some of the major issues in this dilemma? How should the clinic director attempt to facilitate a change in the off-campus supervisor's style? Should she intervene or coach the student in the use of certain interpersonal skills? What are the university's, supervisor's and supervisee's expectations and have they been shared? Would tools such as Larson's Expectations (Appendix 4A) and Needs (Appendix 4B) scales, Tihen's Scale (Appendix 4C), and/or Broyles et al. instruments (Appendix 4D) enable Mia and her supervisor to "safely" discuss the problem?

Observing.   Here is a case where the supervisee has the opportunity to modify the supervisor's behavior by using a systematic approach in collecting and analyzing data. What initial steps in self-observation would you recommend? How can Mia "turn the tables" and be more active and decrease the supervisor's directive style without creating a conflict?

Analyzing.   If Mia employs a systematic approach in collecting and analyzing data, she would demonstrate an unexpected level of competence that would likely effect some change in the supervisor's behavior. What kinds of analyses would provide the most powerful evidence of Mia's competence to her supervisor? That is, how can she demonstrate therapeutic efficiency and effectiveness? How can Mia demonstrate that she is capable of managing the caseload without all of the supervisor's "constructive criticism"?

Integrating. The power differential between Mia and her on-site supervisor makes this a very sensitive situation. Here is a time when the university coordinator can collaborate with Mia and make a difference. In a conference, the two can develop a plan of action. First, they should review the kinds of communication behaviors that decrease defensiveness, such as use of "I statements."

Next, they should practice or role play. For example, at a time when you know your supervisor is fairly relaxed, ask if you can talk about feedback. Let her know that you appreciate her suggestions—but feel awkward and uncomfortable with the method she is using to provide feedback. Use "I statements" and focus on *how you feel* for example, I feel embarrassed in front of the students when you give me feedback during my sessions, or I feel like I must not be a very competent intern when you tell me how to do something in the middle of an activity, or I really want to do the best job possible with the students but I get rattled and find it hard to refocus when you tell me what to do while the students are in the room.

Then, provide solutions and convert the problem to goals. After you've shared some feelings, let her know that you've thought about some alternative strategies. Make sure your initial solution is tied to one of your personal goals. For example, tell her that you want to become more skilled in self-analysis and evaluating therapy outcomes and ask if she'd be willing to try a different strategy for sharing feedback. For example, she could write her comments in a stenographer's notebook (on half the page). Later that evening, you could reflect, listen to taped segments of your sessions, and review data collected during your session (list a variety of strategies) to formulate ideas about what could have been done differ-

ently or better. You'll write those on the other half of the page—opposite her feedback. She can look at your ideas and suggestions in the morning before you see any kids and you could have a brief conference (15–20 minutes) to discuss which you'll implement. You can decide how to share in collecting data to assess the outcomes.

Lastly, focus on some positive things. Ask her to assist you in identifying some of the behaviors and techniques you use that are affecting the desired results. Again propose ways to collect and analyze data to determine effectiveness.

CASE VI, SLP IN SCHOOL SETTING

You are the school supervisor in a rural county, and your primary responsibility is that of program manager for 27 speech-language specialists in your district. Your duties include: budget development and administration, scheduling assignments for your staff, collaborating with them in planning in-services, completing annual performance reviews for each of them, mentoring nontenured clinicians, being the administrator of record in IEP meetings for communicative handicapped students, monitoring the paperwork required by state and federal governments, keeping abreast of the state and federal issues impacting service delivery in the schools and communicating those to your staff, and serving as the liaison between them and the SELPA Director and district superintendent. You do *not* have the power to hire and fire; that responsibility belongs to the superintendent. Further, your district is regulated by a closed-shop collective bargaining agreement.

Jodie is a speech-language specialist who has worked in your district for twenty years. She has a state teaching certificate, which required a bachelor's degree and some additional coursework and practicum as part of a fifth year experience, but does not hold a Master's degree and thus is not an ASHA certified clinician. She was permitted to "grandfather" into her tenured position when the district began to require a Master's degree ten years ago. Jodie perceives herself to be an excellent clinician and readily shares that perception with teachers in her two schools and with the 26 other clinicians in the district. Although they are too polite to tell her, most of the other clinicians have told you they think Jodie is a professional dinosaur and an embarrassment to the district. She hasn't changed how she conducts therapy in years and is using some techniques and strategies that have no demonstrated validity, but she boasts that her kids love coming to therapy and have great fun in their sessions with her. While she isn't doing any harm, you aren't convinced that what she is doing is *therapeutic*. Further, you suspect that some of the students in her caseload have residual problems that would self-correct without direct intervention. As an advocate of quality services for students, you wonder what you can do to motivate Jodie to change.

Applications

Understanding.   How can this supervisor attempt to persuade Jodie to change? What supervisory competencies seem most essential in this situation? What are some of the inherent risks in this kind of problem? How can they be minimized?

Observing.   Jodie's level of motivation to change is an issue here and makes this a difficult case. Here is a case where group dynamics and vicarious learning might be positive influential forces. What kinds of self-observation and data collection initiatives might yield the desired outcomes here? (Think about peer coaching or mentoring.)

Analyzing.   In an attempt to modify Jodie's performance, peers may be able to exert positive influence. What kinds of self-analyses, with opportunities for revising client management plans, might motivate Jodie to want to change her behavior and increase therapeutic efficiency and effectiveness? (Think about peer supervision, mentoring, etc.)

Integrating.   This could be an opportune time for implementing a new staff development plan. For example, every other week, on Friday afternoons from 2:00–3:00 p.m., your staff will participate in Teaching Clinics. You are going to modify the format a bit by dividing the clinicians in your district in half so that each group of 13 will participate in two clinics each month. This addresses the need expressed by many of the clinicians for increased opportunity to interact and get assistance from peers for some of their difficult cases. With the goal of demonstrating evidence-based practice, the problem solving and critical thinking that occurs in the clinics ought to provide the opportunity for Jodie to learn vicariously. In addition, you might ask each clinician to formulate one or two professional development goals and to share those goals with their peers, as a way to indirectly nudge Jodie to change while demonstrating a collective commitment to continued professional growth (12.9).

By treating all of your staff the same, you don't risk a grievance for singling out an individual. Individual rights stipulated in the collective bargaining agreement are maintained.

REFERENCES

Acheson, K., & Gall, M. (1980). *Techniques in the clinical supervision of teachers.* New York: Longman, Inc.

Alfonso, R., Firth, G., & Neville, R. (1975). *Instructional supervision.* Boston: Allyn & Bacon.

American Speech and Hearing Association. (1970). Report of Committee on Supportive Personnel. Guidelines on the role, training, and supervision of the communication aide. *ASHA, 12,* 78–80.

American Speech and Hearing Association. (1978a). Committee on Supervision in Speech-Language-Pathology and Audiology. Current status of supervision of speech-language pathology and audiology [Special report]. *ASHA, 20,* 478–486.

American Speech and Hearing Association. (1978b). Principles underlying the requirements for the Certificate of Clinical Competence adopted. *ASHA, 20,* 331–333.

American Speech-Language Hearing Association. (1981). Employment and utilization of supportive personnel in audiology and speech-language pathology. *ASHA, 23,* 165–169.

American Speech-Language Hearing Association. (1982). Committee on Supervision in Speech-Language-Pathology and Audiology. Minimum qualifications for supervisors and suggested competencies for effective clinical supervision. *ASHA, 24,* 339–342.

American Speech-Language Hearing Association. (1985a). ASHA demographic update. *ASHA, 27,* 55.

American Speech-Language Hearing Association. (1985b). Committee on Supervision in Speech-Language-Pathology and Audiology. Clinical supervision in speech-language pathology and audiology. A position statement. *ASHA, 27,* 57–60.

American Speech-Language Hearing Association. (1987). Legislative council report. *ASHA, 29,* 38.

American Speech-Language Hearing Association. (1988). Utilization and employment of speech-language pathology supportive personnel with underserved populations. *ASHA, 30,* 55–56.

American Speech-Language Hearing Association. (1989). Bilingual speech-language pathologists and audiologists. *ASHA, 31,* 93.

American Speech-Language Hearing Association. (1992). Technical report. Support personnel: Issues and impact on the professions of speech-language pathology and audiology. Rockville, MD: American Speech-Language Hearing Association.

American Speech-Language Hearing Association. (1994). ASHA policy regarding support personnel. *ASHA, 36* (Supple.13), 24.

American Speech-Language Hearing Association. (1995). *Practical tools and forms for supervising speech-language pathology assistants.* Rockville, MD: American Speech-Language Hearing Association.

American Speech-Language Hearing Association. (1996). Guidelines for the training, credentialing, use and supervision of speech-language pathology assistants. *ASHA, 38*(16), 21–34.

American Speech-Language Hearing Association. (1997). *ASHA membership and certification handbook.* Rockville, MD: American Speech-Language Hearing Association.

American Speech-Language Hearing Association. (1999). *Practical tools and forms for supervising speech-language pathology assistants.* Rockville, MD: American Speech-Language Hearing Association.

American Speech-Language Hearing Association. (2000a). *Background information and standards and implementation for the certificate of clinical competence in speech-language pathology* [Special report]. Rockville, MD: American Speech-Language Hearing Association, Council on Professional Standards in Speech-Language Pathology and Audiology.

American Speech-Language Hearing Association. (2000b). *Council on Academic Accreditation in Audiology and Speech-Language Pathology: Criteria for approval of associate degree technical training programs for speech-language pathology assistants.* Rockville, MD: American-Speech-Language Hearing Association.

American Speech-Language Hearing Association. (2000c). *Council of Professional Standards in Speech-Language Pathology and Audiology: Background information and criteria for registration of speech-language pathology assistants.* Rockville, MD: American Speech Language Hearing Association.

American Speech-Language Hearing Association. (2001a). Code of Ethics. Rockville, MD: American Speech-Language Hearing Association.

American Speech-Language Hearing Association. (2001b). *Demographic profile of ASHA constituents for the period of January 1 through June 30, 2001.* Rockville, MD: Author.

American Speech-Language Hearing Association (2001c). *Knowledge and skills for supervisors of speech-language pathology assistants.* Rockville, MD: Author.

American Speech-Language Hearing Association. (2001d). *American Speech-Language Hearing Association summary of membership and affiliation counts for the period January 1 through June 30, 2001.* Rockville, MD: Author.

Amidon, E., & Flanders, N. (1967). *The role of the teacher in the classroom.* Minneapolis, MN: Association for Productive Teaching.

Andersen, C. (1981). The effect of supervisor bias on the evaluation of student clinicians in speech/language pathology and audiology (Doctoral dissertation, Indiana University, 1981). *Dissertation Abstracts International, 41,* 4479B. (University Microfilms No. 81-12, 499)

Anderson, J. (Ed.). (1970). *Proceedings of Conference on Supervision of Speech and Hearing Programs in the Schools.* Bloomington: Indiana University.

Anderson, J. (1972). Status of supervision in speech, hearing and language programs in the schools. *Language, Speech and Hearing Services in Schools, 3,* 12–23.

Anderson, J. (1973a). Status of college and university programs of practicum in the schools. *ASHA, 15,* 60–68.

Anderson, J. (1973b). Supervision: The neglected component of the profession. In L. Turton (Ed.), *Proceedings of a Workshop on Supervision in Speech Pathology.* Ann Arbor, MI: University of Michigan.

Anderson, J. (1974). Supervision of school speech, hearing and language programs—An emerging role. *ASHA, 16,* 7–10.

Anderson, J. (Ed.). (1980). *Proceedings—Conference on Training in the Supervisory Process in Speech-Language Pathology and Audiology.* Bloomington: Indiana University.

Anderson, J. (1981). Training of supervisors in speech-language pathology and audiology. *ASHA, 23,* 77–82.

Anderson, J. (1982). *Report of survey of speech-language pathologists and audiologists in public schools of Indiana.* Unpublished manuscript.

Anderson, J. (1985). Doctoral level emphasis. In K. Smith (Moderator), *Preparation and training models for the supervisory process.* Short course presented at the annual convention of the American Speech-Language-Hearing Association, Washington, DC.

Anderson, J. (1988). *The supervisory process in speech-language pathology and audiology.* Boston: College-Hill.

Anderson, J., Brasseur, J., Casey, P., Roberts, J., & Smith, K. (1979, November). *Studying the supervisory process.* Short course presented at the annual convention of the American Speech and Hearing Association, Atlanta, GA.

Anderson, J., & Milisen, R. (1965). *Report on pilot project in student teaching in speech and hearing.* Bloomington: Indiana University.

Anderson, S. (1993). A report of supervisory preparation at a rehabilitation hospital. In R. Gillam (Ed.), *The Supervisor's Forum, 1,* 1–5. Council of Supervisors in Speech-Language Pathology and Audiology.

Anderson, P., & Guerrero, L. (1998). *Handbook of communication and emotion: Research, theory, applications, and contexts.* San Diego, CA: Academic Press.

Andrews, J. (1971). Operationally written therapy goals in supervised clinical practicum. *ASHA, 13,* 385–387.

Argyris, C. (1962). *Interpersonal competence and organizational effectiveness.* Homewood, IL: Richard D. Irwin.

Baker, E., & Popham, W. J. (1973). *Expanding dimensions of instructional objectives.* Englewood Cliffs, NJ: Prentice-Hall.

Bales, R. (1950). *Interaction process analysis: A method for the study of small groups.* Reading, MA: Addison-Wesley.

Bales, R. (1951). *Interaction process analysis.* Reading, MA: Addison-Wesley.

Barbara, D. A. (1958). *The art of listening.* Springfield, IL: Charles C. Thomas.

Barlett, S. (2001). *Supervisory Action Plan.* Presented in Supervision 102: Short Course conducted with J. Brasseur, E. McCrea, W. Newmann, J. Rassi, B. Solomon, & B. Weinrich at annual convention of the American Speech-Language-Hearing Association, Washington, DC.

Barrows, H., & Pickell, G. (1991). *Developing clinical problem-solving skills: A guide to more effective diagnosis and treatment.* New York: W. W. Norton.

Battle, D. (1993). *Communication disorders in multicultural populations.* Boston: Butterworth-Heinemann.

Battle, D. (1995). Variations in learning styles: Implications for clinical supervision. In R. Gillam (Ed.), *The supervisors' forum, 2,* 46–51. Council of Supervisors in Speech-Language Pathology and Audiology.

Belenky, M. F., Clinchy, B. M., Goldberger, N. R., & Tarule, J. M. (1986). *Women's ways of knowing: The development of self, voice, and mind.* New York: Basic Books.

Berne, E. (1964). *Games people play.* New York: Ballantine.

Berne, E. (1966). *Principles of group treatment.* New York: Oxford University Press.

Bernthal, J. (2001). Focused initiative on web-based and advanced technology. *ASHA Leader, 6*(4), 23.

Bernthal, J., & Beukelman, D. (1975). Self-evaluation by the student clinician. *National Student Speech and Hearing Association Journal,* 39–44.

Biddle, B., & Thomas, E. (1966). *Role theory: Concepts and research.* New York: John Wiley.

Block, F. (1982). The preconference observation system: Supervisor's point of view. *SUPERvision, 6,* 1–6.

Blodgett, E., Schmitt, J., & Scudder, R. (1987). Clinical session evaluation: The effect of familiarity with the supervisee. *The Clinical Supervisor, 5,* 33–43.

Blumberg, A. (1968, Spring). Supervisory behavior and interpersonal relations. *Educational Administration, 34–35.*

Blumberg, A. (1974). *Supervisors and teachers: A private cold war.* Berkeley, CA: McCutchan Publishing.

Blumberg, A. (1980). *Supervisors and teachers: A private cold war* (2nd ed.). Berkeley, CA: McCutchan Publishing.

Blumberg, A., & Amidon, E. (1965). Teacher perceptions of supervisor-teacher interaction. *Administrator's Notebook, 14,* 1–4.

Blumberg, A., Amidon, E., & Weber, W. (1967). *Supervisor-teacher interaction as seen by supervisors.* Unpublished manuscript, Temple University.

Blumberg, A., & Cusick, P. (1970). Supervisor-teacher interaction: An analysis of verbal behavior. *Education, 91,* 126–134.

Blumberg, A., & Weber, W. (1968). Teacher morale as a function of perceived supervisor behavior style. *Journal of Educational Research, 62,* 109–113.

Boone, D. (1970). A close look at the clinical process. In J. Anderson (Ed.), *Proceedings of Conference on Supervision of Speech and Hearing Programs in the Schools.* Bloomington: Indiana University.

Boone, D., & Goldberg, A. (1969). An experimental study of the clinical acquisition of behavioral principles by videotape self-confrontation. *Final Report* (Project No. 4071-Grant No. OEG-8-071319-2814). Washington, DC: U.S. Department of Health, Education, and Welfare.

Boone, D., & Prescott, T. (1972). Content and sequence analysis of speech and hearing therapy. *ASHA, 14,* 58–62.

Boone, D., & Stech, E. (1970). The development of clinical skills in speech pathology by audiotape and videotape self-confrontation. *Final Report* (Project No. 1381-Grant No. OEG-9-071318-2814). Washington, DC: U.S. Department of Health, Education, and Welfare.

Bowline, W., Bunce, B., Polmanteer, K., & Wegner, J. (1996). There's no "I" in team. In B. Wagner (Ed.), *Proceedings of the 1996 Conference on Clinical Supervision-Partnerships in Supervision: Innovative and Effective Practices* (pp. 127–131). Council of Supervisors in Speech-Language Pathology and Audiology, Cincinnati, OH.

Boyer, E. (1990). *Scholarship reconsidered.* Princeton, NJ: Carnegie Foundation for the Advancement of Teaching.

Brammer, L. (1985). *The helping relationship.* Englewood Cliffs, NJ: Prentice-Hall.

Brammer, L., & Wassmer, A. (1977). Supervision in counseling and psychotherapy. In D. Kurpius, R. Baker, & I. Thomas (Eds.), *Supervision of applied training.* Westport, CT: Greenwood Press.

Brasseur, J. (1978). *Personal model of consultation.* Unpublished manuscript.

Brasseur, J. (1980a). The observed differences between direct, indirect, and direct/indirect videotaped supervisory conferences by speech-language pathology supervisors, graduate students, and undergraduate students (Doctoral dissertation, Indiana University, 1980). *Dissertation Abstracts International, 41,* 2131B. (University Microfilms No. 80-29, 212)

Brasseur, J. (1980b). System for analyzing supervisor-teacher interaction—Arthur Blumberg. In J. Anderson (Ed.), *Proceedings—Conference on Training in the Supervisory Process in Speech-Language Pathology and Audiology,* (pp. 71–73). Bloomington: Indiana University.

Brasseur, J. (1985). External-internal practicum. In K. Smith (Moderator), *Preparation and training models for the supervisory conference.* Short course presented at the annual convention of the American Speech-Language Hearing Association, Washington, DC.

Brasseur, J. (1987a). Preparation of supervisees for the supervisory process. In S. Farmer (Ed.), *Proceedings of a National Conference on Supervision—Clinical Supervision: A Coming of Age* (pp. 144–163). Council of University Supervisors of Practicum in Speech-Language Pathology and Audiology, Jekyll Island, GA.

Brasseur, J. (1987b). A descriptive case study of direct-indirect supervisory behaviors. In S. Farmer (Ed.), *Proceedings of a National Conference on Supervision—Clinical Supervision: A Coming of Age* (pp. 57–65). Council of University Supervisors of Practicum in Speech-Language Pathology and Audiology, Jekyll Island, GA.

Brasseur, J. (1989). The supervisory process: A continuum perspective. *Language, Speech, and Hearing Services in Schools, 20,* 274–295.

Brasseur, J. (1994). Women and men on top—Getting or being a mentor. In M. Bruce (Ed.), *Proceedings of the 1994 International & Interdisciplinary Conference on Clinical Supervision: Toward the 21st Century* (pp. 236–243). Council of Supervisors in Speech-Language Pathology and Audiology, Cape Cod, MA.

Brasseur, J., & Anderson, J. (1983). Observed differences between direct, indirect, and direct/indirect videotaped supervisory conferences. *Journal of Speech and Hearing Research, 26,* 349–355.

Brasseur, J., & Jimenez, B. (1994). Supervisee self-analysis and changes in clinical behavior. In M. Bruce

(Ed.), *Proceedings of the 1994 International & Interdisciplinary Conference on Clinical Supervision: Toward the 21st Century* (pp. 111–125). Council of Supervisors in Speech-Language Pathology and Audiology, Cape Cod, MA.

Brasseur, J., & Jimenez, B. (1996). Novice supervisees' attitude changes after active participation in the supervisory process. In B. Wagner (Ed.), *Proceedings of the 1996 Conference on Clinical Supervision—Partnerships in Supervision: Innovative and Effective Practices* (pp. 80–89). Council of Supervisors in Speech-Language Pathology and Audiology, Cincinnati, OH.

Brooks, R., & Hannah, E. (1966). A tool for clinical supervision. *Journal of Speech and Hearing Disorders, 31,* 383–387.

Brookshire, R. (1967). Speech pathology and the experimental analysis of behavior. *Journal of Speech and Hearing Disorders, 32,* 215–227.

Brookshire, R., Nicholas, L., & Krueger, K. (1978). Sampling of speech pathology treatment activities: An evaluation of momentary and interval sampling procedures. *Journal of Speech and Hearing Research, 21,* 652–666.

Brookshire, R., Nicholas, L., Krueger, K., & Redmond, K. (1978). The Clinical Interaction Analysis System: A system for observational recording of aphasia treatment. *Journal of Speech and Hearing Disorders, 43,* 437–447.

Broyles, S., McNeice, E., Ishee, J., Ross, S., & Lance, D. (1999). *Influence of selected factors on the perceived effectiveness of various supervision strategies.* Poster session presented at the annual convention of the American Speech-Language Hearing Association, San Francisco.

Butler, K. (1976). *The supervision of clinicians: The three C's…competition, complaints and competencies.* Paper presented at the annual convention of the American Speech and Hearing Association, Houston, TX.

Byng-Hall, J., & Whiffen, R. (1982). Evolution of supervision: An overview. In R. Whiffen & J. Byng-Hall (Eds.), *Family Therapy Supervision.* New York: Grune and Stratton.

Camarata, M. (1992). Facilitating self-analysis of videotaped treatment: A generalization effect. In S. Dowling (Ed.), *Proceedings of the 1992 National Conference on Supervision—Total Quality Supervision: Effecting Optimal Performance* (pp. 46–52). Council of Supervisors in Speech-Language Pathology and Audiology, Nashville, TN.

Camarata, M., & Rassi, J. (1991). Facilitating self-analysis of videotaped treatment: Supervision efficacy factors. Paper presented at the annual convention of the American Speech-Language Hearing Association, Atlanta, GA.

Campbell, D., & Stanley, J. (1963). *Experimental and quasi-experimental designs for research.* Chicago: Rand McNally.

Caracciolo, G. (1977). Perceptions by speech pathology student-clinicians and supervisors of interpersonal conditions and professional growth during the supervisory conferences (Doctoral dissertation, Columbia University Teachers College, 1976). *Dissertation Abstracts International, 37,* 4411B. (University Microfilms No. 77-04, 183)

Caracciolo, G., Rigrodsky, S., & Morrison, E. (1978a). A Rogerian orientation to the speech-language pathology supervisory relationship. *ASHA, 20,* 286–290.

Caracciolo, G., Rigrodsky, S., & Morrison, E. (1978b). Perceived interpersonal conditions and professional growth of master's level speech-language pathology students during the supervisory process. *ASHA, 20,* 467–477.

Carin, A., & Sund, R. (1971). *Developing questioning techniques.* Columbus, OH: Charles E. Merrill.

Carkhuff, R. (1967). Toward a comprehensive model of facilitative processes. *Journal of Counseling Psychology, 14,* 67–72.

Carkhuff, R. (1969a). *Helping and human relations: A primer for lay and professional helpers—I.* New York: Holt, Rinehart and Winston.

Carkhuff, R. (1969b). *Helping and human relations—II.* New York: Holt, Rinehart and Winston.

Carkhuff, R., & Berenson, B. (1967). *Beyond counseling and therapy.* New York: Holt, Rinehart and Winston.

Carkhuff, R., & Truax, C. (1964). Concreteness: A neglected variable in research in psychotherapy. *Journal of Clinical Psychology, 20,* 264–267.

Cartwright, C., & Cartwright, G. (1984). *Developing observation skills.* New York: McGraw-Hill Book.

Cartwright, D., & Zander, A. (1960). *Group dynamics* (2nd ed.). New York: Harper and Row.

Casey, P. (1980). The validity of using small segments for analyzing supervisory conferences with McCrea's Adapted System (Doctoral dissertation, Indiana University, 1980). *Dissertation Abstracts International, 41,* 1729B. (University Microfilms No. 80-24, 566)

Casey, P. (1985). *Supervisory skills self-assessment.* Whitewater: University of Wisconsin.

Casey, P., Smith, K., & Ulrich, S. (1988). *Self supervision: A career tool for audiologists and speech-language pathologists* (Clinical Series No. 10). Rockville, MD: National Student Speech Language Hearing Association.

Champagne, D., & Morgan, J. (1978). *Supervision—A study guide for educational administrators.* Ft. Lauderdale, FL: Nova University.

Chan, J., Carter, S., & McAllister, L. (1994). Anxiety related to clinical education in speech-language pathology students. In M. Bruce (Ed.), *Proceedings of the 1994 International & Interdisciplinary Conference on Clinical Supervision: Toward the 21st Century* (pp. 126–132). Council of Supervisors in Speech-Language Pathology and Audiology, Cape Cod, MA.

Chomsky, N. (1968). Language and mind. NY: Harcourt, Brace.

Cogan, M. (1973). *Clinical supervision.* Boston: Houghton Mifflin.

Condon, J. (1977). *Interpersonal communication.* New York: Macmillan Publishing.

Connell, P., & Thompson, C. (1986). Flexibility of single-subject experimental design. Part III: Using flexibility to design or modify experiments. *Journal of Speech and Hearing Disorders, 51,* 214–215.

Conover, H. (1979). *Conover Analysis System.* Unpublished manuscript. Athens, OH: Ohio University.

Cooper, H., & Good, T. (1983). *Pygmalion grows up: Studies in the expectation communication process.* New York: Longman.

Copeland, W. (1980). Affective dispositions of teachers in training toward examples of supervisory behavior. *Journal of Educational Research, 74,* 37–42.

Copeland, W. (1982). Student teachers' preference for supervisory approach. *Journal of Teacher Education, 33,* 32–36.

Copeland, W., & Atkinson, D. (1978). Student teachers' perceptions of directive and nondirective supervisory behavior. *Journal of Educational Research, 71,* 123–226.

Costa, A., & Garmston, R. (1985a, February). Supervision for intelligent teaching. *Educational Leadership,* 70–80.

Costa, A., & Garmston, R. (1985b). *The art of cognitive coaching: Supervision for intelligent teaching.* Sacramento, CA: The Institute for Intelligent Behavior.

Costello, J. (1977). Programmed instruction. *Journal of Speech and Hearing Disorders, 42,* 3–28.

Council of Academic Programs in Communication Sciences and Disorders. (2000). *Annual report.* Retrieved January 22, 2001 from the World Wide Web: http://www.capscd.org

Crago, M. (1987). Supervison and self-exploration. In M. Crago & M. Pickering (Eds.), *Supervision in human communication disorders: Perspectives on a process.* San Diego, CA: Little Brown-College Hill Press.

Crago, M., & Pickering, M. (Eds.). (1987). *Supervision in human communication disorders: Perspectives on a process.* San Diego, CA: Little Brown-College Hill Press.

Culatta, R., Colucci, S., & Wiggins, E. (1975). Clinical supervisors and trainees: Two views of a process. *ASHA, 17,* 152–157.

Culatta, R., & Seltzer, H. (1976). Content and sequence analysis of the supervisory session. *ASHA, 18,* 8–12.

Culatta, R., & Seltzer, H. (1977). Content and sequence analysis of the supervisory session: A report of clinical use. *ASHA, 19,* 523–526.

Cunningham, R. (1971). Developing question-asking skills. In J. Weigand (Ed.), *Developing teacher competencies.* Englewood Cliffs, NJ: Prentice-Hall.

Danish, S. J., & Kagan, N. (1971). Measurement of affective sensitivity: Toward a valid measurement of interpersonal perception. *Journal of Counseling Psychology, 18,* 51–54.

Darley, F., & Spriestersbach, D. C. (1978). *Diagnostic methods in speech pathology* (2nd ed.). New York: Harper and Row.

Davies, I. (1981). *Instructional techniques.* New York: McGraw-Hill.

Deetz, S., & Stevenson, S. (1986). *Managing interpersonal communication.* New York: Harper and Row.

DeVane, G. (1992). Multicultural strategies for quality improvement in the supervisory process. In S. Dowling (Ed.), *Proceedings of the 1992 National Conference on Supervision—Total Quality Supervision: Effecting Optimal Performance* (pp. 150–155). Council of Supervisors in Speech-Language Pathology and Audiology, Nashville, TN.

Diedrich, W. (1969). Assessment of the clinical process. *Journal of Kansas Speech and Hearing Association.*

Diedrich, W. (1971a). Functional description of therapy and revised multidimensional scoring system. In T. Johnson (Ed.), *Clinical interaction and its measurement.* Logan: Utah State University.

Diedrich, W. (1971b). Procedures for counting and charting a target phoneme. *Language, Speech and Hearing Services in Schools, 2,* 18–32.

Dopheide, W., Thornton, B., & McCready, V. (1984). *A preliminary validation of a practicum performance assessment scale.* Paper presented at the annual convention of the American Speech-Language-Hearing Association.

Douglas, R. (1983). Defining and describing clinical accountability. *Seminars in Speech and Language, 4,* 107–119.

Dowling, S. (1977). A comparison to determine the effects of two supervisory styles, conventional and teaching clinics, in the training of speech pathologists (Doctoral dissertation, Indiana University, 1977). *Dissertation Abstracts International, 37,* 889B. (University Microfilms No. 77-01, 883)

Dowling, S. (1979). Developing student self-supervisory skills in clinical training. *Journal of National Student Speech and Hearing Association, 7,* 37–41.

Dowling, S. (1981). Observation analysis: Procedures for training coders and data collection. *Journal of*

National Student Speech and Hearing Association, 9, 82–88.

Dowling, S. (1982). Supervisor and supervisee responsibilities in the supervisory process. *Tejas Journal of Audiology and Speech Pathology, 7,* 26–29.

Dowling, S. (1983a). An analysis of conventional and teaching clinic supervision. *The Clinical Supervisor, 1,* 15–29.

Dowling, S. (1983b). Teaching clinic conference participant interactions. *Journal of Communication Disorders, 16,* 385–397.

Dowling, S. (1986). Supervisory training: Impetus for clinical supervision. *The Clinical Supervisor, 4,* 27–35.

Dowling, S. (1987). Teaching clinic participation: Impact on conference perceptions. In S. Farmer (Ed.), *Proceedings of A National Conference on Supervision—Clinical Supervision: A Coming of Age* (pp. 72–77). Council of University Supervisors of Practicum in Speech-Language Pathology and Audiology, Jekyll Island, GA.

Dowling, S. (1992). *Implementing the supervisory process: Theory and practice.* Englewood Cliffs, NJ: Prentice Hall.

Dowling, S. (1993). Supervisory training, objective setting, and grade contingent performance. *Language, Speech, and Hearing Services in Schools, 24,* 92–99.

Dowling, S. (1994). Supervisory training effects of grade contingent/non-contingent objective setting. In M. Bruce (Ed.), *Proceedings of the 1994 International & Interdisciplinary Conference on Clinical Supervision: Toward the 21st Century* (pp. 180–183). Council of Supervisors in Speech-Language Pathology and Audiology, Cape Cod, MA.

Dowling, S. (1995). Conference question usage: Impact of supervisory training. In R. Gillam (Ed.) *The supervisors' forum, 2,* 11–14. Council of Supervisors in Speech-Language Pathology and Audiology.

Dowling, S. (2001). *Supervision: Strategies for successful outcomes and productivity.* Boston: Allyn & Bacon.

Dowling, S. & Biskyni, R. (1993). Effects of supervisory training and a practicum: A case study. In R. Gillam (Ed.), *The supervisor's forum, 1,* 9–12. Council of Supervisors in Speech-Language Pathology and Audiology.

Dowling, S., & Bliss, L. (1984). Cognitive complexity, rhetorical sensitivity: Contributing factors in clinical skill? *Journal of Communication Disorders, 7,* 9–17.

Dowling, S., Glaser, A., Shapiro, D., Mawdsley, B., & Sbaschnig, K. (1992). Implementing the teaching clinic. In S. Dowling (Ed.), *Proceedings of the 1992 National Conference on Supervision—Total Quality Supervision: Effecting Optimal Performance* (pp. 156–161). Council of Supervisors in Speech-Language Pathology and Audiology, Nashville, TN.

Dowling, S., Sbaschnig, K., & Williams, C. (1982). Culatta & Seltzer. Content and analysis of the supervisory session: Question of reliability and validity. *Journal of Communication Disorders, 15,* 353–362.

Dowling, S., Sbaschnig, K., & Williams, C. (1991). *Supervisory training, objective setting and grade contingent performance.* Paper presented at the annual convention of the American Speech-Language-Hearing Association, Atlanta, GA.

Dowling, S., & Shank, K. (1981). A comparison of the effects of two supervisory styles, conventional and teaching clinic, in the training of speech and language pathologists. *Journal of Communication Disorders, 14,* 51–58.

Dowling, S., & Wittkopp, M. (1982). Students' perceived supervisory needs. *Journal of Communication Disorders, 15,* 319–328.

Duck, S. (Ed.). (1997). *Handbook of personal relationships: Theory, research, and interventions* (2nd ed.). New York: John Wiley.

Dussault, G. (1970). *Theory of supervision in teacher education.* New York: Teachers College, Columbia University.

Elbert, M., & Geirut, J. (1986). *Handbook of clinical phonology.* San Diego, CA: College-Hill Press.

Emerich, L., & Hatten, J. (1979). *Diagnosis and evaluation in speech pathology.* Englewood Cliffs, NJ: Prentice-Hall.

Engnoth, G. (1974). A comparison of three approaches to supervision of speech clinicians in training (Doctoral dissertation, University of Kansas, 1973). *Dissertation Abstracts International, 34,* 6261B. (University Microfilms No. 74-12, 552)

Ervin-Tripp, S. (1970). Discourse agreement: How children answer questions. In J. Hayes (Ed.), *Cognitions and the development of language.* New York: John Wiley.

Evertson, C., & Green, J. (1986). Observation as inquiry and method. In M. Wittrock (Ed.), *Handbook of research on teaching.* New York: Macmillan.

Faiver, C., Eisengart, S., & Colonna, R. (2000). *The counselor intern's handbook* (2nd ed.). Belmont, CA: Brooks/Cole.

Farmer, S. (1980). *Interview Analysis System.* Paper presented at the annual convention of the American Speech-Language-Hearing Association, Detroit, MI.

Farmer, S. (1984). Supervisory conferences in communicative disorders: Verbal and non-verbal interpersonal communication pacing (Doctoral dissertation, University of Colorado, 1983). *Dissertation Abstracts International, 44,* 2715B. (University Microfilms No. 84-00, 891)

Farmer, S. (1987a). The art and science of conferences: Tessellations. In S. Farmer (Ed.), *Proceedings of A National Conference on Supervision—Clinical Supervision: A Coming of Age* (pp. 176–189). Council of University Supervisors of Practicum in Speech-Language Pathology and Audiology, Jekyll Island, GA.

Farmer, S. (1987b). Visual literacy and the clinical supervisor. *The Clinical Supervisor, 5,* 45–73.

Farmer, S. (1994). Team supervision in communication disorders: A key to professional development. In M. Bruce (Ed.), *Proceedings of the 1994 International & Interdisciplinary Conference on Clinical Supervision: Toward the 21st Century* (pp. 141–149). Council of Supervisors in Speech-Language Pathology and Audiology, Cape Cod, MA.

Farmer, S., & Farmer, J. (1989). *Supervision in communication disorders.* Columbus, OH: Merrill.

Farmer, S., & Farmer, J. (1995). SMART supervision: Theory and application to dyadic and team supervision. In R. Gillam (Ed.), *The Supervisors' Forum, 2,* 36–45. Council of Supervisors in Speech-Language Pathology and Audiology.

Farris, G. F. (1974). Leadership and supervision in formal organizations. In J. G. Hunt & L. L. Larson (Eds.), *Contingency approaches to leadership.* Carbondale: Southern Illinois University Press.

Feltham, C. (2000). *Handbook of counseling and psychotherapy.* Thousand Oaks, CA: Sage.

Fiedler, F. E. (1967). *A theory of leadership effectiveness.* New York: McGraw Hill.

Filter, M., Brandell, M., Smith, J., & Kopin, M. (1989). Reliability of counting supervisee responses/errors during a treatment session. In D. Shapiro (Ed.), *Proceedings of the 1989 National Conference on Supervision: Supervision Innovations* (pp. 84–86). Council of Supervisors in Speech-Language Pathology and Audiology.

Fish, D., & Twinn, S. (1997). *Quality clinical supervision in the health care professions: Principled approaches to practice.* Oxford, England: Butterworth-Heinemann.

Fisher, L. (1982). Supervision. In R. Van Hattum (Ed.), *Speech-language programming in the schools.* Springfield, IL: Charles C. Thomas.

Fishler, A. S. (1971). Confrontations: Changing teacher behavior through clinical supervision. In L. Rubin (Ed.), *Improving in-service education.* Boston: Allyn & Bacon.

Flanders, N. (1967). Teacher influence in the classroom. In E. Amidon & J. Hough (Eds.), *Interaction analysis: Theory, research, and application.* Reading, MA: Addison-Wesley.

Flanders, N. (1969). *Classroom interaction patterns, pupil attitudes, and achievement in the second, fourth and sixth grades* (Cooperative Research Project No. 5-1055 [OE 4-10-243]). Ann Arbor: The University of Michigan.

Flanders, N. (1970). *Analyzing teacher behavior.* Reading, MA: Addison-Wesley.

Flower, R. (1984). *Delivery of speech-language pathology and audiology services.* Baltimore, MD: Williams and Wilkins.

Fox, R. (1983). Contracting in supervision: A goal oriented process. *The Clinical Supervisor, 1,* 37–49.

Francis, B. (1993). *Effects of speech-language pathology students' interaction analyses on clinical behaviors.* Unpublished master's thesis, California State University, Chico.

Freeman, G. (1982). Consultation. In R. Van Hattum, *Speech-Language programming in the schools.* Springfield, IL: Charles C. Thomas.

Gallagher, T., & Prutting, C. (1983). *Pragmatic assessment and intervention issues in language.* San Diego, CA: College Hill Press.

Ganz, C., & Hunt-Thompson, J. (1985). Speech-language intern supervisor training program. In K. Smith (Moderator), *Preparation and training models for the supervisory process.* Short course presented at the annual convention of the American Speech-Language-Hearing Association, Washington, DC.

Gardner, H. (1983). *Frames of the mind: The theory of multiple intelligences.* New York: Basic Books.

Gardner, H. (1993). *Multiple intelligences: The theory in practice.* New York: Basic Books.

Gardner, H. (1999). *Intelligence reframed: Multiple intelligences for the 21st century.* New York: Basic Books.

Gazda, G. (1974). *Human relations development—A manual for educators.* Boston: Allyn & Bacon.

Geertz, C. (1973). *The interpretation of cultures.* New York: Basic Books.

Geoffrey, V. (1973). *Report on supervisory practices in speech and hearing.* Unpublished report, College Park, MD: University of Maryland, Department of Hearing and Speech Sciences.

George, R., & Cristiani, T. (1981). *Theory, methods, and processes of counseling and psychotherapy.* Englewood Cliffs, NJ: Prentice-Hall.

Gerstman, H. (1977). Supervisory relationships: Experiences in dynamic communication. *ASHA, 19,* 527–529.

Getzel, J., & Guba, E. (1954). Role, role conflict and affectiveness: An empirical study. *American Sociological Review, 19,* 164–175.

Ghitter, R. (1987). Relationship of interpersonal and background variables to supervisee clinical effectiveness. In S. Farmer (Ed.), *Proceedings of A National*

Conference on Supervision—Clinical Supervision: A Coming of Age (pp. 49–56). Council of University Supervisors of Practicum in Speech-Language Pathology and Audiology, Jekyll Island, GA.

Gibb, J. (1969). Defensive communication. *Journal of Communication, 11,* 141–148.

Gillam, R. (1999). ISSUE III: Models of clinical instruction. Adopting an integrated apprenticeship model in a university clinic. In P. Murphy (Ed.), *Proceedings of the Annual Conference on Graduate Education* (pp. 97–99). Minneapolis, MN: Council of Academic Programs in Speech-Language Pathology and Audiology.

Gillam, R., & Pena, E. (1995). Clinical education: A social constructivist perspective. In R. Gillam (Ed.), *The Supervisor's Forum, 2,* 24–29. The Council of Supervisors in Speech-Language Pathology and Audiology.

Gillam, R., Strike, C., & Anderson, J. (1987). *Facilitating change in clinical behaviors: An investigation of supervisory effectiveness.* Unpublished manuscript, Indiana University, Bloomington: Indiana University.

Gillam, R., Strike-Roussos, C., & Anderson, J. (1990). Facilitating changes in supervisees' clinical behaviors: An experimental investigation of supervisory effectiveness. *Journal of Speech and Hearing Disorders, 55,* 729–739.

Glaser, A., & Donnelly, C. (1994). The development of a competency based assessment for supervisors. In M. Bruce (Ed.), *Proceedings of the 1994 International and Interdisciplinary Conference on Clinical Supervision: Toward the 21st Century.* (pp. 173–183). Cape Cod, MA.

Goldman, D. (1995). *Emotional intelligence.* New York: Bantam.

Goldberg, S. (1997). *Clinical skills for speech-language pathologists.* San Diego, CA: Singular.

Goldhammer, R. (1969). *Clinical supervision.* New York: Holt, Rinehart and Winston.

Goldhammer, R., Anderson, R., & Krajewski, R. (1980). *Clinical supervision* (2nd ed.). New York: Holt, Rinehart and Winston.

Golper, L., McMahon, J., & Gordon, M. (1976). *The use of interaction analysis for training in observation.* Paper presented at the annual convention of the American Speech-Language-Hearing Association.

Goodman, R. (1985). The live supervision model in clinical training. *The Clinical Supervisor, 3,* 43–59.

Goodwin, W. (1977). The frequency of occurrence of specified therapy behaviors of student speech clinicians following three conditions of supervisory conferences (Doctoral dissertation, Indiana University, 1976). *Dissertation Abstracts International, 37,* 3889B. (University Microfilms No. 77-01, 892)

Gorham, J. (1988). The relationship between verbal teacher immediacy behaviors and student learning. *Communication Education, 37,* 40–53.

Gouran, D. (1980). Leadership skills for supervisors. In J. Anderson (Ed.), *Conference on Training in the Supervisory Process in Speech-Language Pathology and Audiology* (pp. 87–110). Bloomington, IN.

Gunter, C. (1985). Clinical reports in speech-language pathology: Nature of supervisory feedback. *Australian Journal of Human Communication Disorders, 13,* 37–51.

Hackney, H., & Nye, S. (1973). *Counseling strategies and objectives.* Englewood Cliffs, NJ: Prentice-Hall.

Hagler, P. (1986). *Effects of verbal directives, data, and contingent social praise on amount of supervisor talk during speech-language pathology supervision conferencing.* Unpublished dissertation, Indiana University, Bloomington.

Hagler, P., Casey, P., & DesRochers, C. (1989). Effects of feedback on facilitative conditions offered by supervisors during conferencing. In D. Shapiro (Ed.), *Proceedings of the 1989 National Conference on Supervision: Supervision Innovations* (pp. 155–158). Council of Supervisors in Speech-Language Pathology and Audiology, Sonoma, CA.

Hagler, P., & Fahey, R. (1987). The validity of using short segments for analyzing supervisory conferences in speech pathology. *Human Communication Canada.*

Hagler, P., & Holdgrafer, G. (1987). Effects of supervisory feedback on clinician and client discourse participation. In S. Farmer (Ed.), *Proceedings of A National Conference on Supervision—Clinical Supervision: A Coming of Age* (pp. 106–111). Council of University Supervisors of Practicum in Speech-Language Pathology and Audiology, Jekyll Island, GA.

Hagler, P., & McFarlane, L. (1994). Teaching and working with interdisciplinary groups in clinical education. In M. Bruce (Ed.), *Proceedings of the 1994 International & Interdisciplinary Conference on Clinical Supervision: Toward the 21st Century* (pp. 253–257). Council of Supervisors in Speech-Language Pathology and Audiology, Cape Cod, MA.

Hagler, P., & McFarlane, L. (1997). *Collaborative Service Delivery by Assistants and Professionals (Revised).* Edmonton, Alberta, Canada: Alberta Rehabiliation Coordinating Council.

Hagler, P., Warren, & Pain. (1993). Personal communication.

Halfond, M. (1964). Clinical supervision—stepchild in training. *ASHA, 6,* 441–444.

Hall, A. (1971). The effectiveness of videotape recordings as an adjunct to supervision of clinical practicum by speech pathologists. (Doctoral dissertation, Ohio

State University, 1970). *Dissertation Abstracts International, 32,* 612B. (University Microfilms No. 71-18, 014)

Hampton, D. R., Summer, C. E., & Webber, R. A. (1982). *Organizational behavior and the practice of management.* Glenview, IL: Scott Foresman.

Hardick, E., & Oyer, H. (1987). Administration of speech-language-hearing programs within the university setting. In H. Oyer (Ed.), *Administration of programs in speech-language pathology and audiology.* Englewood Cliffs, NJ: Prentice-Hall.

Harris, B. (1975). *Supervisory behavior in education.* Englewood Cliffs, NJ: Prentice-Hall.

Harris, H., Ludington, J., Roberts, J., Hooper, C., & Ringwalt, S. (1992). A documentation of the effectiveness of instruction in the supervisory process. In S. Dowling (Ed.), *Proceedings of the 1992 National Conference on Supervision—Total Quality Supervision: Effecting Optimal Performance* (pp. 58–61). Council of Supervisors in Speech-Language Pathology and Audiology, Nashville, TN.

Hart, G. (1982). *The process of clinical supervision.* Baltimore: University Park Press.

Hatten, J. (1966). A descriptive and analytical investigation of speech therapy supervisors-therapist conferences (Doctoral dissertation, University of Wisconsin, 1965). *Dissertation Abstracts International, 26,* 5595–5596. (University Microfilms No. 71-18, 014)

Hatten, J., Bell, J., & Strand, J. (1983). *A comparative study of supervisor evaluation of a clinical session.* Paper presented at the annual convention of the American Speech-Language-Hearing Association, Washington, DC.

Haverkamp, K. (1983). The orientation experience for the adult learner. In R. Smith (Ed.), *Helping adults learn how to learn.* San Francisco: Jossey-Bass.

Hawthorne, L. (1975). Games supervisors play. *Social Work, 20,* 179–183.

Hegde, M., & Davis, D. (1995). *Clinical methods and practicum in speech-language pathology* (2nd ed.). San Diego, CA: Singular.

Heidelbach, R. (1967). The development of a tentative model for analyzing and describing the verbal behavior of cooperating teachers engaged in individualized teaching with student teachers (Doctoral dissertation, Columbia University, 1967). *Dissertation Abstracts, 28,* 1326-A. (University Microfilms No. 67-12, 689)

Henri, B. (2001, June). *Performance review and emotional intelligence: A necessary synthesis.* Paper presented at ASHA Special Interest Division 11 Leadership Conference: Power Tools for Leadership and Supervision, Chicago.

Herbert, J., & Attridge, C. (1975). A guide for developers and users of observation systems and manuals. *American Educational Research Journal, 12,* 1–20.

Hersey, P., & Blanchard, K. (1982). *Management of organizational behavior* (4th ed.). Englewood Cliffs, NJ: Prentice-Hall.

Herson, M., & Barlow, D. (1976). *Single case experimental design: Strategies for studying behavioral change.* New York: Pergamon.

Hoffman, S., & Willie, P. (1992). Comparative analysis of supervisees' needs and expectations ratings. In S. Dowling (Ed.), *Proceedings of the 1992 National Conference on Supervision—Total Quality Supervision: Effecting Optimal Performance* (pp. 62–69). Council of Supervisors in Speech-Language Pathology and Audiology, Nashville, TN.

Hunt, J., & Kauzlarich, M. (1979). *Enhancing the effectiveness of the supervisory process.* Paper presented at the annual convention of the American Speech-Language-Hearing Association, Atlanta, GA.

Hutchinson, D., Uhl, S., & Weinrich, B. (1987). A comparative study of student clinician performance under two types of supervisory conditions. In S. Farmer (Ed.), *Proceedings of A National Conference on Supervision—Clinical Supervision: A Coming of Age* (pp. 131–137). Council of University Supervisors of Practicum in Speech-Language Pathology and Audiology, Jekyll Island, GA.

Inglebret, E. (1996). Meeting the needs of a diverse student population: Application of cooperative learning. In B. Wagner (Ed.), *Proceedings of the 1996 Conference on Clinical Supervision—Partnerships in Supervision: Innovative and Effective Practices* (pp. 73–79). Council of Supervisors in Speech-Language Pathology and Audiology, Cincinnati.

Ingrisano, D., & Boyle, K. (1973). *A study of effectiveness and efficiency variables in a supervisory interaction.* Unpublished manuscript, University of Wisconsin, Madison.

Irwin, R. (1948). Ohio looks ahead in speech and hearing therapy. *Journal of Speech and Hearing Disorders, 13,* 55–60.

Irwin, R. (1949). Speech and hearing therapy in the public schools of Ohio. *Journal of Speech and Hearing Disorders, 14,* 63–68.

Irwin, R. (1972). *Microsupervision—A study of the behaviors of supervisors of speech clinicians.* Unpublished manuscript, Ohio State University, Columbus.

Irwin, R. (1975, Spring). Microcounseling interview skills of supervisors of speech clinicians. *Human Communication, 4,* 5–9.

Irwin, R. (1976). Verbal behavior of supervisors and speech clinicians during microcounseling. *Central States Speech Journal, 26,* 45–51.

Irwin, R. (1981a). Training speech pathologists through microtherapy. *Journal of Communication Disorders, 14,* 93–103.

Irwin, R. (1981b). Video self-confrontation on speech pathology. *Journal of Communication Disorders, 14,* 235–243.

Irwin, R., & Hall, A. (1973). Microtherapy—A study of the behaviors of speech clinicians. *Central States Speech Journal, 24,* 297–303.

Irwin, R., Van Riper, C., Breakey, M., & Fitzsimmons, R. (1961). Professional standards in training. In F. Darley (Ed.), Public school speech and hearing services. *Journal of Speech and Hearing Disorders.* (Monograph Suppl. 8)

Ivey, A. E. (1971). *Microcounseling.* Springfield, IL: Charles C. Thomas.

James, S., & Seebach, M. (1982). The pragmatic function of children's questions. *Journal of Speech and Hearing Research, 25,* 2–11.

Jans, L., Hagler, P., & McFarlane, L. (1994). Effects of agenda use over time on participants' level of involvement in supervisory conferences. In M. Bruce (Ed.), *Proceedings of the 1994 International & Interdisciplinary Conference on Clinical Supervision: Toward the 21st Century* (pp. 102–106). Council of Supervisors in Speech-Language Pathology and Audiology, Cape Cod, MA.

Jans, L., Hagler, P., McFarlane, L., McCrea, E., & Casey, P. (1994). Effects of supervisors' written session comments on their verbal feedback during supervisory conference. In M. Bruce (Ed.), *Proceedings of the 1994 International & Interdisciplinary Conference on Clinical Supervision: Toward the 21st Century* (pp. 107–110). Council of Supervisors in Speech-Language Pathology and Audiology, Cape Cod, MA.

Johnson, C., & Fey, S. (1983). Comparative effects of teaching clinic versus traditional supervision methods. *SUPERvision, 7,* 2–4.

Johnson, S. (1998). *Who moved my cheese? An amazing way to deal with change in your work and life.* New York: Putnam.

Johnson, T. (1970). The development of a multidimensional scoring system for observing the clinical process in speech pathology (Doctoral dissertation, University of Kansas, 1970). *Dissertation Abstracts International, 30,* 5735B-5736B. (University Microfilms No. 70-11, 036)

Johnson, T. (Ed.). (1971). *Clinical interaction and its measurement.* Utah State University, Department of Communicative Disorders, Logan.

Johnson, W., Darley, F., & Spriestersbach, D. (1963). *Diagnostic methods in speech pathology.* New York: Harper and Row.

Jones, M. (1993). A comparison of perceived supervisory needs and expectations of audiology versus speech pathology student clinicians. In R. Gillam (Ed.), *The Supervisors' Forum, 1,* 54–56. Council of Supervisors in Speech-Language Pathology and Audiology.

Kadushin, A. (1968). Games people play in supervision. *Social Work, 13,* 23–32.

Kadushin, A. (1976). *Supervision in social work.* New York: Columbia University Press.

Kagan, N. (1970). Human relationships in supervision. In J. Anderson (Ed.), *Conference on Supervision of Speech and Hearing Programs in the Schools.* Bloomington: Indiana University.

Kagan, N., & Werner, A. (1977). Supervision in psychiatric education. In D. Kurpius, R. Baker, & I. Thomas (Eds.), *Supervision of applied training.* Westport, CT: Greenwood Press.

Kaslow, F. (1977). Training of marital and family therapists. In F. Kaslow & Associates (Ed.), *Supervision, consultation, and staff training in the helping professions.* San Francisco, CA: Jossey-Bass.

Kayser, H. (1993). Supervision of the Hispanic speech language pathology graduate student. In R. Gillam (Ed.), *The supervisors' forum, 1,* 18–23. Council of Supervisors in Speech-Language Pathology and Audiology.

Kearns, K. (1986). Flexibility of single-subject experimental design. Part II: Design selection and arrangement of experimental phases. *Journal of Speech and Hearing Disorders, 51,* 204–214.

Keeney, B. (1983). *Aesthetics of change.* New York: The Guilford Press.

Kelly, J. (1980). *Organizational behavior.* Homewood, IL: Richard D. Irwin.

Kelman, M., & Whitmire, K. (1994). Simultaneous training of students and supervisors: Improving field-based practicum experiences. In M. Bruce (Ed.), *Proceedings of the 1994 International & Interdisciplinary Conference on Clinical Supervision: Toward the 21st Century* (pp. 249–252). Council of Supervisors in Speech-Language Pathology and Audiology, Cape Cod, MA.

Kendall, P. C., & Norton-Ford, J. D. (1982). *Scientific and professional dimensions.* New York: John Wiley.

Kennedy, K. (1981). The effect of two methods of supervisor preconference written feedback on the verbal behaviors of participants in individual speech pathology supervisory conferences (Doctoral dissertation, University of Oregon, 1981). *Dissertation Abstracts International, 42,* 2071A. (University Microfilms No. 81-23, 492)

Kent, L. P. (1977). *Problem-oriented record for clinical service and supervision in speech pathology and audiology.* Paper presented at the annual convention of the American Speech and Hearing Association, Chicago.

Kent, L. P., & Chabon, S. (1980). Problem-oriented record in a university speech and hearing clinic. *ASHA, 22,* 151–155.

Khami, A. (1995). Defining, developing, and teaching clinical expertise. In R. Gillam (Ed.), *The Supervisor's Forum, 2,* 30–35. Council of Supervisors in Speech-Language Pathology and Audiology.

Kleffner, F. (Ed.). (1964). *Seminar on guidelines for the internship year.* Washington, DC: American Speech and Hearing Association.

Klevans, D., & Volz, H. (1974). Development of a clinical evaluation tool. *ASHA, 16,* 489–491.

Klevans, D., Volz, H., & Friedman, R. (1981). A comparison of experimental and observational approaches for enhancing the interpersonal communication skills of speech-language pathology students. *Journal of Speech and Hearing Disorders, 46,* 208–213.

Knapp, M. (1972). *Nonverbal communication in human interaction.* New York: Holt, Rinehart and Winston.

Knight, H., Hahn, E., Ervin, J., & McIsaac, G. (1961). The public school clinician: Professional definition and relationships. In F. Darley (Ed.), Public school speech and hearing services. *Journal of Speech and Hearing Disorders.* (Monograph Suppl. 8)

Knowles, M. (1984). *The adult learner: A neglected species.* Houston, TX: Gulf Publishing.

Kooper, R. (1994). Professional Liability. In R. Lubinski & C. Frattalli (Eds.), *Professional issues in speech-language pathology and audiology* (pp. 166–172). San Diego, CA: Singular.

Korner, I., & Brown, W. (1952). The mechanical third ear. *Journal of Consulting Psychology, 16,* 81–84.

Kunze, L. (1967). Program for training in behavioral observation. In A. Miner, A symposium: Improving supervision of clinical practicum. *ASHA, 9,* 473–497.

Kurpius, D. (1976). Implementing interpersonal communication in school environments. In J. Weigand (Ed.), *Implementing teacher competencies.* Englewood Cliffs, NJ: Prentice-Hall.

Kurpius, D. (1978). Consultation theory and process: An integrated model. *The Personnel and Guidance Journal, 56,* 335–338.

Kurpius, D., Baker, R., & Thomas, I. (Eds.). (1977). *Supervision of applied training.* Westport, CT: Greenwood Press.

Kurpius, D., & Christie, S. (1978). A systematic and collaborative approach to problem solving. In D. Kurpius (Ed.), *Learning: Making learning environments more effective.* Muncie, IN: Accelerated Development.

Kurpius, D., & Robinson, S. (1978). An overview of consultation. *Personal and Guidance Journal, 3,* 231–233.

Laccinole, M., & Shulman, B. (1985). Clinical effectiveness for the student clinician. *SUPERvision, 9*(3), 23–26.

Laney, M. (1982). Research and evaluation in the public schools. *Language, Speech and Hearing Services in Schools, 13,* 53–60.

Langellier, K. M., & Natalle, E. J. (1987). Gender, interpersonal communication, and supervision. In S. Farmer (Ed.), *Proceedings of A National Conference on Supervision—Clinical Supervision: A Coming of Age* (pp. 14–37). Council of University Supervisors of Practicum in Speech-Language Pathology and Audiology, Jekyll Island, GA.

Larkins, P. (1992). Women's ways of supervising: What's your type? In S. Dowling (Ed.), *Proceedings of the 1992 National Conference on Supervision—Total Quality Supervision: Effecting Optimal Performance* (pp. 38–40). Council of Supervisors in Speech-Language Pathology and Audiology, Nashville.

Larson, L. (1982). Perceived supervisory needs and expectations of experienced vs. inexperienced student clinicians (Doctoral dissertation, Indiana University, 1981). *Dissertation Abstracts International, 42,* 4758B. (University Microfilms No. 82-11, 183)

Larson, L., Hoag, L., & Schraeder-Neidenthal, J. (1987). Supervisee satisfaction with a contract-based system for grading practicum. In S. Farmer (Ed.), *Proceedings of A National Conference on Supervision—Clinical Supervision: A Coming of Age* (pp. 117–124). Council of University Supervisors of Practicum in Speech-Language Pathology and Audiology, Jekyll Island, GA.

Leach, E. (1972). Interrogation: A model and some implications. *Journal of Speech and Hearing Disorders, 37,* 33–46.

Lemmer, E., & Drake, M. (1983). Client management and professional development. *ASHA, 25,* 33–39.

Levert, M. (2000). Leadership skills needed to manage complex change. In P. Hargrove, R. McGuire, C. O'Rourke, & W. Swisher (Eds.), *Proceedings of the Annual Conference—The Challenge of Change* (pp. 48–53). Council of Academic Programs in Communication Sciences and Disorders, Minneapolis, MN.

Lincoln, M., McLeod, S., McAllister, L., Maloney, D., Purcell, A., & Eadie, P. (1994). Learning styles of speech-language pathology students: A longitudinal investigation. In M. Bruce (Ed.), *Proceedings of the 1994 International & Interdisciplinary Conference on Clinical Supervision: Toward the 21st Century* (pp. 133–140). Council of Supervisors in Speech-Language Pathology and Audiology, Cape Cod, MA.

Lincoln, Y., & Guba, E. (1985). *Naturalistic inquiry.* Beverly Hills, CA: Sage.

Lindsey, M. (1969). *Inquiry into teaching behavior of supervisors in teaching education laboratories.* New York: Teachers College Press, Columbia University.

Link, C. (1971). Teacher-supervisor conference interaction: A study of perceptions and their relation in selected variables (Doctoral dissertation, Western Michigan University, 1970). *Dissertation Abstracts International, 31,* 3824A. (University Microfilms No. 71-4376)

Loewenstein, S., & Reder, P. (1982). The consumers' response: Trainees' discussion of the experience of live supervision. In R. Whiffen & J. Byng-Hall (Eds.), *Family therapy supervision.* New York: Grune and Stratton.

Lougeay-Mottiger, J., Harris, M., & Stillman, R. (1987). Use of a videotaped coding system to change clinician behavior. In S. Farmer (Ed.), *Proceedings of A National Conference on Supervision—Clinical Supervision: A Coming of Age* (pp. 86–91). Council of University Supervisors of Practicum in Speech-Language Pathology and Audiology, Jekyll Island, GA.

Lowery, L. (1970). *Learning about instruction: Questioning strategies: A personal workshop.* (ERIC Research Document No. ED113 297).

Lubinski, R., & Frattali, C. (2001). *Professional issues in speech-language pathology and audiology* (2nd ed.). San Diego, CA: Singular Thompson Learning.

Lubinsky, J., & Hildebrand, S. (1996). Journal keeping to help students attain personal goals in practicum. In B. Wagner (Ed.), *Proceedings of the 1996 Conference on Clinical Supervision—Partnerships in Supervision: Innovative and Effective Practices* (pp. 235–242). Council of Supervisors in Speech-Language Pathology and Audiology, Cincinnati, OH.

Luft, J. (1969). *Of human interaction.* Palo Alto, CA: National Press Books.

Lund, N., & Duchan, J. (1993). *Assessing children's language in naturalistic contexts* (3rd ed.) Englewood Cliffs, NJ: Prentice-Hall.

Luterman, D. (1984). *Counseling the communicatively disordered and their families.* Boston: Little, Brown.

Mager, R. (1962). *Preparing instructional objectives.* Palo Alto, CA: Fearon.

Mager, R. (1972). *Goal analysis.* Belmont, CA: Fearon.

Mager, R., & Pipe, P. (1970). *Analyzing performance problems.* Belmont, CA: Fearon.

Maloney, D. (1994). Client-centered student journaling: A way of reflecting on clinical learning. In M. Bruce (Ed.), *Proceedings of the 1994 International & Interdisciplinary Conference on Clinical Supervision: Toward the 21st Century* (pp. 191–195). Council of

Supervisors in Speech-Language Pathology and Audiology, Cape Cod, MA.

Maslow, A. H. (1954). *Motivation and personality.* New York: Harper and Bros.

Mastriano, B., Gordon, T., & Gottwald, S. (1999). Expectations in the supervisory process: An analysis of attitudes II. Poster session presented at the annual convention of the American Speech-Language-Hearing Association, San Francisco.

Mawdsley, B. (1985a). *The integrative task-maturity model of supervision.* Presentation at the annual meeting of the American Speech-Language-Hearing Association, Washington, DC.

Mawdsley, B. (1985b). *Kansas inventory of self-supervision.* Paper presented at the annual convention of the American Speech-Language-Hearing Association, Washington, DC.

May, et al. (1995, Spring). Model of ability-based assessment in physical therapy educations. *Journal of Physical Therapy Education, 9*(1), 3–6.

Mayo, E. (1933). *The human problems of an industrial civilization.* New York: MacMillan.

McAllister, L. (2000). Where are we going in clinical education? A review of current status and some theoretical and philosophical guideposts for new directions. *Proceedings of the Council of Academic Programs in Communication Sciences and Disorders 2000 Conference.* Minneapolis, MN: The Council of Academic Programs in Communication Sciences and Disorders.

McCrea, E. (1980). Supervisee ability to self-explore and four facilitative dimensions of supervisor behavior in individual conferences in speech-language pathology (Doctoral dissertation, Indiana University, 1980). *Dissertation Abstracts International, 41,* 2134B. (University Microfilms No. 80-29, 239)

McCrea, E. (1985). Supervision component in undergraduate clinical management class. In K. Smith (Moderator), *Preparation and training models for the supervisory process.* Short course presented at the annual convention of the American Speech-Language-Hearing Association, Washington, DC.

McCrea, E. (1994). Supervision as a Master's degree thesis option. In M. Bruce (Ed.), *Proceedings of the 1994 International & Interdisciplinary Conference on Clinical Supervision: Toward the 21st Century* (pp. 221–229). Council of Supervisors in Speech-Language Pathology and Audiology, Cape Cod, MA.

McCready, V., Roberts, J., Bengala, D., Harris, H., Kingsley, G., & Krikorian, C. (1996). A comparison of conflict tactics in the supervisory process. *Journal of Speech and Hearing Research, 39,* 191–199.

McCready, V., Shapiro, D., & Kennedy, K. (1987). Identifying hidden dynamics in supervision: Four scenarios. In M. Crago & M. Pickering (Eds.), *Supervision in human communication disorders: Perspectives on a process.* San Diego, CA: College Hill Press.

McFarlane, L., & Hagler, P. (1992a). An experimentally-based peer supervision component in a university clinic. In S. Dowling (Ed.), *Proceedings of the 1992 National Conference on Supervision—Total Quality Supervision: Effecting Optimal Performance* (pp. 78–84). Council of Supervisors in Speech-Language Pathology and Audiology, Nashville, TN.

McFarlane, L., & Hagler, P. (1992b). Effects of a supervisee-prepared agenda on conference interaction. In S. Dowling (Ed.), *Proceedings of the 1992 National Conference on Supervision—Total Quality Supervision: Effecting Optimal Performance* (pp. 85–91). Council of Supervisors in Speech-Language Pathology and Audiology, Nashville, TN.

McGregor, D. M. (1960). *The human side of enterprise.* New York: McGraw-Hill.

McReynolds, L., & Kearns, K. (1983). *Single-subject experimental designs in communicative disorders.* Baltimore: University Park Press.

McReynolds, L., & Thompson, C. (1986). Flexibility of single-subject experimental designs. Part I: Review of the basics of single-subject designs. *Journal of Speech and Hearing Disorders, 51,* 194–203.

Mehrabian, A. (1969). Significance of posture and position in the communication of attitude and status relationships. *Psychological Bulletin, 71,* 359–372.

Mehrabian, A. (1981). Silent messages: Implicit communication of emotions and attitudes (2nd ed.). Belmont, CA: Wadsworth.

Messick, C. (1999). ISSUE III: Models of clinical instruction. Clinical Network: The challenges of establishing a new training model. In P. Murphy (Ed.), *Council of Academic Programs in Communication Sciences and Disorders Proceedings of the Annual Conference on Graduate Education* (pp. 90–96). Minneapolis, MN: Council of Academic Programs in Communication Sciences and Disorders.

Michalak, D. (1969). Supervisory conferences improve teaching. *Florida Educational Research and Development Council Research Bulletin, 5.*

Miller, J. (1996). Research opportunities for undergraduate students. In C. Scott (Ed.), *Council of Graduate Programs in Communication Sciences and Disorders Proceedings of the Annual Conference on Graduate Education* (pp. 56–59). Minneapolis, MN: Council of Academic Programs in Communication Sciences and Disorders.

Miner, A. (1967). A symposium: Improving supervision of clinical practicum. *ASHA, 9,* 471–482.

Molyneaux, D., & Lane, V. (1982). *Effective interviewing: Techniques and analysis.* Boston: Allyn & Bacon.

Monnin, L., & Peters, K. (1981). *Clinical practice for speech-pathologists in the schools.* Springfield, IL: Charles C. Thomas.

Moon Meyer, S. (1998). *Survival guide for the beginning speech-language clinician.* Gaithersburg, MD: Aspen.

Mosher, R., & Purpel, D. (1972). *Supervision: The reluctant profession.* Boston: Houghton Mifflin.

Mournot, C., Siegle, D., & Solomon, B. (1985). *Which competencies are important for clinical supervision?* Paper presented at the annual convention of the American speech-Language-Hearing Association, Washington, DC.

Mowrer, D. (1969). Evaluating speech therapy through precision recording. *Journal of Speech and Hearing Disorders, 34,* 239–245.

Mowrer, D. (1977). *Methods of modifying speech behaviors.* Columbus, OH: Charles E. Merrill.

Munson, C. (1983). *An introduction to clinical social work supervision.* New York: The Haworth Press.

Murray, M., & Owen, M. (1991). *Beyond the myths and magic of mentoring.* San Francisco, CA: Jossey-Bass.

Myers, F. (1980). Clinician needs in the practicum setting. *SUPERvision, 4.*

Naremore, R. (1984). *Research methodologies for the supervisory process.* Presentation with J. Anderson, G. DeVane, M. Laccinole, W. Kennan, E. McCrea, D., Ingrisano, & K. Smith at the annual convention of the American Speech-Language Hearing Association, San Francisco.

Nelson, G. (1974). *Does supervision make a difference?* Paper presented at the annual convention of the American Speech and Hearing Association, Las Vegas, NV.

Newman, W. (2001, June/July). The ethical and legal aspects of clinical supervision. *CSHA [California Speech-Language-Hearing Association] Magazine, 30*(1) 10–11, 27.

Nilsen, J. (1983). Supervisor's use of direct/indirect verbal conference style and alteration of clinical behavior (Doctoral dissertation, University of Illinois, 1983). *Dissertation Abstracts International, 43,* 3935B. (University Microfilms No. 83-09, 991)

Olswang, L. (1990). Treatment efficacy research, a path to quality assurance. *ASHA, 32*(1), 45–47.

O'Neil, J. (1985). The clinical supervisor—proctor or accountant? *ASHA, 27,* 23–24.

Oratio, A. (1977). *Supervision in speech pathology: A handbook for supervisors and clinicians.* Baltimore: University Park Press.

Pannbacker, M., Middleton, G., & Lass, N. (1993). Am I a good supervisor? That depends on who's asking! *The Supervisors' Forum, 1,* 57.

Pascale, R. T., & Athos, A. G. (1981). *The art of Japanese management.* New York: Warner Books.

Paul-Brown, D., & Goldberg, L. (2001). Current policies and directions for speech-language pathology assistants. *Language, Speech, and Hearing Services in the Schools, 32,* pp. 4–17.

Peaper, R. (1984). An analysis of student perceptions of the supervisory conference and student developed agendas for that conference. *The Clinical Supervisor, 2,* 55–64.

Peaper, R., & Mercaitis, P. (1987). The nature of narrative written feedback provided to student clinicians: A descriptive study. In S. Farmer (Ed.), *Proceedings of a National conference on Supervision—Clinical Supervision: A Coming of Age.* Council of University Supervisors of Practicum in Speech-Language Pathology and Audiology, Jekyll Island, GA.

Peaper, R., & Mercaitis, P. (1989a). Satisfactory and unsatisfactory supervisory experiences: Contributing factors. In D. Shapiro (Ed.), *Proceedings of the 1989 National Conference on Supervision: Supervision Innovations* (pp. 126–140). Council of Supervisors in Speech-Language Pathology and Audiology, Sonoma, CA.

Peaper, R., & Mercaitis, P. (1989b). Strategies for helping supervisees to participate actively in the supervisory process. In D. Shapiro (Ed.), *Proceedings of the 1989 National Conference on Supervision: Supervision Innovations* (pp. 20–28). Council of Supervisors of Practicum in Speech-Language Pathology and Audiology, Sonoma, CA.

Peaper, R., & Wener, D. (1984). A comparison of perceptions of written clinical plans and reports. *ASHA, 26,* 37–41.

Pederson, P. B., & Ivey, A. (1993). *Culture-centered counseling and interviewing skills: A practical guide.* Westport, CT: Praeger.

Peters, T. J., & Waterman, R. H. (1982). *In search of excellence: Lessons from America's best-run companies.* New York: Harper and Row.

Pickering, M. (1977). An examination of concepts operative in the supervisory process and relationship. *ASHA, 19,* 607–610.

Pickering, M. (1979). Interpersonal communication in speech-language pathology clinical practicum: A descriptive humanistic perspective (Doctoral dissertation, Boston University School of Education, 1979). *Dissertation Abstracts International, 40,* 2140B. (University Microfilms No. 79-23, 892)

Pickering, M. (1980). *Introduction to qualitative research methodology: Purpose, characteristics, procedures, examples.* Paper presented at the annual convention of the American Speech-Language Hearing Association, Detroit, MI.

Pickering, M. (1981a). Supervising student teachers: How to provide non-threatening feedback. *Journal of Childhood Communication Disorders, 5*(2), 150–153.

Pickering, M. (1981b). *Supervisory interaction: The subjective side.* Paper presented at the CUSPSPA meeting during the annual convention of the American Speech-Language Hearing Association, Los Angeles, CA.

Pickering, M. (1982). *Interpersonal communication in student-conducted therapy sessions.* Paper presented at the annual convention of the American Speech-Language-Hearing Association, Los Angeles, CA.

Pickering, M. (1984). Interpersonal communication in speech-language pathology supervisory conferences: A qualitative study. *Journal of Speech and Hearing Disorders, 49,* 189–195.

Pickering, M. (1986). Communication. *Explorations—A journal of research at the University of Maine.* Orono: University of Maine.

Pickering, M. (1987a). Interpersonal communication and the supervisory process: A search for Ariadne's thread. In M. Crago & J. Pickering, (Eds.), *Supervision in human communication disorders: Perspectives on a process.* San Diego, CA: College-Hill Press.

Pickering, M. (1987b). Supervision: A person-focused process. In J. Crago & M. Pickering (Eds.), *Supervision in human communication disorders: Perspectives on a process.* San Diego, CA: College-Hill Press.

Pickering, M. (1990). Establishing and maintaining an effective working relationship: The first task of supervision. In *Clinical Supervision Across Settings: Communication and Collaboration* (pp. 36–44). Rockville, MD: American Speech-Language Hearing Association.

Pickering, M. (1992). A feminist vision for clinical education. In S. Dowling (Ed.), *Proceedings of the 1992 National Conference on Supervision—Total Quality Supervision: Effecting Optimal Performance* (pp. 41–45). Council of Supervisors in Speech-Language Pathology and Audiology, Nashville, TN.

Pickering, M. (2001). Scholarship and the clinical educator. *Administration and Supervision, 11*(1), 11–15.

Pickering, M., & McCready, V. (1983). Supervisory journals: An 'inside' look at supervision. *SUPERvision, 7,* 5–7.

Pickering, M., & McCready, V. (1990). Interpersonal communication skills: A process in action. In *Clinical Supervision Across Settings: Communication and Collaboration* (pp. 23–35). Rockville, MD: American Speech-Language Hearing Association.

Pittinger, A. (1972). An analysis of the patterns of verbal interaction and their relationship to self-reported satisfaction ratings and a measure of empathic accuracy in selecting secondary student teaching supervisory conferences (Doctoral dissertation, University of Maryland, 1971). *Dissertation Abstracts International, 32,* 5658A. (University Microfilms No. 72-12, 847)

Popham, W. J., & Baker, E. (1970). *Establishing instructional goals.* Englewood Cliffs, NJ: Prentice-Hall.

Powell, R. G., & Harville, B. (1990). The effects of teacher immediacy and clarity on instructional outcomes: An intercultural assessment. *Communication Education, 39,* 369–379.

Powell, T. (1987). A rating scale for measurement of attitudes toward clinical supervision. *SUPERvision, 11,* 31–34.

Prather, E. (1967). An approach to clinical supervision. *ASHA, 9,* 471–482.

Prescott, T. (1971). The development of a methodology for describing speech therapy. In T. Johnson (Ed.), *Clinical interaction and its measurement.* Logan: Utah State University.

Rao, P. (1990). Evaluating clinical performance on the job: A sequential process approach. In *Clinical Supervision Across Settings: Communication and Collaboration* (pp. 87–95). Rockville, MD: American Speech-Language Hearing Association.

Rassi, J. (1978). *Supervision in audiology.* Baltimore: University Park Press.

Rassi, J. (1985). Supervision in audiology. In K. Smith (Moderator), *Preparation and training models for the supervisory process.* Short course presented at the annual convention of the American Speech-Language Hearing Association, Washington, DC.

Rassi, J. (1987). The uniqueness of audiology supervision. In M. Crago & M. Pickering (Eds.), *Supervision in human communication disorders: Perspectives on a process* (pp. 31–54). San Diego, CA: Singular.

Rassi, J. (June/July 2001). A comparison of supervision practices in audiology and speech-language pathology. *California Speech-Language-Hearing Association (CSHA) Magazine, 30*(1), 12–13.

Rassi, J., Dodd, J., & Baer, J. (1993). The instructional value of joint clinical practicum-clinical research activity. In R. Gillam (Ed.), *The Supervisor's Forum, 1,* 29–32. Council of Supervisors in Speech-Language Pathology and Audiology.

Rassi, J., Hoffman, S., & Willie, P. (1991). *Comparative analysis of supervisees' expectations and needs ratings.* Presentation at the annual convention of the American Speech-Language-Hearing Association, Atlanta, GA.

Rassi, J., & McElroy, M. (1992). Clinical teaching: Delineating competencies and planning strategies. In J. A. Rassi & M. D. McElroy (Eds.), *The educa-*

tion of audiologists and speech-language pathologists (pp. 301–335). Timonium, MD: York Press.

Rassi, J., Rao, P., & Hicks, P. (1995). Preparing and retaining leaders for the professions. In R. Gillam (Ed.), *The Supervisors' Forum, 2,* 82–85. Council of Supervisors in Speech-Language Pathology and Audiology.

Reitz, J. (1981). *Behavior in organizations.* Homewood, IL: Richard D. Irwin.

Richardson, A., & Gillam, R. (1994). Efficacy research in university settings: Supervisory issues. In In M. Bruce (Ed.), *Proceedings of the 1994 International & Interdisciplinary Conference on Clinical Supervision: Toward the 21st Century* (pp. 202–206). Council of Supervisors in Speech-Language Pathology and Audiology, Cape Cod, MA.

Roberts, J. (1980). Content and sequence analysis system. In J. Anderson, *Proceedings—Conference on Training in the Supervisory Process in Speech-Language Pathology and Audiology.* Bloomington: Indiana University.

Roberts, J. (1982). An attributional model of supervisors' decision-making behavior in speech-language pathology (Doctoral dissertation, Indiana University, 1981). *Dissertation Abstracts International, 42,* 2794B. (University Microfilms No. 81-28, 040)

Roberts, J., & Naremore, R. (1983). An attributional model of supervisors' decision-making behavior in speech-language pathology. *Journal of Speech and Hearing Research, 26,* 537–549.

Roberts, J., & Smith, K. (1982). Supervisor-supervisee role differences and consistency of behavior in supervisory conferences. *Journal of Speech and Hearing Research, 25,* 428–434.

Rocchio, C., & Iacarino, J. (1990). *Written feedback provided to student clinicians.* Poster session presented at the annual convention of the American Speech-Language Hearing Association, Seattle, WA.

Rockman, B. (1977). *Supervisor as clinician: A point of view.* Paper presented at the annual convention of the American Speech and Hearing Association, Chicago.

Rogers, C. (1951). *Client-centered therapy.* Boston: Houghton-Mifflin.

Rogers, C. (1957). The necessary and sufficient conditions of therapeutic personality change. *Journal of Consulting Psychology, 21,* 95–103.

Rogers, C. (1961). *On becoming a person: A therapist's view of psychotherapy.* Boston: Houghton Mifflin.

Rogers, C. (1962). The interpersonal relationship: The core of guidance. *Harvard Educational Review, 32,* 116–129.

Rogers, C. (1980). *A way of being.* Boston: Houghton Mifflin.

Rosenshine, B. (1970). Evaluation of classroom instruction. *Review of Educational Research, 40,* 282.

Rosenshine, B. (1971). Research on teacher performance criteria. In B. Smith (Ed.), *Research in teacher education.* Englewood Cliffs, NJ: Prentice-Hall.

Rosenshine, B., & Furst, N. (1973). The use of direct observation to study teaching. In R. Travers (Ed.), *Second handbook of research on teaching.* Chicago: Rand McNally.

Ruder, K., Simpson, K., Ruder, C., Smith, L., Trammel, R., & Landes, T. (1996). Laptop computer aids for supervision. In B. Wagner (Ed.), *Proceedings of the 1996 Conference on Clinical Supervision—Partnerships in Supervision: Innovative and Effective Practices* (pp. 106–118). Council of Supervisors in Speech-Language Pathology and Audiology, Cincinnati, OH.

Runyan, S., & Seal, B. (1985). A comparison of supervisors' ratings while observing a language remediation session. *The Clinical Supervisor, 3,* 61–75.

Rushakoff, G., & Farmer, S. (1989). Supervision applications of microcomputer technology. In S. Farmer & J. Farmer, *Supervision in communication disorders* (pp. 250–272). Columbus, OH: Merrill.

Russell, L. (1976). *Aspects of supervision.* Unpublished manuscript, Temple University, Philadelphia.

Russell, L., & Engle, B. (1977). *A study of the supervisory process.* Paper presented at the convention of the New Jersey Speech and Hearing Association.

Russell, L., & Halfond, M. (1985). *An expanded view of the evaluative component of clinical supervision.* Paper presented at the annual convention of the American Speech-Language Hearing Association, Washington, DC.

Sanders, N. (1966). *Classroom questions: What kinds?* New York: Harper and Row.

Sbaschnig, K., Dowling, S., & Williams, C. (1992). Agenda planning, talk time and question usage in the conference. In S. Dowling (Ed.), *Proceedings of the 1992 National Conference on Supervision—Total Quality Supervision: Effecting Optimal Performance* (pp. 92–96). Council of Supervisors in Speech-Language Pathology and Audiology, Nashville, TN.

Sbaschnig, K., & Williams, C. (1983). *A reliability audit for supervisors.* Paper presented at the annual meeting of the American Speech-Language Hearing Association, Cincinnati, OH.

Schiavetti, N., & Metz, D. (1997). *Evaluating research in communicative disorders* (3rd ed.). Boston: Allyn & Bacon.

Schill, M. (1992). Quality supervision: Beginning with observation. In S. Dowling (Ed.), *Proceedings of the 1992 National Conference on Supervision—Total Quality Supervision: Effecting Optimal Performance* (pp. 53–57). Council of Supervisors in Speech-Language Pathology and Audiology, Nashville, TN.

Schill, M., & Glick, A. (1994). Use of a portfolio review process to enhance self-evaluation by student clinicians. In M. Bruce (Ed.), *Proceedings of the 1994 International & Interdisciplinary Conference on Clinical Supervision: Toward the 21st Century* (pp. 207–212). Council of Supervisors in Speech-Language Pathology and Audiology, Cape Cod, MA.

Schill, M., & Swanson, D. (1993). Use of an audiotaped dialogue journal in the supervisory process: A case study. In R. Gillam (Ed.), *The supervisor's forum, 1,* 33–35. Council of Supervisors in Speech-Language Pathology and Audiology.

Schneider, D., Hastorf, A., & Ellsworth, P. (1979). *Person perception.* Reading, MA: Addison-Wesley.

Schubert, G. (1978). *Introduction to clinical supervision.* St. Louis, MO: W. H. Green.

Schubert, G., & Aitchison, C. (1975). A profile of clinical supervisors in college and university speech and hearing training programs. *ASHA, 17,* 440–447.

Schubert, G., & Glick, A. (1974). A comparison of two methods of recording and analyzing student clinician-client interaction: ABC system and the "Boone" system. *Acta Symbolica, 5,* 39–56.

Schubert, G., & Gudmundson, P. (1976, November). *Effects of videotape feedback and interaction upon nonverbal behavior of student clinicians.* Paper presented at the annual convention of the American Speech-Language Hearing Association, Houston, TX.

Schubert, G., & Laird, B. (1975, December). The length of time necessary to obtain a representative sample of clinician-client interaction. *Journal of National Student Speech and Hearing Association,* 26–32.

Schubert, G., Miner, A., & Till, J. (1973). *The analysis of behavior of clinicians (ABC) system.* Unpublished manuscript, University of North Dakota, Grand Forks.

Schubert, G., & Nelson, J. (1976). *Verbal behaviors occurring in speech pathology supervisory conferences.* Paper presented at the annual convention of the American Speech-Language Hearing Association, Houston, TX.

Scott, C. (1996). Research at the master's level. In C. Scott (Ed.), *Council of Graduate Programs in Communication Sciences and Disorders Proceedings of the Annual Conference on Graduate Education* (pp. 60–66). Minneapolis, MN: Council of Academic Programs in Communication Sciences and Disorders.

Seymour, C. (1992). Women's ways of supervising: Juggling, balancing, and walking a tightrope life under the big top. In S. Dowling (Ed.), *Proceedings of the 1992 National Conference on Supervision—Total Quality Supervision: Effecting Optimal Performance* (pp. 32–37). Council of Supervisors in Speech-Language Pathology and Audiology, Nashville, TN.

Shadden, B., & Aslin, L. (1993). Facilitating clinical observation skills through interactive computer/laser disc technology. In R. Gillam (Ed.), *The Supervisor's Forum, 1,* 37–43. Council of Supervisors in Speech-Language Pathology and Audiology, Nashville, TN.

Shapiro, D. (1985a). Clinical supervision: A process in progress. *National Student Speech-Language-Hearing Association Journal.*

Shapiro, D. (1985b). An experimental and descriptive analysis of supervisees' commitments and follow-through behaviors as one measure of supervisory effectiveness in speech-language pathology and audiology (Doctoral dissertation, Indiana University, 1984). *Dissertation Abstracts International, 45,* 2889B. (University Microfilms No. 84-26, 682)

Shapiro, D., & Anderson, J. (1988). An analysis of commitments made by student clinicians in speech-language pathology and audiology. *Journal of Speech and Hearing Disorders, 53,* 202–210.

Shapiro, D., & Anderson, J. (1989). One measure of supervisory effectiveness in speech-language pathology and audiology. *Journal of Speech and Hearing Disorders, 54,* 549–557.

Sharpe, T., Koperwas, J., & Wood, D. (1994). Behavioral evaluation system and taxonomy [Computer software]. Lincoln, NE: Educational Consulting. Cited in Ruder, K., Simpson, K., Ruder, C., Smith, L., Trammel, R., & Landes, T. (1996). Laptop computer aids for supervision. In B. Wagner (Ed.), *Proceedings of the 1996 Conference on Clinical Supervision—Partnerships in Supervision: Innovative and Effective Practices* (pp. 106–118). Council of Supervisors in Speech-Language Pathology and Audiology, Cincinnati, OH.

Shipley, K. (1997). *Interviewing and counseling in communicative disorders—Principles and procedures* (2nd ed.). Boston: Allyn & Bacon.

Shipley, K., & McAfee, J. (1998). *Assessment in speech-language pathology: A resource manual* (2nd ed.). San Diego, CA: Singular.

Shriberg, L., Filley, F., Hayes, D., Kwiatkowski, J., Shatz, J., Simmons, K., et al. (1974). *The Wisconsin procedure for appraisal of clinical competence (W-PACC).* Madison: Department of Communicative Disorders, University of Wisconsin-Madison.

Shriberg, L., Filley, F., Hayes, D., Kwiatkowski, J., Shatz, J., Simmons, K., et al. (1975). The Wisconsin procedure for appraisal of clinical competence (W-PACC): Model and data. *ASHA, 17,* 158–165.

Silverman, F. (1998). *Research design and evaluation in speech-language pathology and audiology.* Boston: Allyn & Bacon.

Simon, A., & Boyer, E. (Eds.). (1970a). *Mirrors for behavior: An anthology of classroom observation instruments* (Vol. A). Philadelphia: Research for Better Schools.

Simon, A., & Boyer, E. (Eds.). (1970b). *Mirrors for behavior: An anthology of classroom observation instruments* (Vol. B). Philadelphia: Research for Better Schools.

Simon, A., & Boyer, E. (1974). *Mirrors for Behavior III.* Wyncote, PA: Communications Materials Center.

Skinner, B. F. (1954). The science of learning and the art of teaching. *Harvard Educational Review, 24,* 86–97.

Sleight, C. (1984). Games people play in clinical supervision. *ASHA, 26,* 27–29.

Sleight, C. (1985). Confidence and anxiety in student clinicians. *The Clinical Supervisor, 3,* 25–48.

Smith, K. (1978). Identification of perceived effectiveness components in the individual supervisory conference in speech pathology and an evaluation of the relationship between ratings and content in the conference (Doctoral dissertation, Indiana University, 1977). *Dissertation Abstracts International, 39,* 680B. (University Microfilms No. 78-13, 175)

Smith, K. (1979). *Supervisory conferences questions: Who asks them and who answers them.* Paper presented at the annual convention of the American Speech and Hearing Association, Atlanta, GA.

Smith, K. (1980a). Examples of data collected during therapy sessions. *Clinical supervision: What does it mean?* Presentation at the annual convention of the American Speech-Language Hearing Association, Detroit, MI.

Smith, K. (1980b). Multidimensional Observational System for the Analysis of Interactions in Clinical Supervision (MOSAICS). In J. Anderson (Ed.), *Proceedings—Conference on Training in the Supervisory Process in Speech-Language Pathology and Audiology.* Bloomington: Indiana University.

Smith, K. (Moderator). (1985). *Preparation and training models for the supervisory process.* Short course presented at the annual convention of the American Speech-Language Hearing Association, Washington, DC.

Smith, K., & Anderson, J. (1982a). Development and validation of an individual supervisory conference rating scale for use in speech-language pathology. *Journal of Speech and Hearing Research, 25,* 252–261.

Smith, K., & Anderson, J. (1982b). Relationship of perceived effectiveness to content in supervisory conferences in speech-language pathology. *Journal of Speech and Hearing Research, 25,* 243–251.

Sorensen, D. (1992). Communicator style characteristics of speech-language pathology students. *ASHA, 34,* 67–71.

Spahr, F. (1995). The impact of external forces on educational reforms in higher education.). *Proceedings of the Annual Conference— Restructure* (pp. 37–43). Council of Academic Programs in Communication Sciences and Disorders, Minneapolis, MN.

Stace, A., & Drexler, A. (1969). Special training for supervisors of student clinicians: What private speech and hearing centers do and think about training their supervisors. *ASHA, 11,* 318–320.

Starkweather, C. W. (1974). Behavior modification in training speech clinicians: Procedures and implications. *ASHA, 16,* 607–611.

Stewart, J., & D'Angelo, G. (1975). *Together: Communicating interpersonally.* Reading, MA: Addison-Wesley.

Strike, C., & Gillam, R. (1988). Toward practical research in supervision. Chapter 15 in J. Anderson, *The supervisory process in speech-language pathology and audiology,* 273–298. Boston: College-Hill.

Strike-Roussos, C. (1988). Supervisors' implementation of trained information regarding broad questioning and discussion of supervision during their supervisory conferences in speech-language pathology (Doctoral dissertation, Indiana University, Bloomington). *Dissertation Abstracts International, 44,* 3048B. (University Microfilms No. DEW 8824185, 3710)

Strike-Roussos, C. (1995). Supervisor questions and supervisee responses: Is there agreement? In R. Gillam (Ed.), *The supervisors' forum, 2,* 15–17. Council of Supervisors in Speech-Language Pathology and Audiology.

Strike-Roussos, C., Brasseur, J., Jimenez, B., O'Connor, L., & Boggs, T. (1991). *Analysis and evaluation in supervision: An ongoing process.* Presentation at the conference of the California Speech-Language Hearing Association, Long Beach, CA.

Tanck, M. (1980). *A cooperative approach to improving instruction through supervision.* Presentation at the Conference on Administration of Special Education. Bloomington: Indiana University.

Tannen, D. (1990). *You just don't understand: Women and men in conversation.* New York: William Morrow, Ballantine.

Tannen, D. (1994). *Talking from 9 to 5.* New York: William Morrow.

Tannenbaum, A. (1966). *Social psychology of the work organization.* Belmont, CA: Wadsworth.

Taylor, F. (1911). *The principles of scientific management.* New York: Harper and Bros.

Tihen, L. (1984). Expectations of student speech/language clinicians during their clinical practicum (Doctoral dissertation, Indiana University, 1983). *Dissertation Abstracts International, 44,* 3048B. (University Microfilms No. 84-01, 620)

Trow, R. (1960). Role functions of the teacher in the instructional group. In *Dynamics of instructional groups.* National Society for the Study of Education Yearbook.

Tufts, L. (1984). A content analysis of supervisory conferences in communicative disorders and the relationship of the content analysis system to the clinical experience of supervisees (Doctoral dissertation, Indiana University, 1983). *Dissertation Abstracts International, 44,* 3048B. (University Microfilms No. 84-01, 588)

Turton, L. (Ed.). (1973). *Proceedings of a Workshop on Supervision in Speech Pathology.* Ann Arbor: University of Michigan, Institute for the Study of Mental Retardation and Related Disabilities.

Tyack, D., & Ingram, D. (1977). Children's production and comprehension of questions. *Journal of Child Language, 4,* 211–224.

Uffen, E. (1998). Where the jobs are: Keeping an eye on the future. *ASHA,* 25–28.

Ulrich, S. (1985). Continuing education model of training. In K. Smith (Moderator), *Preparation and training models for the supervisory process.* Short course presented at the annual convention of the American Speech-Language Hearing Association, Washington, DC.

Ulrich, S. (1990). The supervisory process: Tasks basic to effective clinical supervision. In *Clinical Supervision Across Settings: Communication and Collaboration* (pp. 9–22). Rockville, MD: American Speech-Language Hearing Association.

Underwood, J. (1973). Interaction analysis between the supervisor and the speech and hearing clinician (Doctoral dissertation, University of Denver, 1973). *Dissertation Abstracts International, 34,* 2995B. (University Microfilms No. 73-29, 608)

Underwood, J. (1979). *Underwood category system.* Unpublished manuscript, University of Northern Colorado, Greeley.

Van Dersal, C. (1974, September). The relationship of personality, values, and race to anticipation of the supervisory relationship. *Rehabilitation Counseling Bulletin,* 41–46.

Van Riper, C. (1965). Supervision of clinical practice. *ASHA, 3,* 75–77.

Vargus, I. (1977). Supervision in social work. In D. Kurpius, R. Baker, & I. Thomas (Eds.), *Supervision of applied training.* Westport, CT: Greenwood Press.

Ventry, I. M., & Schiavetti, N. (1980). *Evaluating research in speech pathology and audiology.* Reading, MA: Addison-Wesley.

Villareal, J. (Ed.). (1964). *Seminar on guidelines for supervision of clinical practicum.* Washington, DC: American Speech and Hearing Association.

Volz, H. (1976). The effects on clinician performance, client progress, and client satisfaction of two programs to enhance the helping skills of undergraduate students in speech pathology (Doctoral dissertation, University of Pennsylvania, 1976). *Dissertation Abstracts International, 37,* 716B. (University Microfilms No. 76-17, 239)

Volz, H., Klevans, D., Norton, S., & Putens, D. (1978). Interpersonal communication skills of speech-language pathology undergraduates: The effects of training. *Journal of Speech and Hearing Disorders, 43,* 524–541.

Vygotsky, L. S. (1978). *Mind in society: The development of higher psychological processes.* Cambridge, MA: Harvard University Press.

Wagner, B., McCrea, E., & Spigarelli, K. (1992). Supervisory conferences in speech-language pathology through computer electronic mail. In S. Dowling (Ed.), *Proceedings of the 1992 National Conference on Supervision—Total Quality Supervision: Effecting Optimal Performance* (pp. 97–105). Council of Supervisors in Speech-Language Pathology and Audiology, Nashville, TN.

Ward, L., & Webster, E. (1965a). The training of clinical personnel: I. Issues in conceptualization. *ASHA, 7,* 38–41.

Ward, L., & Webster, E. (1965b). The training of clinical personnel: II. A concept of clinical preparation. *ASHA, 7,* 103–106.

Webster's II New Riverside University Dictionary. (1984). Boston: Riverside Publishing.

Wegner, J. (1999). K-TEAM: Empowering students. In P. Murphy (Ed.), *Proceedings of the Annual Conference on Graduate Education—New Horizons,* (pp. 100–106). Minneapolis, MN: Council of Academic Programs in Communication Sciences and Disorders.

Weller, R. (1969). An observational system for analyzing clinical supervision of teachers (Doctoral dissertation, Harvard University, 1969). *Dissertation Abstracts, 29,* 1904A. (University Microfilms No. 69-18, 245)

Weller, R. (1971). *Verbal Communication in Instructional Supervision.* New York: Teachers College Press, Columbia University.

Whalen, T. (2001, June). *Incorporating professional behavior expectations into performance appraisals.* Paper presented at ASHA Special Interest Division 11 Leadership Conference: Power Tools for Leadership and Supervision, Chicago.

Whiffen, R., & Byng-Hall, J. (1982). *Family therapy supervision.* New York: Grune & Stratton.

Whitelaw, G., & Donohue, J. (1996). The 'town-gown' connection: An advisory board for external site supervisors. In B. Wagner (Ed.), *Proceedings of the 1996 Conference on Clinical Supervision—Partnerships in Supervision: Innovative and Effective Practices* (pp. 90–99). Council of Supervisors in Speech-Language Pathology and Audiology, Cincinnati, OH.

Whitelaw, G., & Wynne, M. (1996). Developing partnerships: Crafting the externship practicum experience. In B. Wagner (Ed.). *Proceedings of the 1996 Conference on Clinical Supervision—Partnerships in Supervision: Innovative and Effective Practices* (pp. 132–140). Council of Supervisors in Speech-Language Pathology and Audiology, Cincinnati, OH.

Whiteside, J. (1981). *Analysis of question type in supervisory conferences and classroom in speech-language pathology.* Unpublished manuscript, Indiana University, Bloomington.

Wilson, J., Welch, N., & Welling, R. (1996). Interactive supervision system: A tool for clinical teaching. In B. Wagner (Ed.), *Proceedings of the 1996 Conference on Clinical Supervision—Partnership in Supervision: Innovative and Effective Practices* (pp. 196–198). Council of Supervisors in Speech-Language Pathology and Audiology, Cincinnati, OH.

Wolf, K. (2000). Managing the impact of market-driven changes in communication sciences and disorders: The health care setting. In P. Hargrove, R. McGuire, C. O'Rourke, & W. Swisher (Eds.), *Proceedings of the Annual Conference—The Challenge of Change* (pp. 70–90). Council of Academic Programs in Communication Sciences and Disorders, Minneapolis, MN.

Wollman, I. L., & Conover, H. B. (1979). The student clinician's reception of the supervisory process. *Ohio Journal of Speech and Hearing, 14,* 192–201.

Young, M. (2001). *Learning the art of helping: Building blocks and techniques* (2nd ed.). Upper Saddle River, NJ: Prentice-Hall.

NAME INDEX

SUBJECT INDEX